Gait in Rehabilitation

CLINICS IN PHYSICAL THERAPY

EDITORIAL BOARD

Otto D. Payton, Ph.D., **Chairman**

Louis R. Amundsen, Ph.D.

Suzann K. Campbell, Ph.D.

Jules M. Rothstein, Ph.D.

**This book is to be returned on or before
the last date stamped below.**

Smidt, g.h

90-711

Forthcoming Volumes in the Series

Gait in Rehabilitation

Edited by

Gary L. Smidt, Ph.D., P.T., F.A.P.T.A.

Professor and Former Director
Physical Therapy Graduate Program
College of Medicine
University of Iowa
Iowa City, Iowa

CHURCHILL LIVINGSTONE

NEW YORK, EDINBURGH, LONDON, MELBOURNE

Library of Congress Cataloging-in-Publication Data

Gait in rehabilitation / edited by Gary L. Smidt.
      p.   cm. — (Clinics in physical therapy)
    Includes bibliographical references.
    ISBN 0-443-08663-X
    1. Gait disorders—Patients—Rehabilitation. I. Smidt, Gary L.
II. Series.
    [DNLM: 1. Gait. 2. Rehabilitation. W1 CL831CN / WE 103
G144]
RC376.5.G35   1990
616.7—dc20
DNLM/DLC
for Library of Congress   90-1702
                                                CIP

Distributed in the United Kingdom by Churchill Livingstone, Robert Stevenson House, 1–3 Baxter's Place, Leith Walk, Edinburgh EH1 3AF, and by associated companies, branches, and representatives throughout the world.

Accurate indications, adverse reactions, and dosage schedules for drugs are provided in this book, but it is possible that they may change. The reader is urged to review the package information data of the manufacturers of the medications mentioned.

The Publishers have made every effort to trace the copyright holders for borrowed material. If they have inadvertently overlooked any, they will be pleased to make the necessary arrangements at the first opportunity.

Acquisitions Editor: *Kim Loretucci*
Copy Editor: *Elizabeth Bowman*
Production Designer: *Angela Cirnigliaro*
Production Supervisor: *Jeanine Furino*

Printed in the United States of America

First published in 1990

I dedicate this book to almighty God
and to Jesus Christ, His Son.

He has commanded
all people to walk
humbly in His ways (Micah 6:8)
and to walk in love as
Christ has loved us (Ephesians 5:2).

Contributors

Thomas D. Cahalan, P.T.
Adjunct Faculty, Physical Therapy Program, Mayo School of Health Related Sciences; Physical Therapist, Orthopedic Biomechanics Laboratory, Department of Orthopedics, Mayo Foundation/Mayo Clinic, Rochester, Minnesota

Edmund Y.S. Chao, Ph.D.
Professor of Bioengineering in Medical Education, Mayo Medical School; Director, Orthopedic Biomechanics Laboratory, Department of Orthopedics, Mayo Foundation/Mayo Clinic, Rochester, Minnesota

Joan E. Edelstein, M.A., P.T.
Senior Research Scientist and Clinical Assistant Professor, Department of Orthopedic Surgery, New York University School of Medicine and Post-Graduate Medical School; Adjunct Professor of Physical Therapy and of Prosthetics and Orthotics, New York University School of Education, Health, Nursing and Arts Professions, New York, New York

Carol A. Giuliani, Ph.D., P.T.
Assistant Professor, Division of Physical Therapy, Department of Medical Allied Health Professions, University of North Carolina at Chapel Hill School of Medicine, Chapel Hill, North Carolina

Elizabeth L. Leonard, Ph.D., P.T.
Children's Health Center, St. Joseph's Hospital and Medical Center; Affiliate Staff, Division of Neurobiology, Barrow Neurological Institute, Phoenix, Arizona

Elisabeth C. Olsson, Dr. Med. Sci., P.T.
Research Physical Therapist, Department of Orthopaedics, Karolinska Hospital, Stockholm, Sweden

Claire Peel, Ph.D., P.T.
Associate Professor and Chairman, Department of Physical Therapy, School of Allied Health Sciences, University of Texas Medical Branch at Galveston, Galveston, Texas

Richard Shiavi, Ph.D.
Professor, Department of Biomedical Engineering, Vanderbilt University School of Medicine; Research Engineer, Research Service, Veterans Administration Medical Center, Nashville, Tennessee

Gary L. Smidt, Ph.D., P.T., F.A.P.T.A.
Professor and former Director, Physical Therapy Graduate Program, College of Medicine, University of Iowa, Iowa City, Iowa

Robert Waters, M.D.
Medical Director, Clinical Professor, Orthopedic Surgery, University of Southern California School of Medicine, Rancho Los Amigos Medical Center, Downey, California

Marilynn Patten Wyatt, M.A., P.T.
Supervisor, Motion Analysis Laboratory, Children's Hospital and Health Center, San Diego, California

Joy Yakura, M.S., P.T.
Research Associate, Regional Spinal Cord Injury Care System, Rancho Los Amigos Medical Center, Downey, California

Foreword

It is a pleasure to be invited to compose the foreword to this book for two reasons. First, I applaud the effort to create a comprehensive treatise on gait. I am not aware of any similar work on this subject of great importance to both practitioners and students of orthopaedic surgery, physical medicine, physical therapy, and rheumatology. The authors are recognized leaders in their fields and have performed admirably in compiling a complete summary of existing knowledge in each of their various sections. This book fills a "void." It certainly will be used in our orthopaedic training program.

Secondly, on a personal level, it is gratifying to witness the "maturing" of the editor, Dr. Gary Smidt. We are both cornhusker born and bred. I was closely associated with Dr. Smidt at the University of Iowa in the early, or "salad," days of our careers. He has dedicated his professional life to the study of human locomotion and movement—and a productive life it has been. It is a common opinion that only old men and women write books. This cannot be in Dr. Smidt's case—as we are of an age. I'm certain that he has a good deal of productive investigation left in him. Congratulations, Gary, and many thanks for providing this valuable text to those of us interested in health and disease of the musculoskeletal system.

Richard Stauffer, M.D.
Department of Orthopedic Surgery
Mayo Clinic
Rochester, Minnesota

Preface

This book is intended to be a comprehensive treatise on gait. Heretofore works have in an isolated manner dealt with fundamental or applied aspects of normal and/or abnormal gait. Thanks to the contributions from several investigators of gait, a broad spectrum of areas relevant to rehabilitation are knowledgeably addressed in this book.

Chapter 1 is foundational in the sense that the basic nomenclature for the temporal and distance factors is defined and illustrated. A brief historical overview is provided as a launching pad for the refinements, expansion, and application of concepts and methods that appear in subsequent chapters. Chapters 2 through 5 present methodologies, concepts, and descriptions for gait for the primary areas of gait study: temporal and distance factors, kinematics (motion), kinetics (forces and moments of force), energy expenditure, and electromyography. In these chapters the emphasis is on normal gait. In addition, Chapter 4 addresses pathologic gait. Chapter 6, on early motor development and control, and Chapter 7, on assistive devices, provide a transition from normal gait to clinically relevant topics. A scheme for standardly reporting the various types of assisted gaits is proposed for universal use in Chapter 7. Chapter 6 and Chapter 8 focus on pediatrics while geriatric issues are considered in Chapter 9. Pathologic gait frequently results from sequelae or trauma effects on the musculoskeletal, neuromuscular, and cardiopulmonary systems, topics that are covered in Chapters 10 through 12. Chapter 13 is on prosthetics and orthotics, a specialty topic that deserves separate consideration.

I did not originally intend to have a chapter on gait assessment and training in clinical practice (Chapter 14). However, some controversy and misconceptions concerning observation of a patient's gait are apparent in the literature. Chapter 14 attempts to clarify these issues. In addition, gait investigators have yielded one important physiologic indicator of abnormal gait, that of physiologic efficiency. Another important clinically meaningful index of walking ability is proposed in Chapter 14. The index, called the *Smidt Number,* is obtained from a simple equation based on forward walking velocity, a consensus-discriminating factor for walking ability.

Wherever possible clinical implications, suggestions, and questions pertinent to physical rehabilitation are presented. It is my hope that this book will be of interest to all who are interested in the topic of walking, especially those clinicians dealing with patients who walk abnormally. I remind investigators of gait that a large number of unresolved clinical and theoretical problems associated with gait yet remain. To this end my final hope is that the book will serve as an idea generator for fostering improved physical rehabilitation outcomes for gait abnormalities.

Gary L. Smidt, Ph.D., P.T., F.A.P.T.A.

Acknowledgements

To my wife, Elaine, and three sons, Russell, Wesley, and Alexander, and daughter-in-law, Susan, who are a continuous source of encouragement to me.

To my mother and late father, who from their rural Nebraska environment saw to it that I had an opportunity to pursue higher education.

To Judy Biderman and Carol Lipsius for typing the manuscript.

To Physical Therapy Graduate Students, in particular my advisees, at The University of Iowa for their stimulation of creative thoughts and tolerance of my demanding nature.

To Physical Therapy Faculty at The University of Iowa who during an extended period of accelerated departmental change, graciously allowed me to be productive in research concurrently with 15 years of administrative service as a Director.

To Carroll Larson, M.D., former Head of Orthopaedic Surgery, and Richard Johnston, M.D., at The University of Iowa, who gave me a start in academic life in the College of Medicine, and as such to act on a vision to advance physical therapy as a science. Also to several noteworthy orthopaedic surgeons with whom I had the opportunity to collaborate on research projects.

To Gene Asprey, Ph.D., my M.A. and Ph.D. advisor, who patiently taught me the art of scientific writing.

To Al Burstein, Ph.D. (formerly from Case Western Reserve University), Edmund Chao, Ph.D., Gary Fischer, Ph.D., Jasbir Arora, Ph.D., and Don Bartel, Ph.D. (all formerly from The University of Iowa) who freely shared with me their knowledge of engineering mechanics.

To Bonita Lin and Gayatri Desai, physical therapy graduate students who assisted with literature searches and preparation of selected figures.

To professionals outside the borders of the United States who willingly welcomed me at their respective institutions and helped expand my understanding of gait and the world.

Contents

1 | Rudiments of Gait

Gary L. Smidt

DEFINITION OF GAIT

The term *gait* within the context of this book is defined as the manner of moving the body from one place to another by alternately and repetitively changing the location of the feet, with the condition that at least one foot is in contact with the walking surface. Since numerous types of descriptions and analytical approaches are included in this book, gait is considered the most appropriate as a title. In the strict sense, this book addresses walking gait, whereby one foot is always in contact with the supporting surface. By contrast, running gait, whereby both feet are cyclically airborne, is only considered in brief. Unless otherwise stated, the terms *gait* and *walk* or *walking* are used interchangeably.

Locomotion is defined as movement from one place to another.[1] I view this term in a broad, general way. There are obviously a number of ways to move from one place to another. In addition to gait or walking, use of a wheelchair, bicycle, bus, airplane, and train are examples of locomotion. Even in our high-technology era, walking is no doubt the most common mode of locomotion used by people.

GENERAL DESCRIPTION OF NORMAL WALKING

A locomotor process involving a morphologic object of inexhaustible complexity, walking is one of the most frequently performed motor acts.[2] Congruently, this motor act is probably the most complex automatic activity accomplished by the human body. In walking, a complex synergy of the nervous and muscular systems synchronously move 206 bones, dozens of organs, gallons of body fluid, hundreds of sensing structures, thousands of communication circuits, and 636 muscles.[3] In the process, work is accomplished and energy is expended.

To walk, one foot is alternately placed ahead of the other during which time multiple superincumbent body segments move about joint articulations. Most of these articulations have six degrees of freedom (i.e., rotate and translate in each of three planes). Thus, an incredible number of these movement combinations occur about the base of support at the feet and the entire body moves forward. In so doing, relatively small extremity joint rotations occur in the transverse and coronal planes, while large angular excursions take place in the sagittal plane. This sagittal plane movement is contralaterally reciprocal between the upper and lower extremities. Ideally, translational movement at the joints is small, thus a minor contributor. Whole body translation, as reflected by movement of the center of gravity, is quite small from side to side and up to down, while the large continuous translation in forward progression is accomplished. In normal walking, all people display the same qualitative patterns of movement. Minor quantitative movement differences among people account for the various distinctive ways in which people walk.[4]

REASONS FOR STUDYING GAIT

The topic of gait has captivated interest for a variety of reasons. Fundamental processes of movement from a mechanical and physiological point of view are advantageously studied in gait because (1) walking is cyclic in nature and is among the most highly automated movements, (2) movements display widespread synergy involving interaction between central and peripheral nervous system processes in the context of whole body musculature and the entire moving skeleton, (3) movements have generality in a way that the motor act is mastered more completely than any other skill, and (4) it is stable and typical insofar as the details of normal walking are found in normal adults with differences showing up only in rhythms and amplitudes.[2]

In addition to using the motor act of gait to study underlying movement principles, there are good reasons to be concerned from a clinical perspective. Patients are justifiably afraid of impaired or lost vision, hearing, and movement. Gait as a primary means of locomotion is understandably a primary movement concern. Within this context, inquiry of gait is important to (1) unequivocally clarify levels and types of gait abnormality; (2) prevent, alleviate, or control abnormalities; (3) measure the degree and extent of departure from normal; (4) determine progressive changes resulting from therapeutic intervention; and (5) evaluate the end clinical result as compared with initial impairment or disability.[3]

TEMPORAL AND DISTANCE FACTORS

Gait by definition involves location of foot placement. Temporal (time) and distance (length) factors are used to reflect foot placements. Since humans use two feet to walk, some factors are unique to each foot, while others are associations of one foot to the other. For example, each foot has a longer stance and shorter swing phase, which occur with recurring gait cycles. Twice during the cycle, there is a double-stance phase when overlap between the left and right stance phases occurs. Also during a portion of the cycle, each foot independently provides exclusive weightbearing or single support.

In normal walking, the start of the cycle is most easily conceptualized at heel strike on one side. Subsequently, the swinging opposite foot strikes the walking surface at which time one step is completed. A stride is completed when the heel strike on the stance side recurs. Thus, in the normal case, a step is one-half of a stride (Fig. 1-1).

In abnormal walking, the heel may not be the first part of the foot to make floor contact, in which case "initial foot contact" would be more accurate than heel strike. In either the normal or abnormal cases, temporal and distance factors are appropriate, and indeed fundamental, for describing gait. In so doing stance, swing, and single support can be reported as time measures and either the right or left side should be designated. The side of the stride should also be designated and can be measured as a time or length.

A distinction of double stance and steps is that the chronologic association of both feet is necessary to completely describe these events. For example in a gait cycle there are time measures for a period when the left stance is succeeded and concurrent with the right (double stance left-right) and a period when right stance is succeeded and concurrent with the left (double stance right-left). A step can be measured in terms of either time or length. For example, if the measure refers to the initial right heel strike and the subsequent left heel strike, the appropriate designation is step time right-left or step length right-left (Fig. 1-2).

Humans are capable of walking backward and laterally as well as forward. These multiple possibilities ideally necessitate the use of the term *walking velocity*, which permits designation of direction. The term *speed* is less desirable because it connotes a scalar quantity that includes magnitude but does not allow for direction of movement. The forward walking velocity is simply a function of stride length and stride time. The range of forward walking velocity is large for the normal reaching 363 cm/s or 8.12 mph for race walking.[5] In Northeast

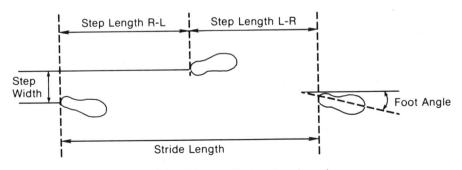

Fig. 1-1.   Distance factors in gait cycle.

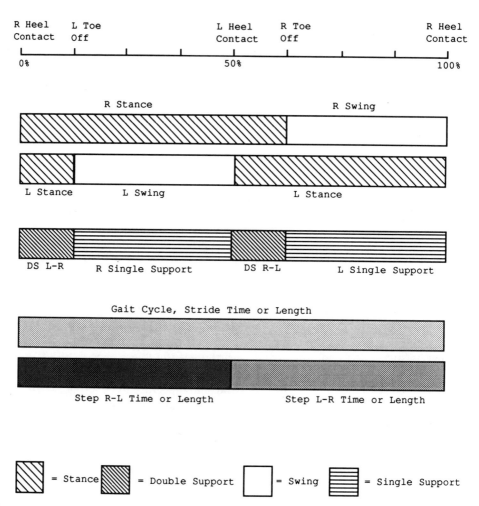

Fig. 1-2.   Basic temporal and distance factors in gait cycle.

England I evaluated a 4-foot, 11-inch female World Class race walker whose walking velocity was measured at 437 cm/s (9.8 mph). Her stride length was 236 cm (94 in.), cadence was 3.8 steps/s (225 steps/min), and cycle time was 0.55 seconds. Walking velocity is influenced by a variety of factors such as the objective for walking and walking environment. Therefore, a commonly used general figure of 135 cm/s or 3.0 mph for walking velocity has little more than academic meaning. An incremental range of forward walking velocities represented by five commonly used measurement units is provided in Table 1-1. For purposes of standardization and clinical reporting, suggested categories for the range of forward-walking velocities are presented in Table 1-2.

Table 1-1. Converted Values for Six Commonly Used Measurement Units for a Range of Walking Velocities

cm/s	m/min	in./s	ft/s	km/h	mph
5	3	1.97	0.16	0.18	0.11
10	6	3.94	0.33	0.36	0.22
15	9	5.91	0.49	0.54	0.34
20	12	7.87	0.66	0.72	0.45
25	15	9.84	0.82	0.90	0.56
30	18	11.81	0.98	1.08	0.67
35	21	13.78	1.15	1.26	0.78
40	24	15.75	1.31	1.44	0.89
45	27	17.72	1.48	1.62	1.01
50	30	19.69	1.64	1.80	1.12
55	33	21.65	1.80	1.98	1.23
60	36	23.62	1.97	2.16	1.34
65	39	25.59	2.13	2.34	1.45
70	42	27.56	2.30	2.52	1.57
75	45	29.53	2.46	2.70	1.68
80	48	31.50	2.62	2.88	1.79
85	51	33.46	2.79	3.06	1.90
90	54	35.43	2.95	3.24	2.01
95	57	37.40	3.12	3.42	2.13
100	60	39.37	3.28	3.60	2.24
105	63	41.34	3.44	3.78	2.35
110	67	43.31	3.61	3.96	2.46
115	70	45.28	3.77	4.14	2.57
120	73	47.24	3.94	4.32	2.68
125	76	49.21	4.10	4.50	2.80
130	79	51.18	4.27	4.68	2.91
135	82	53.15	4.43	4.86	3.02
140	85	55.12	4.59	5.04	3.13
145	87	57.90	4.75	5.22	3.24
150	90	59.06	4.92	5.40	3.36
155	93	61.02	5.09	5.58	3.47
160	96	62.99	5.25	5.76	3.58
165	99	64.96	5.41	5.94	3.69
170	102	66.93	5.58	6.12	3.80
175	105	68.90	5.74	6.30	3.91
180	108	70.87	5.91	6.48	4.03
185	111	72.83	6.07	6.66	4.14
190	114	74.80	6.23	6.84	4.25
195	117	76.77	6.40	7.02	4.36
200	120	78.74	6.56	7.20	4.47
205	123	80.71	6.73	7.38	4.59
210	126	82.68	6.89	7.56	4.70
215	129	84.65	7.05	7.74	4.81
220	132	86.61	7.22	7.92	4.92
225	135	88.58	7.38	8.10	5.03
230	138	90.55	7.55	8.28	5.15
235	141	92.52	7.71	8.46	5.26
240	144	94.49	7.87	8.64	5.37
245	147	96.46	8.04	8.82	5.48
250	150	98.43	8.20	9.00	5.59

(continued)

Table 1-1. *(continued)*. Converted Values for Six Commonly Used Measurement Units for a Range of Walking Velocities

cm/s	m/min	in./s	ft/s	km/h	mph
255	153	100.39	8.37	9.18	5.70
260	156	102.36	8.53	9.36	5.82
265	159	104.33	8.69	9.53	5.93
270	162	106.30	8.86	9.72	6.04
275	165	108.26	9.02	9.90	6.15
280	168	110.41	9.19	10.08	6.26
285	171	112.38	9.35	10.26	6.38
290	174	114.34	9.52	10.44	6.49
295	177	116.31	9.68	10.62	6.60
300	180	118.27	9.85	10.80	6.71
305	183	120.24	10.01	10.98	6.83
310	186	122.20	10.18	11.16	6.94
315	189	124.17	10.34	11.34	7.05
320	192	126.13	10.51	11.52	7.16
325	195	128.10	10.67	11.70	7.27
330	198	130.06	10.84	11.88	7.39
335	201	132.03	11.00	12.06	7.50
340	204	133.99	11.17	12.24	7.61
345	207	135.96	11.33	12.42	7.72
350	210	137.92	11.50	12.60	7.83
355	213	139.89	11.68	12.78	7.94
360	216	141.85	11.85	12.96	8.06
365	219	143.82	12.01	13.14	8.17
370	222	145.78	12.18	13.32	8.28
375	225	147.75	12.34	13.50	8.39

Walking velocity is important to report for any patient or, in the case of group investigations, it is an independent variable for which control should be made. It has been clearly demonstrated that angular joint movement,[6] floor reaction force,[7] joint reaction force and movements,[8] stride length,[6,9] and energy expenditure[10] are all related to walking velocity. Therefore, the faster

Table 1-2. Range of Forward-Walking Velocity

Rate	Velocity (cm/s)
Very slow	≤40
Slow	41–70
Slow-moderate	71–100
Moderate	101–130
Moderate-fast	131–160
Fast	161–190
Very fast	>190

you walk, the greater the tendency for the temporal factor values to decrease and the requirements for the distance factors and biomechanical and physiologic requirements to increase. As such in group studies, unless the walking velocity is similar among the subjects, differences between groups or changes in one group over time may simply be due strictly to changes in walking velocity alone. Cadence, the rate of taking steps over time, is often wrongly used to standardize walking among subjects. To illustrate this point, it is possible to walk or march in place, as in the military, at a rate of 120 steps/min and never advance in any direction.

Derivations of some previously identified temporal and distance factors have been used to provide, in one number, associations between two different variables. This approach is quite important when with linear type measures are used for comparisons among subjects. Examples of such measures are step or stride length. Since tall subjects with long extremities would be expected to use longer strides than used by their counterparts of shorter stature, the step or stride lengths have been normalized to standing height[9] or more appropriately to the lower extremity length.[6,11] In the latter case, the derived variable is a stride length/lower-extremity length ratio. Another example of a derived variable is the swing/stance ratio.

Classically, the stance phase consumes 60 percent of the gait cycle and swing phase 40 percent. In reality, this 60:40 breakdown seems to hold primarily for the moderate-fast and fast walking velocities with stance percentages being larger at the slowest walking velocities (Fig. 1-3). Cycle times range from as long as 3 seconds for very slow walking to less than 1 second for very fast walking, race walking, and running (Fig. 1-3). As walking velocity increases, the double stance time progressively diminishes to near zero for race walking. For running neither foot is on the walking surface for a portion of the cycle and swing time exceeds stance time.

In effect, four primary stance support surfaces are provided by forefoot and hindfoot on each side. The number of these four support surfaces used at any instant during the gait cycle might provide an indication of relative mechanical stability. All four points are used during erect standing. To examine this dynamic stability concept, foot switches were used to subdivide each stance phase into three component periods: heel strike/foot flat, foot flat/heel-off, and heel-off/toe-off.[12] With increasing walking velocities, the percentage of the cycle for heel strike/foot flat and heel-off/toe-off remains essentially the same while the two-point support from the foot-flat/heel-off component of stance phase decreases (Fig. 1-4). The number of the four available foot support points used decreases with incremented walking velocity.

For the very slow rate, at least two points are always in contact with the walking surface, and during a sizable portion of the cycle, three points are in contact. By contrast, and over a much shorter time interval, only one foot contact point is operational for a considerable period during the gait cycle for the moderate walking velocity (Fig. 1-4).

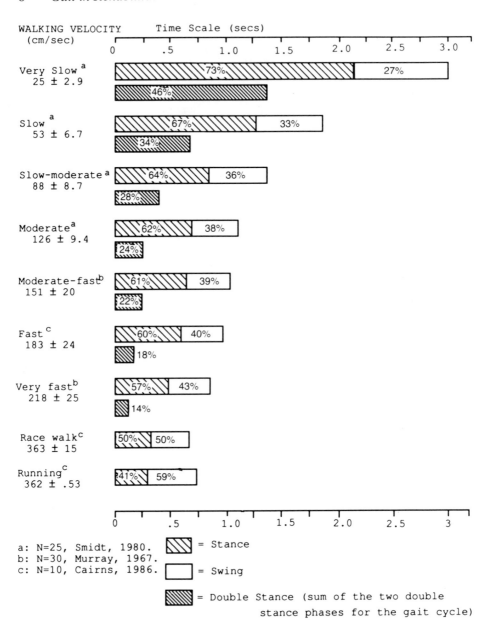

Fig. 1-3. Influence of walking velocity on swing, stance, and double-stance times.

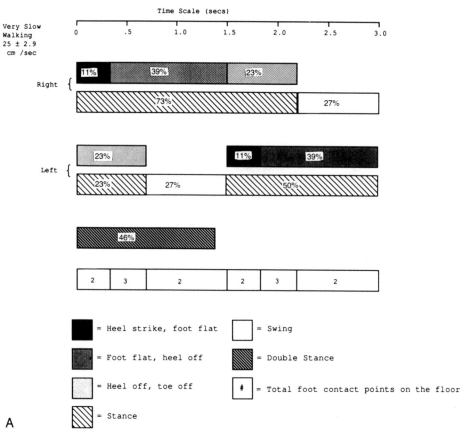

Fig. 1-4. Influence of walking velocity on the number of foot support sites during the gait cycle. (**A**) Very slow walking velocity. (*Figure continues.*)

DEFINITIONS OF COMMONLY USED TEMPORAL AND DISTANCE FACTORS

Forward-walking velocity: the rate of linear forward motion of the body. This is the product of distance and time walked; for example, it can be calculated by measuring the distance between the location of an initial right-foot placement (e.g., heel or toe) and a subsequent right foot placement and then divide the distance by the associated elapsed time. Another method of calculation is to multiply the average step length by cadence in steps per second or to multiply the stride length by strides per second. Walking velocity is typically reported in centimeters per second (cm/s) or meters per second (m/s). Centimeters may be preferred because a decimal is avoided

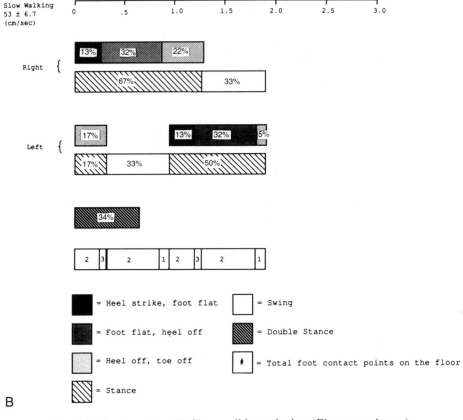

Fig. 1-4 (*Continued*).   (B) Slow walking velocity. (*Figure continues.*)

Gait cycle: usually considered the interval between successive ipsilateral foot contact on the walking surface but can be accurately considered as the interval between any recurring event that delineates a sequential equivalent of two steps

Cycle time: the elapsed time during an entire gait cycle (measured in seconds)

Stance time: during one gait cycle, the elapsed time that one foot is in contact with the walking surface (measured in seconds)

Swing time: during one gait cycle, the elapsed time that one foot is not in contact with the walking surface (measured in seconds)

Single support time: during one gait cycle, the elapsed time when one foot is the only contact point on the walking surface (measured in seconds)

Double-stance time: during one gait cycle, the sum of the time both feet are concurrently in contact with the walking surface. The two double-stance

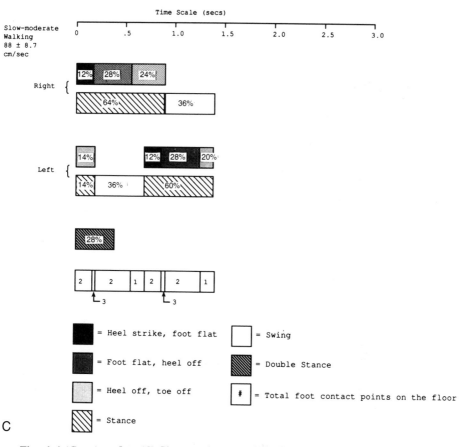

Fig. 1-4 (*Continued*).   (**C**) Slow-moderate walking velocity. (*Figure continues.*)

events in the cycle can be reported separately and as such designated by trail foot-lead foot, e.g., double-stance time left-right (measured in seconds).

Step time: the elapsed time between consecutive walking surface contacts by opposite feet. For one gait cycle, there are two step times, designated R-L and L-R (measured in seconds).

Stride length: in the line of walking progression, the linear distance between two consecutive ipsilateral foot contacts on the walking surface (measured in centimeters or meters)

Step length: in the line of walking progression, the linear distance between two consecutive contralateral foot contacts with the walking surface. For one gait cycle, there are two step lengths, designated by R-L and L-R (measured in centimeters or meters).

Foot angle: the angle bounded by the line of walking progression and a line representing the long axis of the foot while in the foot flat portion of the gait cycle. Outward- and inward-turned foot locations might be designated as positive (+) and negative (−) respectively (measured in degrees).

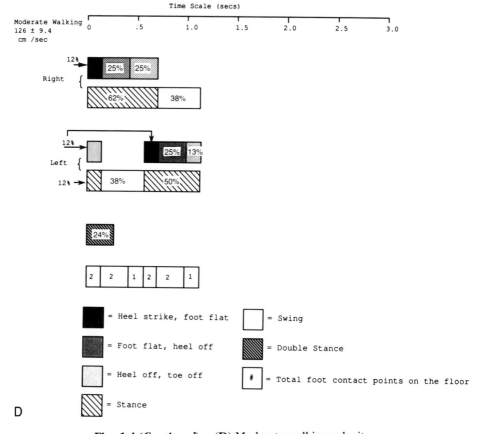

Fig. 1-4 (Continued).   (D) Moderate walking velocity.

Walking distance: simply a total designated walking length or total length a subject has walked

Cadence: the number of strides or steps per unit of time. By counting the number of steps and dividing this number by the elapsed time, cadence can be reported in steps per second; alternatively, strides can be counted and cadence reported in strides per second; cadence is also frequently reported as steps per minute

Functional lower-extremity length: with the subject in the standing position, the distance between the length from the femoral head center (can use tip of the greater trochanter) to the floor (measured in centimeters or meters)

Stride length/lower-extremity length ratio: stride length divided by functional lower-extremity length (measurement unit is dimensionless)

Step width: relative to the line of walking progression, the perpendicular distance between consecutive midheel placement locations. If midheel locations are apart, the measure is positive (+), and if the consecutive heel locations cross over, the measure should be designated as negative (−) (measured in centimeters or meters).

Swing/stance ratio: swing time divided by stance time (measurement unit is dimensionless)

Indices of symmetry: using selected aforementioned temporal and distance factors, mathematically derived quotients obtained by dividing a measurement associated with one side of the body by a measurement for the same variable associated with the other side of the body, e.g., swing time ratio L-R, step length ratio L-R/R-L (measurement unit is dimensionless)

TEMPORAL AND DISTANCE FACTORS
IN THE DAILY ENVIRONMENT

This section presents samples of temporal and distance factor data obtained from non-laboratory settings. This information provides a general orientation framework as a backdrop against which predominantly laboratory-based studies in subsequent chapters might be related.

Walking velocity needs to be standardized for investigative purposes, but the wide range of walking velocities available to the human are no doubt used in daily life. For example, walking velocity may be impacted by environmental conditions such as hurrying to work, walking in the park, or shopping leisurely.[13] In this vein, Bowerman[14] has demonstrated that people in crowded conditions leaving a major league baseball game walked faster than people who traversed the same location after the crowd had dissipated.[13]

Based on extrapolations from pedometer generated data, a U.S. citizen will walk approximately 115,000 miles in a lifetime.[15] This estimate is based on data obtained for 30 consecutive days for 30 subjects aged 23 to 45 years. The average distance walked per day was 4.3 miles. Using an electromagnetic step counter, Marsden and Montgomery[16] investigated the number of steps taken during the day by a wide variety of employees who were measured for 6 h/day to more than 12 h/day. In this study, a step is actually a stride so for the report in this paragraph results were doubled to reflect the number of steps. The range of steps taken per hour was 0 to 300 in the lowest range and 2400 to 2700 in the highest range. The rate most frequently used by those monitored over a 12-hour period was 300 to 600 steps/h. Using the same standard values (16-hour day and 26-inch step length) as Bates and Gorecki,[15] the people in the lowest range walked approximately 2 miles/day or less, while the highest range was 16 to 18 miles/day. Most of the people walked approximately 2 to 4 miles/day.

Finley and Cody[17] acquired temporal and distance factors in four different settings (shopping center, small commercial area, residential area, and business area) for 1,106 pedestrians (534 men and 572 women). On average, the range of walking velocities used among the four settings was small (2.8 mph or 124 cm/s to 3.1 mph or 135 cm/s). Descriptive data for men and women are shown in Table 1-3. Interestingly, I have personal communication from the backward walking champion, and he states that his most comfortable backward walking

Table 1-3. Descriptive Data for a Walking Velocity, Cadence, and Step Length[a]

	Men		Women	
	Mean	SD	Mean	SD
Walking Velocity (cm/sec)	137	21.8	123	19.2
Cadence (steps/min)	111	10.0	117	11.7
Step length (cm)	74	8.9	64	6.6

[a] N = 534 men and 572 women.
(Calculated from data in Finley and Cody.[17])

velocity was 3 mph. At age 81, he walked backward for 452 miles in celebration of a bicentennial.

Further evidence in favor of the importance of walking velocity as a variable is shown.[17] The coefficient of correlation (r) between walking velocity and (1) step length was high at 0.81, and (2) cadence was 0.59. By contrast, the correlation between cadence and step length was essentially zero (0.02).

Investigators in an erudite fashion have attempted to capitalize on the strong relationship between walking velocity and stride length by developing mathematical equations that might be generalizable to all walking humans.[11,18] Should such an equation permit meaningful consolidation of gait parameters, the potential impact on understanding and assessment of gait abnormalities could be great. Such an equation was developed by Alexander[11] to estimate walking velocity from footprints made by hominids. The equation is

$$L/h = F_3(\mu/\sqrt{gh})$$

where F_3 is the same function for hominids of all statures, L is stride length, h is standing height or preference is to use lower extremity length, μ is walking velocity, and g is gravitational acceleration.

HISTORY OF GAIT STUDY

In my experience with students and general audiences over the years, historical perspectives on any topic including gait have seemingly incited minimal interest. However, because of our contemporary indebtedness, and in some cases, reliance, on the significant and often clever contributions of past investigators of gait, an overview of historical developments is provided.

An interest in science and the human body probably led Hippocrates and Aristotle to make analytical observations of walking in 400 to 300 B.C. Borelli (1608 to 1679) distinguished himself as the forerunner of gait study as he described concepts of propulsion, restraint, and muscle action. Borelli was the first to determine the body's center of gravity.[19] The German investigators Wilhelm and Edward Weber,[20] in 1836, observed and measured the swing and support phases, the relationship between the step duration and length, and the movement patterns for walking and running. Using a pneumatic sole and a kymograph Carlet,[21] in 1872, quantified the length and duration of the step (Fig. 1-5). Concurrent with the advent of photography, Marey,[22] in 1873, was the first to use this method to analyze body movements during gait and to portray the movement pathways for selected points on the body. Muybridge,[23] in 1882, advanced the art of photography as he studied the movement patterns of many animal types.

Photography opened the way to study the mechanics of gait in terms of kinematics (displacement, velocity and acceleration) and kinetics (forces). In 1895, Braune (an anatomist) and Fischer (a mathematician) used a method similar to that of Marey,[22,24] placing illuminated tubes on the subject. The setup time to prepare each subject took 6 to 8 hours. The pathways of 11 points on the body were studied: shoulders, wrists, hips, knees, and ankles. Using trigonometry and calculus, measurements of displacement, velocity, and accelerations of points and limb segments were obtained in three dimensions as the investigators sought to ascertain the moving forces (Fig. 1-6) responsible for the kinematics of the walking subject. Figure 1-7 depicts lower-extremity kinematics during the gait cycle. Also in the mid-1900s, Bresler and Frankel[25] and Paul[26] advanced our understanding of joint forces and moments.

In Moscow, Bernstein and associates[27] studied the mechanics of walking in 65 subjects in a quest to improve measurement accuracy and understand the effects of carrying objects and fatigue. A University of California group headed by Inman [28] studied gait mechanics and made application to one field of prosthetics. Also during the mid-1900s, Scherb[19] first defined the pattern of sequential muscle action during the gait cycle. Initially, he used palpation methods and later electromyography (EMG).

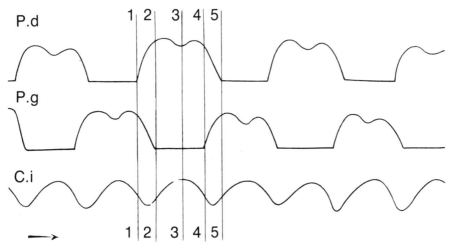

Fig. 1-5. Pneumatic foot-switch pattern for walking. Representation of the sole of the two feet and the count obtained and the parallelogram of inclination. pd, right foot trace; pg, left foot trace; Ci, curve of inclination of body. (From Carlet.[21])

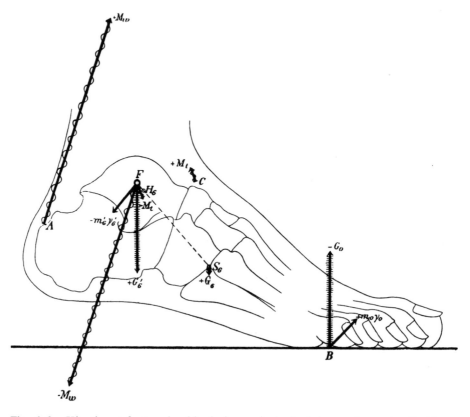

Fig. 1-6. Kinetics at foot and ankle during an instant of stance phase of gait. (From Braune and Fischer,[29] with permission.)

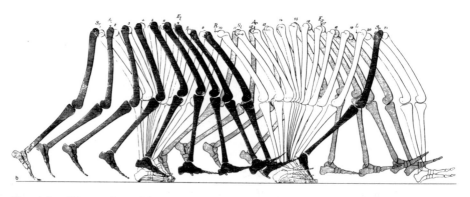

Fig. 1-7. Kinematics of lower extremity during the gait cycle. (From Braune and Fischer,[29] with permission.)

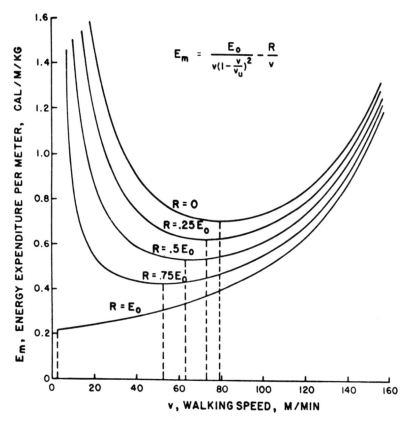

$$E_m = \frac{E_0}{v(1 - \frac{v}{v_u})^2} - \frac{R}{v}$$

Fig. 1-8. Energy expenditure and optimal walking velocity. (From Ralston,[10] with permission.)

As the muscles contract during gait, energy is expended. This aspect of gait has been studied using measurement of oxygen consumption. Ralston[10] was a pioneer in this area. Using experimentally based data, he claims that the most efficient walking velocity is about 80 m/min, or 3.0 mph, or 132 cm/s (Fig. 1-8).

SUMMARY

The definition of gait is the manner of moving the body from one place to another by alternately and repetitively changing the location of the feet with the condition that at least one foot is in contact with the walking surface at all times. A fundamental understanding of gait requires a knowledge of the temporal and distance factors defined and illustrated in this chapter.

An overview of significant pioneering contributions to the topic of gait is provided. Virtually all the major methodologic and conceptual subcategories of gait study emanated from the period 1836 to 1950. Subcategories such as temporal and distance factors, kinematics, kinetics, electromyography, and energy expenditure are mentioned and selectively illustrated. The forthcoming chapters in this book build on the fundamental temporal and distance factor information presented in this chapter and the significant contributions of our predecessors. The result is a comprehensive view of both normal and abnormal human gait.

REFERENCES

1. Dorlands Illustrated Medical Dictionary. WB Saunders, Philadelphia, 1988
2. Bernstein N: Biodynamics of locomotion. p. 60. In Bernstein N (ed): The Coordination and Rebulation of Movements. Pergamon, New York, 1967
3. Smidt GL: Methods of studying gait. Phys Ther 54(1):13, 1974
4. Carlsöö S: p. 96, Chap. 5. In Michael WP (transl): Heinemann: How Man Moves. Crane Russak, New York, 1972
5. Cairns MA, Burdett RG, Pisciotta JC, Simon SR: A biomechanical analysis of racewalking gait. Med Sci Sports Exerc 18:446, 1986
6. Smidt GL: Hip motion and related factors in walking. Phys Ther 51:9, 1971
7. Andriacchi TP, Ogle JA, Galante JO: Walking speed as a basis for normal and abnormal gait measurements. J Biomech 10:261, 1977
8. Crowninshield RD, Brand RA, Johnston RC: The effects of walking velocity and age on hip kinematics and kinetics. Clin Orthop 132:140, 1978
9. Grieve DW, Gear RJ: The relationships between length of stride, step frequency, time of swing and speed of walking for children and adults. Ergonomics 9:379, 1966
10. Ralston JH: Energetics of human walking. p. 77. In Herman RM (ed): Neural Control of Human Motion. Plenum Press, New York, 1976
11. Alexander RM: Stride length and speed for adults, children, and fossil hominids. Am J Phys Anthropol 63(1):23, 1984
12. Smidt GL, Mommens MA: System of reporting and comparing influence of ambulatory aids on gait. Phys Ther 60:551, 1980
13. Bornstein MN, Bornstein HG: The pace of life. Nature (Lond) 259:557, 1976
14. Bowerman WR: Ambulatory velocity in crowded and uncrowded conditions. Percept Motor Skills 36:107, 1973
15. Bates JE, Gorecki GA: A study on US lifetime walking distance: Implications and questions. J Am Podiatry Assoc 70(1):19, 1980
16. Marsden JP, Montgomery SR: A general survey of the walking habits of individuals. Ergonomics 15:439, 1972
17. Finley FR, Cody KA: Locomotive characteristics of urban pedestrians. Arch Phys Med Rehabil 51:423, 1970
18. Grieve DW: Gait patterns and the speed of walking. BioMed Eng 3:119, 1968
19. Steindler A: Historical review of the studies and investigations made in relation to gait. J Bone Joint Surg 35A:540, 1953
20. Weber W, Weber EF: Mechanik der menschlichen gehiverkzeuge. Gottingen, Dietrich, 1836
21. Carlet MG: Essai experimental sur la locomotion humaine. Etude March Ann Sci Nat 16:1, 1872
22. Marey EJ: De la locomotion terreste chez les bipedes et les quadripedes. J Am Physiol 9:42, 1873

23. Muybridge E: p. 29. In Brown LS (ed): Animals in Motion. Dover Publications, New York, 1957
24. Braune CW, Fischer O: Der gang des menschen teil versuche unbelastin und belaetin menschen abhandl. Math-Phys C1 Sach Ges Wiss 21:152, 1895
25. Bresler B, Frankel JP: Forces and moments in the leg during level walking. Trans Am Soc Mechan Eng Jan 27, 1950
26. Paul JP: Forces transmitted by joint in the human body. Proc Inst Mech Eng 181:8, 1967
27. Bernstein N, et al: Determination of Masses and Centroids of Segments of Human Body on Live Subjects. VIEM, Moscow, 1936
28. Fundamental Studies of Human Locomotion and other Information Relating to Design of Artificial Limbs. Report to National Research Council for September 1945–June 1947 period
29. Braune CW, Fischer O: The Human Gait. Maquet P, Furlong R (transl). Springer-Verlag, New York, 1987

2 | Methods of Studying Gait

Elisabeth C. Olsson

> Human gait is a constant play between loss and recovery of the equilib-
> rium and therefore a series of narrowly escaped catastrophies.
>
> *A. Steindler, 1955*

Human walking is the most common of all human movements. It is one of
the more difficult movement tasks that we learn but, once learned, it becomes
almost subconscious. Only when walking is disturbed by injury, disease, degeneration, or fatigue do we realize our limited understanding of this complex
biomechanical process.

Gait evaluation in the clinic is generally based on subjective findings, that
is, the patient's answers to questions on walking distance, walking aids, and
pain and the clinician's observation on the patient's gait. Examples of expres-
sions used to describe how a patient walks are slow, fast, long steps, pronounced limp, recurvatum of the knee in the stance phase, three-point gait,
antalgic, spastic, hemiparetic, and drop foot gait. Even the role in scoring
systems concerning gait is based on subjective judgments. The reliability of such
an evaluation is evidently poor.

OBSERVATIONAL GAIT ANALYSIS

Techniques of observational gait analysis, frequently used by physical
therapists, were developed to achieve greater precision in observations of the
motion pattern of each segment during walking.[1-3] According to the method
developed at Rancho Los Amigos Hospital, the occurrence and timing in the gait

21

cycle of any 32 deviations from normal gait are registered on the chart shown in Figure 2-1. By phasically relating the events at one joint to those occurring in adjacent segments, the observer can differentiate primary gait deficits from compensatory actions; thus, therapeutic plans are more easily formulated. The assessment of a complicated gait pattern is time-consuming, making it uncomfortable for the patient. Videotaping the patient's gait gives the observer the time needed for this evaluation. Still, the most experienced clinical observer will have difficulties in differentiating the innumerable details in the walking pattern. The inability to quantitate makes comparison of a patient's walking pattern from one time to another unreliable. Reliability tests of observational gait analysis indicate that it appears to be a convenient but unreliable technique.[4-6] A simple rating system with a known method error is needed, as valid conclusions may be drawn only from reliable instruments. Until this is developed, the assessment of error expectations in observational gait analysis is necessary, and visual observation should be coupled with simple measurement devices, such as a stopwatch.

QUANTITATIVE GAIT ANALYSIS

I often say that when you can measure what you are speaking about and express it in numbers you know something about it; but when you cannot measure it, when you cannot express it in numbers, your knowledge is of a meagre and unsatisfactory kind.

Lord Kelvin, 1891

Consequently, well-defined and clinically meaningful parameters of gait have to be measured and analyzed in quantitative values.

Techniques to evaluate and quantitate gait patterns have been available for about 150 years. During the past 50 years, increasingly accurate methods of studying gait have been developed. The availability of the computer during the past few years has made the collection of gait parameters much easier and made data reduction practical. Today instrumentation is well advanced, and excellent and reliable methods can be used to describe how man walks.

In 1981 Brand and Crowninshield[7] presented six criteria that had to be fulfilled, if gait analysis should gain clinical acceptance.

1. The measured (parameters) must correlate well with the patient's functional capacity.

2. The measured parameter must not be directly observable and semiquantifiable by the physician or therapist. (The ability to add precision to a measurement does not necessarily add to its value in the overall evaluation of the patient, particularly if the measurement is only one of many necessary in the evaluation.)

3. The measured parameters must distinguish clearly between normal and abnormal.

PROFESSIONAL STAFF ASSOCIATION

RANCHO LOS AMIGOS HOSPITAL
PHYSICAL THERAPY DEPARTMENT
GAIT ANALYSIS – FULL BODY

1. Perform gait analysis with least possible bracing and support.
2. Place a check (√) in appropriate box; with bilateral involvement, use (R) or (L) instead of check.
3. To indicate a sustained posture, place a (P) in the appropriate box.

		SWING			STANCE					STEP: (Relationship of heel to opposite foot)
		INITIAL SWING	MID-SWING	TERMINAL SWING	INITIAL CONTACT	LOADING RESPONSE	MID-STANCE	TERMINAL STANCE	PRE-SWING	
TRUNK:	Backward Lean									
	Forward Lean									
	Lateral Lean (R or L)									
	Rotates Back									
	Rotates Forward									
PELVIS:	Hikes									
	Symphysis Up									
	Symphysis Down									
	Lacks Forw. Rotation									
	Lacks Backw. Rotation									
	Excess. Forw. Rot.									
	Excess. Backw. Rot.									WALKING AID: _____
	Ipsilateral Drop									Dependent ▢
	Contralateral Drop									**EXCESSIVE U.E.**
HIP:	Flexion: Limited									**WEIGHT BEARING:**
	Absent									Body Lean ▢
	Excessive									Shld Elevation ▢
	Inadequate Extension									**STANCE RATIO:**
	Past Retracts									Unequal ▢
	External Rotation									**HEAD CONTROL:**
	Internal Rotation									Extraneous Motion ▢
	Abduction									Abnormal Posture ▢
	Adduction									**ARM SWING:**
	Wobbles									Diminished ▢
KNEE:	Flexion: Limited									Absent ▢
	Absent									Abnormal Posture ▢
	Excessive									
	Inadequate Extension									**LIST MAJOR PROBLEMS AND CAUSE(S):**
	Wobbles									**SWING:**
	Hyperextends									_____
	Extension Thrust									_____
	Valgus									_____
	Varus									_____
	Excess. Contral. Flex.									_____
ANKLE:	Forefoot Contact									_____
&	Foot Flat Contact									_____
FOOT:	Foot Slap									_____
	Excessive Plantar Flexion									_____
	Excessive Dorsiflexion									_____
	Varus									**STANCE:**
	Valgus									_____
	Wobbles									_____
	Heel Off									_____
	No Heel Off									_____
	Drag									_____
	Contralateral Vaulting									_____
TOES:	Up									_____
	Clawed									_____

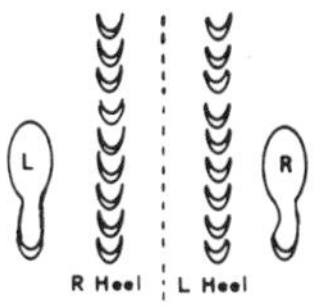

STEP diagram: L — R, R Heel | L Heel

NAME _____ RLAH # _____ DATE _____

DIAGNOSIS _____ RPT _____

Fig. 2-1. Observational gait analysis. (From Rancho Los Amigos Hospital,[1] with permission.)

4. The measurement technique must not significantly alter the performance of the evaluated activity.

5. The measurement must be accurate and reproducible.

6. The results must be communicated in a form that is readily identifiable in a physical or physiological analog.

However, it is no longer enough to describe a walking pattern. To justify the costs associated with gait analysis, the variables that reflect the cause of the pattern must be recognized.

Investigators from a variety of disciplines have been challenged by the complex movement pattern of gait. Clinicians tend to measure what they can visually observe (i.e., time and distance variables and joint angles), neurologists are focusing on electromyelographic (EMG) measurements, biomechanical investigators analyze reaction forces and moments of force, and physiologists look at the oxygen cost of walking.

Exhaustive bibliographies of all the different techniques of studying gait have already been published, most recently in Human Walking, a comprehensive monograph that summarized the knowledge acquired after World War II by investigators at the Biomechanics Laboratory in Berkeley, California.[8-10] The purpose of this chapter is to describe from a clinical point of view a variety of techniques that have demonstrated their use as clinical instruments during the last decades. An apology is given to those whose work have not been reported.

Time-Distance Measurements

Time-distance variables are frequently included in gait analysis because of the importance to relate forces, muscle activity, or joint motion to the phases of the gait cycle (Fig. 2-2). Foot switches have been the most used and least expensive method to study these parameters, such as walking speed, step frequency, step length, the durations of the stance phase, and the pattern of the foot/floor contact. The footswitch is a flexible insole that can either be fitted into a shoe or taped to the subject's foot. It contains compression closing sensors under the areas of the heel, fifth metatarsal head, first metatarsal head, and the great toe (Fig. 2-3). The period in which each individual switch or any combination of switches is active is displayed as a designated voltage level. The foot support pattern is displayed as steps in a staircase. This can then be used to define the stride timing of other data, such as EMG, electrogoniometers, or force data[11] (Fig. 2-4).

The foot-switch stride analyzer (FSSA) is a microprocessor-based computer system developed at the Pathokinesiology Service of Rancho Los Amigos Hospital. The portability of the system facilitates transporting and setting up the system in any convenient walking area.

Almost every gait variable changes with changed walking speed; therefore, gait information is useful only when considered in relationship to walking speed.

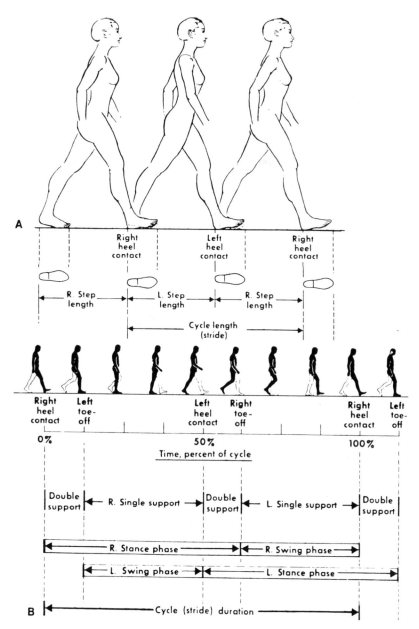

Fig. 2-2.   Distance (**A**) and time (**B**) dimensions of walking cycle. (From Inman et al.,[10] with permission.)

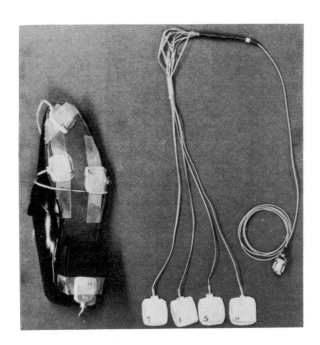

Fig. 2-3. The foot-switch system used at the Biomechanics Laboratory, Mayo Clinic, to measure the foot-floor contact sequences during level walking. The heel switch has a metal tap to provide the measurement of step length and width when it is in contact with the instrumented mats. (From Chao et al.,[46] with permission.)

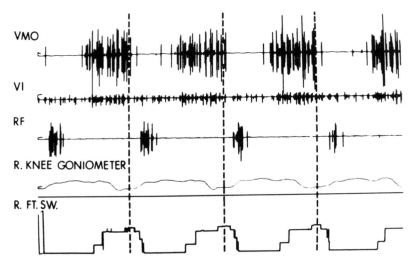

Fig. 2-4. EMG study of a stroke patient with inadequate knee flexion in swing. Causes are out of phase activity of the rectus femoris muscle (RF) and continuous activity of the vastus intermedius muscle (VI). The right foot-switch signal (R:FT.SW.) identifies the intervals of swing (baseline) and stance (irregular staircase). Vertical dashed lines indicate time of contralateral floor contact. (From Gronley and Perry,[11] with permission.)

This important fact, not described until 1966 by Murray et al.[12] and Grieve,[13] makes walking speed a compulsory gait variable to measure. The patient's free walking speed is a measure of overall effectiveness. It has a strong correlation to qualitative and subjective findings, such as weightbearing pain, limp, and stair-climbing and should always be measured first.[14] This can easily be done with a stop watch or photo cells over a known distance.

As speed is the product of step length and step frequency (cadence), many combinations of these can give rise to the same speed. A woman wearing high heels and a tight skirt takes short steps in a fast rate to walk in the same speed as a tall man who takes long steps at a slower rate. Lamoreux[15] found that average velocity was not sufficient but that step frequency and step length should be included in any quantitative examination of walking. The use of metronomes to control step frequency have shown that subjects tend to shorten their stride to accommodate to faster step rates. The proportion between step rate and step length at that particular velocity will then be disturbed. Metronomes are not applicable to subjects with asymmetries of time variables. Andriacchi et al.[16] stated the importance of considering gait measurements over a range of walking speeds in attempting to classify gait abnormalities (Fig. 2-5).

Documentation of treatment effects using time-distance measurements provides useful information concerning the patient's walking ability, which objectively complements and reinforces the clinical evaluation and patient impressions of the procedure. However, time-distance measurements are only end products of a complicated motion pattern that neither explain a gait pattern nor distinguish between the primary gait fault and compensation.

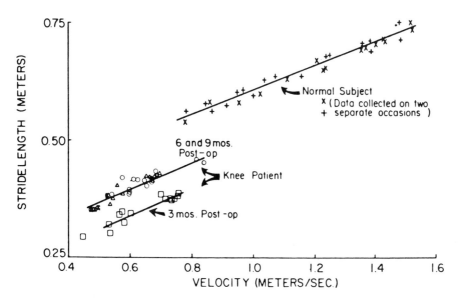

Fig. 2-5. Step length-velocity relationship for a normal subject and a patient treated with a total knee replacement. (From Andriacchi et al.,[16] with permission.)

Stance and swing times are often expressed in percentage of the gait cycle, which does not imply that they are normalized to walking speed. As walking speed increases, both stance and swing time in percentage of gait cycle decrease. Single stance time identifies the weightbearing capability of the limb. This time has proved more accurate than total stance time because the latter measurement is a mixture of single and double stance times. The double stance phase when the leg with a painful hip or knee joint is forward is often longer than the other double stance phase, indicating a hesitation to accept weight on that leg. Weight acceptance of a stroke patient is often shorter indicating a difficulty to synchronize muscle actions.

While mean step length can be calculated by dividing walking speed with step frequency, measurement of individual step length (i.e., of each leg) requires more sophisticated methods, such as a gridded or instrumented walkway.[17] Measuring footprints is not a practical method.

The ratio between the involved and uninvolved leg can be used as a measure of asymmetry or limp, although the ranges of normal symmetry has not yet been identified. The irregularities and asymmetry of time-distance factors have been used in an attempt to find distinct gait abnormalities typical of specific diseases or functional limitations.[18]

Kinematic Factors

Kinematics studies concern movement of the body, of a body segment, or between body segments in different planes. Motion analysis is the appropriate technique for determining what the subject is doing.

Photographic Techniques

Interrupted light photography, also known as *stroboscopy,* indicates that a subject with lights attached to the body, walks across a darkened room in front of a still camera with a rotating shutter, that exposes the film 30 times/sec. The whole motion is shown in one picture, a stick diagram of the subject with the position of the limbs shown at equal intervals of time[19] (Fig. 2-6).

High-speed motion picture film or cinephotography was described by Sutherland and Hagy.[20] The cameras operate at 50 frames/sec in order to freeze the motion of the subject for the analysis portion of the study. The advantages of this method are that no apparatus is attached to the patient, multiple measurements can be made in the same session, EMG may be superimposed on the motion picture film for simultaneous recording, and recording of both legs can be made at the same time. The method is now used less often because data reduction from successive frames is both tedious and time-consuming. TV devices requiring fast computers and large memories but with inferior resolution have replaced the method.[21] In this case, background reflective markers are used for spatial reference, implying that the subject must walk in semidarkness.

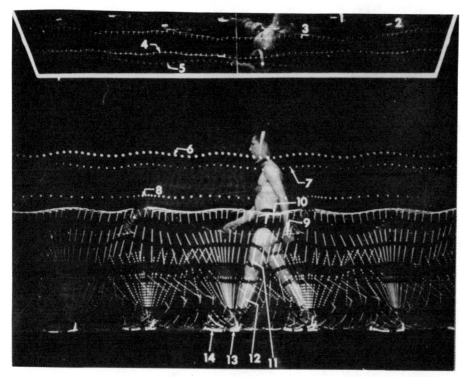

Fig. 2-6.   Interrupted light photography. (From Murray et al.,[19] with permission.)

A tracking cart containing the TV and cinecamera follow the subject along the gait path. This kinematic method used in combination with a force plate and a link segment model can give information of the patterns of generation, absorption, and transfer of mechanical energy at the joints. They involve intersegment transfers of energy through the joint centers, as well as transfers of energy through the muscles in addition to the well-recognized generation and absorption by the muscles.[22]

Goniometric Techniques

Electrogoniometers mounted on an exoskeleton structure attached to the subject describe the position of one body segment relative to another. A great advantage is that they are inexpensive and easy to apply, and the signal is immediately available for analysis. A limiting factor of electrogoniometers is that they do not give absolute angles.

Parallellogram design as described by Lamoreux permits accurate tracking of a joint with a shifting axis of flexion/extension motion but is insensitive to rotation or abduction/adduction[15] (Fig. 2-7). Goniometers are most frequently used to study knee joint motion. In the ankle correspondence between the

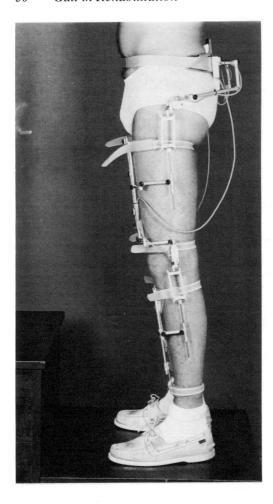

Fig. 2-7. Self-aligning electrogoniometer with parallellogram design.

different axes of motion of the joints and those of the goniometer is unsatisfactory. The validity of some hip goniometers can be questioned, as they do not measure true hip joint motion, but rather a mixture of spine and hip mobility. Polarized light goniometry implies that the subject is illuminated by beams of light. When the beam is reflected by a marker on the subject, this is detected by photodiodes.[23]

Motion analysis systems in which laboratory-fixed detectors measure the position of selected landmarks on the subject are often used in combination with kinetic measurements (Fig. 2-8). The opto-electric Selspot system is an example.[24] Informative motion analysis requires accurate anatomic placement of the skin markers or electrogoniometer. Some of the landmarks are very subtle and pathology can introduce significant change. The physical therapist is well prepared to meet these challenges. Grieve[13] introduced the idea of plotting angle versus angle diagrams as the best way to show segmental interactions. This

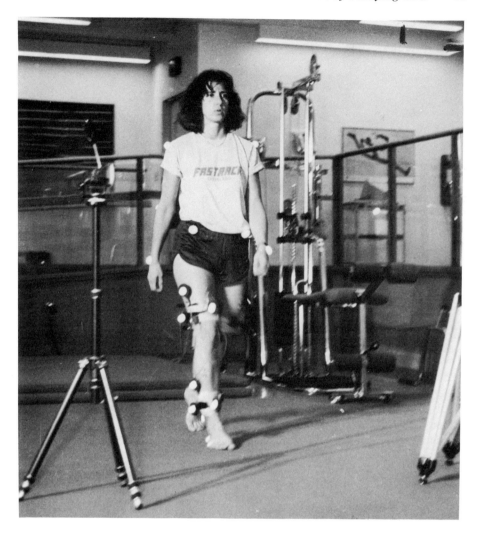

Fig. 2-8. Motion analysis with landmarks on the subject.

way of presenting motion has enjoyed wide clinical and research application (Fig. 2-9).

Kinetic Factors

Kinetics studies concern the causes of the motion, that is, the ground reaction or external forces and the internal forces within the joints. These studies also concern the kinetic energy of the body and body segments.

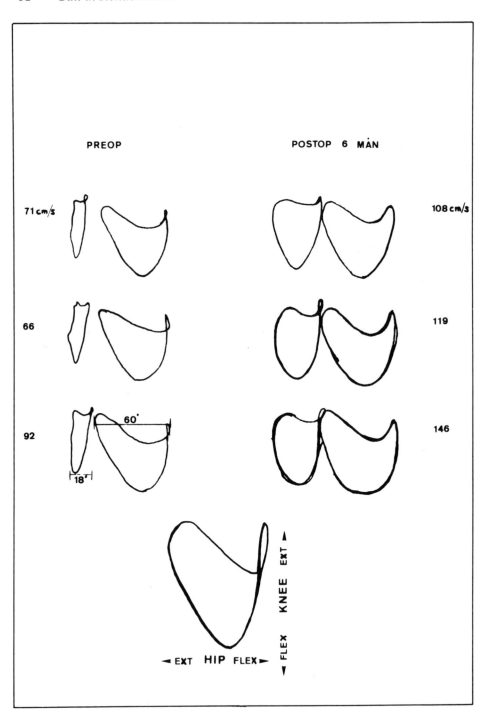

Fig. 2-9. Angle-angle diagram of hip and knee motion during walking before and after a total hip replacement. Shown below is a normal diagram.

Ground Reaction Forces

A ground or floor reaction force is equal in magnitude and opposite in direction to the force that the body applies to the ground through the foot. The ground reaction forces (i.e., the vertical, the horizontal fore and aft and medio-lateral forces) are a direct reflection of the accelerations of the body, a key to the study of human locomotion (Fig. 2-10). The vertical floor reaction force varies above and below the body weight because of vertical upward and downward movement of the centre of gravity, most often determined by walking speed. The development of the force plate has influenced progress in the analysis of body kinetics during locomotion. Increasingly accurate methods have been developed to measure ground reaction forces directly. All of these techniques make use of transducers that change the force into an electric signal. This signal can then be processed in different ways—most often entered into a computer.

The recording instrument can either be attached to the foot, with the attendant risk of disturbing the subject's normal gait, or it can be mounted on the floor. Long force place walkways that register the vertical forces from several consecutive steps from each leg from the unencumbered patient have been described by both Skorecki and Olsson[17,25] (Fig. 2-11). The maximum vertical force percentage of body weight and the vertical impulse for each leg are variables used in addition to time-distance varaibles. Advantages are the clinical applicability and the ease with which a sufficient number of gait cycles can be obtained as a basis for calculations. The methods have shown that the customary double peak pattern found in normal walking disappears in walking speeds of 130 to 100 cm/s. Consequently, time in percentage of the stance phase when a peak occurs is only applicable to subjects walking at almost normal speed (see Fig. 2-10). Floor reaction forces are less sensitive to changes in walking than are time-distance variables.

The widely used Kistler force plate (Kistler Instrumente AG, Winterthur, Switzerland) with piezoelectric force transducers is capable of measuring very rapid changes of forces. It also measures the center of pressure under the foot, necessary for determination of the origin of the force vector. A disadvantage with the small force plate is that it must be hidden to avoid *targeting*. This means that the subject must not be aware that the goal is to step on the plate, as this will alter the normal gait. The numerous repetitions needed to get a sufficient number of steps from each leg on the plate makes the method unapplicable to patients with severe gait disturbances, as they lack the endurance needed.

Internal Forces

Determination of the loads in the joints during normal function and during pathologic conditions is a major aspect of orthopedic biomechanics and is crucial to the design of implants. External forces result from the weight of the body, the ground reaction force acting on the foot, and the acceleration and deceleration of the limb segments. Internal forces act to balance the external

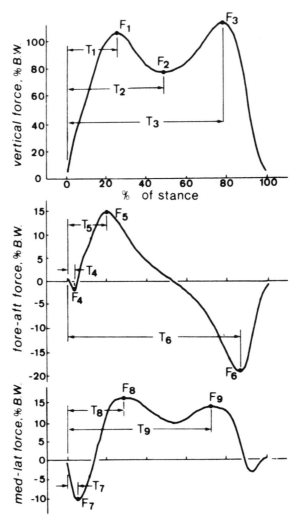

Fig. 2-10. Basic parameters used to describe foot-floor re-action forces. (From Chao et al.,[46] with permission.)

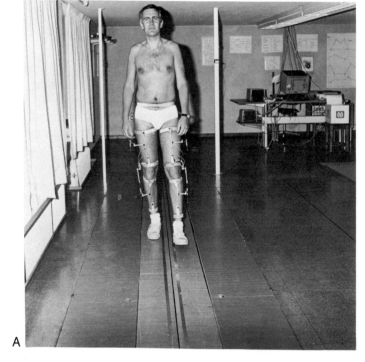

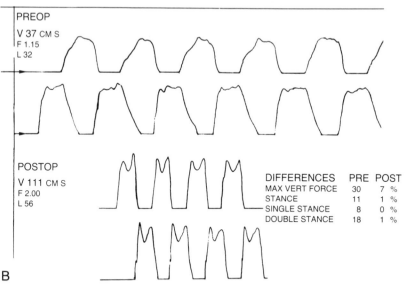

Fig. 2-11. **(A)** Force plate walkway. (From Olsson et al.,[17] with permission.) **(B)** Vertical force curves from several consecutive steps of each leg showing a patient before and 6 months after a total hip replacement. Average walking speed (V), step frequency (F), and step length (L) have increased. The asymmetry between the legs (differences) in maximal vertical force percentage body weight and in duration of the stance phase percentage gait cycle has decreased. Upper curve shows the bad leg. Note the long weight acceptance phase. (From Olsson et al.,[14] with permission.)

forces and are generated by active muscle contraction, ligamentous forces, and joint contact forces.

The only report on intravital measurements was made by Rydell,[26] who registered forces acting on an instrumented femoral head prosthesis while the subject was walking or performing other activities. The recorded values were higher than the theoretical, which was attributed to muscular force.

Because of the difficulties connected with direct force measurements, internal joint forces are determined approximately by measuring the external forces together with a full kinematic description, modeling the body as a system of rigid links and simplifying the representation of joint anatomy.[27-30] This requires advanced technical instrumentation combined with computer data processing; in addition, engineers and technicians are needed to run a gait test. These methods of studying gait are often connected with problems of clinical accessibility.

A gait analysis system to study the biomechanics of the knee joint in terms of prosthesis design and effects of knee surgery was described by Andriacchi et al.[31] Each lower limb is considered to be a three-dimensional linkage with movable joints, assumed to have fixed axes of motion at the hip, knee, and ankle. The position of the joint centers are located and marked on the front and side. Motion of the limbs is determined by measuring the spatial position of light-emitting diodes placed at several points: on the anterior superior iliac spine, at the center of the greater trochanter, over the midpoint of the lateral joint line of the knee, on the lateral aspect of the malleolus, at the base of the calcaneus, and at the fifth metatarsal. An optoelectric system measures the three-dimensional position of each light-emitting diode on the subject. A piezo-electric force plate gives the three components of ground reaction force, the vertical twisting moment, and the location of resultant forces at the foot. Data are collected at the site of the force plate during slow, normal, and fast walking speeds. Kinematic and kinetic measurements are acquired simultaneously. The inertial properties of the segment are approximated from data derived from the literature.[32] Moment magnitudes are normalized to body weight, multiplied by height, and expressed as percentage. A gait test takes approximately 2 hours.

The concept of the *force line visualization,* indicating the alignment of the ground reaction force vector with the supporting limb to be visualized, was described by Cook et al.[33] The vertical and horizontal forces are transposed into a resultant vector that represents the line of body weight. The perpendicular distance between the vector and the joint center marker multiplied by the vector magnitude from each frame of film determines the flexion and extension (or frontal plane abduction and adduction) torques that the muscles must control. This is a good approximation at the ankle joint but should be used with caution at the knee, as the error of the method increases with the distance from the ground.

In single-limb support, the vector remains during 59 percent of the gait cycle anterior to the axis of the ankle, producing a dorsiflexion torque that threatens stance stability and has to be counteracted by the plantar flexors to prevent collapse into excessive dorsiflexion[34] (Fig. 2-12). This technique has contributed to a better understanding of the demands on the muscular system imposed by walking in both normal and pathologic weightbearing patterns.

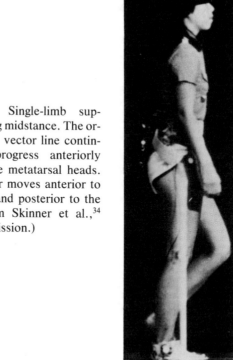

Fig. 2-12. Single-limb support during midstance. The origin of the vector line continues to progress anteriorly toward the metatarsal heads. The vector moves anterior to the knee and posterior to the hip. (From Skinner et al.,[34] with permission.)

Electromyography

The purpose of using EMG during gait is to determine the mode, timing, and intensity of action. Timing within the gait cycle is the most common determination made from the EMG record. Deviations from normal timing are classified as premature, prolonged, or continuous, and out-of-phase action (see Fig. 2-4). This information is used to differentiate normal from abnormal function within muscle groups for final surgical planning of tendon releases or transfers in patients with upper motor neuron lesions. This technique has led to far better clinical results because normal function is not sacrificed and abnormal action is more precisely defined[11] (see Fig. 2-4).

Electromyography is the most frequently used laboratory method of assessing gait of patients with cerebral palsy. At Children's Hospital in San Diego, both indwelling and surface electrodes are used together with high-speed motion picture film and a force plate (for vector analysis and center of pressure indication) to plan and evaluate the effects of treatment and to determine why a particular gait pattern occurs. The method used for many years by Sutherland and his group has demonstrated its clinical relevance and represents one of the best clinical gait analysis methods in use today.[20] Distinctions have been made between primary abnormalities and compensatory mechanisms; gait patterns with common denominators have been identified.

The method has shown that EMGs obtained during walking are more useful in planning treatment than is slow stretch testing and that hip and knee flexion contractures should be relieved prior to heel cord lengthening to prevent the development of crouch gait.[35] Because the value of dynamic EMG depends on the accurate anatomic placement of electrodes and the selection of muscles appropriate to the clinical question, the physical therapist is well suited to contribute to the testing program.

Inman[36] has contributed to the knowledge of the mechanics of gait with an EMG analysis of the hip muscles in their dynamic function. Murray et al.[37] recorded EMG activity in eight muscle groups during slow, free, and fast walking speed. For most of the muscles tested, the amplitude of normalized EMG activity decreased as walking speed decreased. Quantification of the EMG to provide information on the relative intensity of muscle action is reserved for tests involving normal subjects.

Metabolic Energy Expenditure

A fundamental feature of human motor behavior is that a freely chosen rate of activity is preferred that represents minimal energy expenditure per unit task. This also applies to walking. Ralston[38] showed that in natural walking a person chooses an optimal step length and step rate, achieving minimal energy expenditure per unit distance. Consequently, energy costs per distance walked are higher for walking speeds above but also below the "average." However, when a soldier walks in a parade with a stiff-kneed march or a girl walks with very high heels, the aim is clearly not efficient walking.

The purpose of this method is to determine the energy cost, indicated by O_2 uptake, of various modes of ambulation for normal and disabled subjects. When the subject has reached steady state, the expired air is collected for a couple of minutes in a bag carried on the back. The air is then analyzed for O_2 and CO_2 content (Fig. 2-13).

Waters et al.[39] found that nonweightbearing three-point crutch ambulation required exorbitant energy expenditure. He also studied the effort involved in walking versus propelling a wheelchair.[40] The results have made the choice of optimum mode of locomotion for the severely disabled more realistic.

In the study of O_2 consumption after total hip replacement, McBeath et al.[41] found that measurement of self-selected walking speed was a satisfactory indicator of walking efficiency. Treadmills are a convenient means of studying gait. Their use is limited, however, as subjects with impaired limbs either cannot walk on a treadmill at all or must use a velocity that is slower than their customary speed. In studying normal gait, significant differences have been reported between treadmill and overground level walking.

Strathy et al.[72] found that saggital plane knee motion decreased during treadmill walking. When EMG recordings on a treadmill were compared with

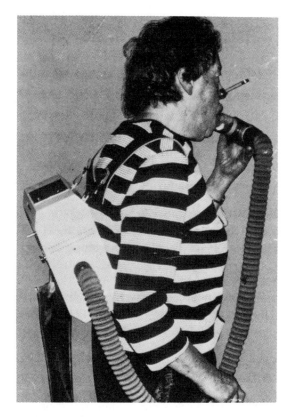

Fig. 2-13. Oxygen consumption measured with the Kofranyi-Michaelis respirometer, showing mouthpiece, connecting tubing, and sample collection bag. (From Macnicol MF, McHardy R, Chalmers J: Exercise testing before and after hip arthroplasty. J Bone Joint Surg 62B:326, 1980, with permission.)

those made on a walkway, Arsenault et al.[43] found a tendency for the treadmill data to indicate slightly larger amplitudes but lower variation. The differences between ground and treadmill locomotion increase with higher speed.

APPLICATION OF GAIT ANALYSIS

Accumulation of Normal Data

Accumulation of normal data is important for the development of a standardized reference base that can be used for comparison with abnormal results. Murray was the first to establish the ranges of normal values for the variables sex, age, weight, and height as a reference for comparison of patients with abnormal gait.[44,45] As gait characteristics tend to vary widely even among normals, sufficient sample sizes must be maintained in order to draw viable conclusions. Chao et al.[46] reported a normative data base, including temporal distance factors, knee joint motion, and ground reaction force patterns for 148 adults. Baseline measures of joint angles, ground reaction forces, joint moment of force, power generated and absorbed, and EMG on normal gait were reported by Winter.[47] Waters et al.[48] established normative standards on the energy cost of walking in 111 young and old adults. Most gait studies continue to be made on normal individuals.

Comparison of Normal and Abnormal Gait Performance

Many investigators have tried to bring out distinct gait abnormalities typical of specific diseases or functional limitations. The irregularities and asymmetry in time-distance factors, in displacement of the body and between body segments typical of coxalgic gait, were described by Murray et al.[18] Chao et al.[49] described eight significant gait variables, providing discriminative power in separating total knee replacement patients from a control group of normals using time-distance, force plate, and the electrogoniometer measurements. Simon et al.[50] compared patients who had excellent results after total knee replacement with normals using high-speed motion cameras, two force plates, and EMG; these workers found that weight acceptance time, cadence, knee flexion in stance, and external moments of the knee joint differentiated between the groups. This application has demonstrated its clinical relevance to the determination of the severity of the disease, to evaluate one parameter of the disease, and to show the effect of the pathology on gait. Still, contemporary high-tech applications to gait have very little clinical explicative capacity. The complexity of human locomotion and our current lack of understanding the relationship between the measurable quantities and the pathologic processes preclude the use of gait analysis as a diagnostic tool in the sense of its capacity to distinguish between diseases.

Evaluation of Treatment Methods

When patients are used as their own control, minute differences in joint functional performance during walking can be determined and quantitated. The documentation of effectiveness of conservative or surgical therapy provides useful information, which objectively complements the clinical evaluation and the patient's own impressions of the procedure.

Assessment of Individual Patients in Clinical Follow-up

The effectiveness of gait analysis in determining treatment strategy and proper timing for children with neurologic deficits has been demonstrated by Sutherland and Cooper.[35] This application has demonstrated the potential value of gait analysis as a clinical tool.

Correlations

For the clinician, the complexity, technical difficulty, and expense of these methods are prohibitive. For this reason, accurate and simple methods of studying gait are essential. Correlations between a thorough clinical examination and gait analysis of time-distance measurements, floor reaction forces, and sagittal motion of hips and knees was used by Olsson et al.[14] as a means of finding simple measurement methods with strong correlations to gait analysis that could be used in the clinic by those who did not have access to a gait laboratory. The results showed that free walking speed and maximal walking speed were the best indicators of a subject's walking function.

CONCLUSIONS

Gait analysis is a young science. During the past several decades, engineers have provided excellent and reliable methods to study walking from a variety of aspects. A number of commercial single-function units are available so that instrumented laboratories can be developed at several levels. The determinants are training, funds, space, and engineering support. Producing meaningful information from the many types of data and methods of processing the outcome depends on including a functional perspective. The physical therapist is well suited to defining the functional problems, can appreciate the functional potential of patients, and can tailor the testing procedure as needed. The skilled physical therapist can also ask the clinical questions, speculate on the phenomenon of a specific gait pattern, and make a strong contribution in determining why a given patient walks the way he or she does, thus, gait analysis can be an accepted clinical tool.

REFERENCES

1. Rancho Los Amigos Hospital: Normal and Pathological Gait Syllabus: Professional Staff Association of Rancho Los Amigos Hospital, Downey, CA, 1981
2. Brunnström S: Recording gait patterns of adult hemiplegic patients. Phys Ther 44:11, 1964
3. Bampton S: A guide to the visual examination of pathological gait. Temple University Rehabilitation Research and Training Centre 8, 1979
4. Goodkin R, Diller L: Reliability among physical therapists in diagnosis and treatment of gait deviations of hemiplegics. Percept Motor Skills 37:727, 1973
5. Krebs DE, Edelstein JE, Fishman S: Reliability of observational kinematic gait analysis. Phys Ther 65:1027, 1985
6. Saleh M, Murdoch G: Indefence of gait analysis. J Bone Joint Surg 67B:237, 1985
7. Brand RA, Crowninshield RD: Comment on criteria for patient evaluation. J Biomech 14:655, 1981
8. Steindler A: A historical review of the studies and investigations made in relation to human gait. J Bone Joint Surg 35A:540, 1953

9. Murray MP: Gait as a total pattern of movement. Am J Phys Med 46:290, 1967
10. Inman VT, Ralston HJ, Todd F: Human Walking. Williams & Wilkins, Baltimore, 1981
11. Gronley J, Perry J: Gait analysis techniques. Rancho Los Amigos Hospital gait laboratory. Phys Ther 64:1831, 1984
12. Murray MP, Kory RC, Clarkson BH, Sepic SB: Comparison of free and fast speed walking patterns of normal men. Am J Phys Med 45:8, 1966
13. Grieve DW: Gait patterns and the speed of walking. J Biomed Eng 3:119, 1968
14. Olsson E, Goldie I, Wykman A: Total hip replacement. A comparison of Charnley (cemented) and HP Garches (non-cemented) fixation. Scand J Rehabil Med 18:107, 1986
15. Lamoreux L: Kinematic measurements in the study of human walking. Bull Prosth Res Spring, 1971
16. Andriacchi TP, Ögle JA, Galante JO: Walking speed as a basis for normal and abnormal gait measurements. J Biomech 10:261, 1977
17. Olsson E, Öberg K, Ribbe T: A computerized method for clinical gait analysis of floor reaction forces and joint angular motion. Scand J Rehabil Med 18:93, 1986
18. Murray MP, Gore DR, Clarkson BH: Walking patterns of patients with unilateral hip pain due to osteoarthritis and avascular necrosis. J Bone Joint Surg 53A:259, 1971
19. Murray MP, Drought B, Kory R: Walking patterns of normal men. J Bone Joint Surg 46A:335, 1964
20. Sutherland DH, Hagy JL: Measurement of gait movements from motion picture film. J Bone Joint Surg 54A:787, 1972
21. Winter DA, Quanbury AO, Hobson DA, et al: Kinematics on normal locomotion. J Biomech 7:479, 1974
22. Winter DA, Robertson DG: Joint torque and energy patterns in normal gait. Biol Cybernet 29:137, 1978
23. Mitchelson DL: Clinical assessment of gait using the polarized light goniometer. Presented at the Orthopaedics Engineering Conference (BES), London, 1974
24. Öberg K, Lanshammar: An investigation of kinematic and kinetic variables for the description of prosthetic gait using the ENOCH system. Prosth Orthop Int 6:43, 1982
25. Skorecki J: The design and construction of a new apparatus for measuring the vertical forces exerted in walking: a gait machine. J Strain Anal 1:429, 1966
26. Rydell NW: Forces acting on the femoral head prosthesis. Acta Orthop Scand (suppl):88, 1966
27. Bresler B, Frankel JP: The forces and moments in the leg during walking. Trans ASME 72:27 (Paper 48-A-62), 1950
28. Paul JP: The biomechanics of the hip joint and its clinical relevance. Proc R Soc Med 59:943, 1966
29. Morrison JB: The mechanics of the knee joint in relation to normal walking. J Biomech 3:51, 1970
30. Crowninshield RD, Johnston RC, Andrews JG, Brand RA: A biomechanical investigation of the human hip. J Biomech 11:75, 1978
31. Andriacchi TP, Hampton SJ, Schultz AB, Galante JO: Three dimensional coordinate data processing in human motion analysis. J Biomech Eng 101:279, 1979
32. Dempster WT, Gaughran GRL: Properties of body segments based on size and weight. Am J Anat 120:33, 1967
33. Cook T, Cozzens B, Kenosian H: Real-time force line visualization. Adv Bioeng. ASME Paper WA/Bio 6:67, 1977

34. Skinner SR, Antonelli D, Perry J, Lester DK: Functional demands on the stance limb in walking. Orthopedics 8:355, 1985
35. Sutherland DH, Cooper L: The pathomechanics of progressive crouch gait in spastic diplegia. Orthop Clin North Am 9:143, 1978
36. Inman V: The abductor muscles of the hip. J Bone Joint Surg 29:607, 1947
37. Murray MP, Mollinger LA, Gardner GM, Sepic SB: Kinematic and EMG patterns during slow, free, and fast walking. J Orthop Res 2:272, 1984
38. Ralston HJ: Energy-speed relation and optimal speed during level walking. Int Z Angew Physiol 17:277, 1958
39. Waters RL, Campbell, J, Perry J: Energy cost of three point crutch ambulation in fracture patients. J Orthop Trauma 1:170, 1987
40. Waters RL, Lunsford BR: Energy cost of paraplegic locomotion. J Bone Joint Surg 67A:1245, 1985
41. McBeath AA, Bahrke MS, Balke B: Walking efficiency before and after total hip replacement as determined by oxygen consumption. J Bone Joint Surg 62A:807, 1980
42. Strathy GM, Chao EY, Laughman RK: Changes in knee function associated with treadmill ambulation. J Biomech 16:517, 1983
43. Arsenault AB, Winter DA, Marteniuk RG: Treadmill versus walkway locomotion in humans: An EMG study. Ergonomics 29:665, 1986
44. Murray MP, Kory R, Sepic SB: Walking patterns of normal women. Arch Phys Med Rehabil 51:637, 1970
45. Murray MP, Kory R, Clarkson B: Walking patterns in healthy old men. J Gerontol 24:169, 1969
46. Chao EY, Laughman RK, Schneider E, Stauffer R: Normative data of knee joint motion and ground reaction forces in adult level walking. J Biomech 16:219, 1983
47. Winter DA: The Biomechanics and Motor Control of Human Gait. University of Waterloo Press, Waterloo, Ontario, Canada, 1987
48. Waters RL, Hislop JH, Perry J, et al: Comparative cost of walking in young and old adults. J Orthop Res 1:73, 1983
49. Chao EY, Laughman RK, Stauffer RN: Biomechanical gait evaluation of pre and postoperative total knee replacement patients. Arch Orthop Traumat Surg 97:309, 1980
50. Simon SR, Trieschmann HW, Burdett RG, et al: Quantitative gait analysis after total knee arthroplasty for monarticular degenerative arthritis. J Bone Joint Surg 65A:605, 1983

3 | Kinematics and Kinetics of Normal Gait

Edmund Y. S. Chao
Thomas D. Cahalan

The gait pattern of each person is as unique to that person as his or her personality. While each person is different, there are certain attributes of gait in healthy subjects that are quite consistent or consistent within a "normal" range. Employment of engineering principles and techniques has allowed for the measurement of human gait, permitting the assignment of values to these attributes. The marriage of engineering and health science has opened a relatively new field of science, *biomechanics,* which strives to understand human musculoskeletal function, both in its normal and pathologic states. With this in mind, this chapter describes the typical kinematics and kinetics, or biomechanics, of human gait.

BIOMECHANICAL CONCEPTS, TERMS, AND DEFINITIONS

Prior to any discussion of the biomechanics of gait, a review of the basic concepts and definitions is necessary. Kinematics is the study of rigid body motion (e.g., displacement, velocity) without concern for the cause of the motion. A *rigid body* is a system of particles for which the mutual distances between all particles remain constant. Regarding biomechanics, or the mechanics of living systems, parts of the anatomy may be considered rigid bodies, such as the lower leg, thigh, and pelvis.

45

There are two basic types of motion. *Translation* occurs when all particles of the rigid body move along parallel paths, or when an object moves in a straight line. *Rotation* occurs when particles of a rigid body move in parallel planes along circles centered on the same axis, or when an object moves in an arc.

Displacement is a vector quantity representing the change of position of a point in space. A *vector* is a physical quantity that possesses magnitude, direction and sense, and a point of application. The displacement vector is independent of the path of motion and can be either linear (along a straight line, measured in meters or inches) or angular (about a rotational axis, measured in degrees or radians).

Velocity is a vector quantity that is the time rate of change of the displacement vector, which may be either linear or angular. A scalar quantity is a physical quantity that has only magnitude, with no direction or sense. *Speed* is a scalar quantity, or simply the magnitude of the velocity vector. *Acceleration* is the vector quantity, which is the time rate of change of velocity.

When a rigid body is moving freely in a plane, it can have both translation and rotation. Because of the translational component of motion, the center of rotation for the body will change throughout the course of motion. At any instant in time, an approximate center of rotation can be determined, which is the instantaneous center of rotation (ICR).

JOINT ANGULAR ROTATION

Human articular joints can be classified as one of three possible types when pure rotation is of primary interest: (1) the 1-degree-of-freedom (DOF) hinge or revolute joint, (2) the 2-DOF universal joint, and (3) the 3-DOF spherical joint.

A special Eulerian angle system is adopted and the finite rotations occur with respect to three localized coordinate axes fixed to the moving body (Fig. 3-1). If a set of unit vector triad (I,J,K) is fixed to an inertial reference frame, and another triad (i,j,k) is fixed locally, the relationship between them, after any arbitrary finite rotation, can be expressed by a rotational matrix in the terms of the Eulerian angles (Φ,Θ,Ω). The Eulerian angles can be calculated on the basis of known orientation of these unit vectors with respect to another global system:

$$\Theta = \sin^{-1} (-i \cdot K) \qquad (-\Pi/2 < \Theta < \Pi/2)$$
$$\Omega = \sin^{-1} (j \cdot K)/\cos \Theta$$
$$\Phi = \sin^{-1} (i \cdot J)/\cos \Theta$$

Usually, an orthogonal axis system is assigned to each bony segment of the lower extremity (Fig. 3-2). The x axis (unit vector i) is pointing anterior, the y axis (unit vector j) is pointing upward, and the z axis (unit vector k) is directed to the right, forming a right-handed triad. Following this convention, angular motion for the hip, knee, and ankle joint can be determined using the above equations. However, joint angular rotation defined in this manner must follow a predetermined sequence, since finite angular displacement is path dependent.

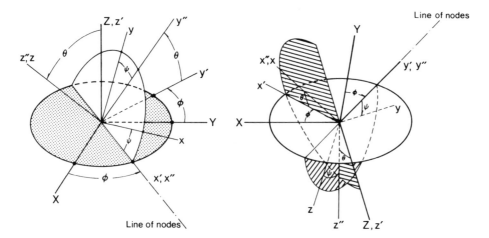

Fig. 3-1. The Eulerian angle system following the three-axis convention. The initial orientation of the local reference axes is XYZ, and the final position is xyz. This convention is similar to the gyroscopic system.

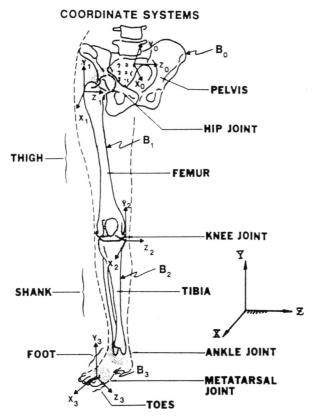

Fig. 3-2. Mechanical model of the lower extremity. The exact procedures to define each of the anatomically based pelvic, femoral, tibial, and foot reference frames vary depending on the specific experimental method used. The inertial reference is expressed by xyz and the unit vectors of each local reference frame to the bone will be expressed in terms of the inertial reference.

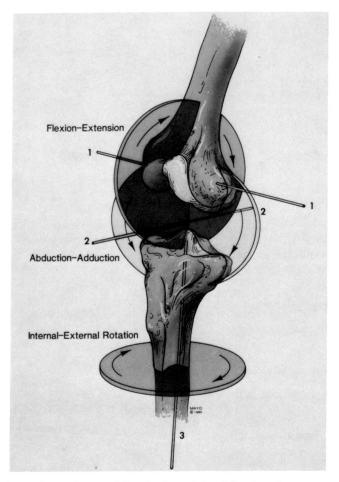

Fig. 3-3. Axes of rotation used for the knee joint following the gyroscopic system. (From Chao and An.[22] By permission of Mayo Foundation.)

Proper selection of axes of rotation between the two bone segments makes these finite rotations sequence independent.[1,2] In the knee joint, for example, the flexion/extension angle occurs about the mediolaterally directed axis fixed to the femoral condyle, and axial rotation is measured about an axis along the shaft of the tibia (Fig. 3-3). The third axis (also defined as the floating axis) is orthogonal to the other axes and defines abduction/adduction. These rotations match the Eulerian angles defined in the above equation, if the localized coordinate axes are used. The advantages of this system are threefold: (1) the rotational sequence can be totally independent, (2) the angular rotations do not have to refer back to the neutral position of the joint, and (3) it can easily be identified with the anatomic structure. In addition, these motion components can be easily measured by a gyroscopic mechanism properly mounted around the joint (Fig. 3-4). This joint motion convention can also be defined as the gyroscopic system.

The same motion convention can also be adopted for the hip and ankle joints (Figs. 3-5 and 3-6). However, when the abduction/adduction angle reaches beyond 90° in either direction, the other two rotational axes may overlap, resulting in a *gimbal-lock* situation, which may occur at the hip joint during extreme range of motion. This complication can be resolved analytically.[3] During both normal and pathologic gait, this situation will not occur. It is important to recognize that two of the rotational axes defined by the present system are nonorthogonal when the joint departs from its neutral position. Consequently, this system is difficult to use in joint force analysis. Angular velocity and acceleration must be transformed into a set of inertial axes in terms of the Eulerian angles defined.

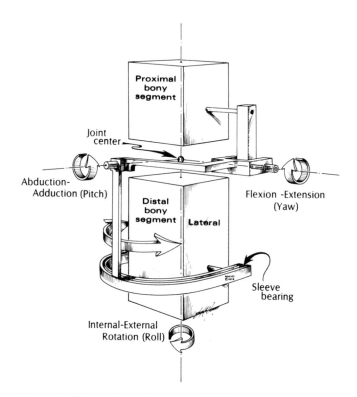

Fig. 3-4. Schematic illustration of an external linkage system used to measure the three-dimensional angular motion of a joint. (From Chao and An.[22] By permission of Mayo Foundation.)

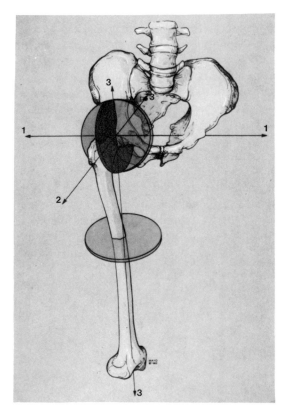

Fig. 3-5. Rotation axes for the hip joint. Axis 1-1 is fixed to the pelvis for flexion/extension measurement; axis 3-3 is fixed to the femur axially for internal/external rotation measurement; axis 2-2 is the floating axis orthogonal to 1-1 and 3-3, used to measure abduction/adduction motion. (By permission of Mayo Foundation.)

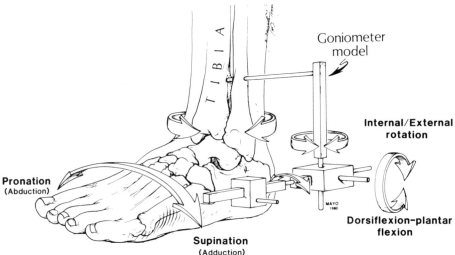

Fig. 3-6. Reference axes and definitions of ankle motion based on the triaxial electrogoniometer attachment and orientation. Plantar/dorsiflexion axis is fixed to the tibia; supination/pronation axis is fixed to the foot, and the internal/external rotation (inversion/eversion) axis is the floating axis. (From Fogal et al.[23] By permission of Mayo Foundation.)

BASIC CONCEPTS OF KINETICS IN GAIT ANALYSIS

Kinetics is the study of the relationship between rigid body motion and the forces causing the motion. Force is a vector quantity that has a point of application, a direction including sense, and a magnitude. It is caused by muscle contraction, gravitational attraction, and other physical and mechanical effects. Force is described by units of a newton (N), which is the force capable of producing an acceleration of 1 m/s² to a mass of 1 kg, or a bf (pound-foot), which is the force capable of producing an acceleration of 32.2 ft/s² (gravitational acceleration of the earth field) to a mass of 1 pound-mass.

Two basic types of forces are described in the biomechanics literature: external and internal. External forces result from direct contact of one body to another (e.g., the foot striking the ground) and from gravitational forces. Internal forces may be applied forces by the muscles and tendons or by constraint forces occurring on the joint contact surface, in the ligamentous structure and within the bone or between bone and prosthetic components.

Newton's *Laws of Motion* apply to particles as well as rigid bodies. The first law states that a body at rest (or in motion) stays at rest (or in constant motion) until a force acts on it. The second law states that force is equal to the product of mass and acceleration (F = ma). The third law holds that for every action there is always an equal and opposite reaction.

A *moment of force* with respect to a point on a rigid body is the product of force and the perpendicular distance (moment arm) between the point and the line of action of the force. The direction of the moment is determined by the *right-handed rule,* and the units are N-m or ft-lb. A torque couple is two noncollinear, equal and opposite forces. The direction of a couple is also defined by the right-handed rule, but it does not have a fixed point of application (free vector). The torque has the same units as the moment. Both moments and torques will produce a tendency of rotating the rigid body with respect to an axis passing through the point of interest. This point is generally referred to as the *point of rotation* for the rigid body.

Reference coordinate systems are needed in order to perform force analysis. On the basis of these systems, externally applied forces can be related to the internal forces of the musculoskeletal system. These relationships form mathematical equations, which we can use to solve for the unknown forces. Gait analysis uses two types of references systems: (1) a global or fixed reference frame, which is nonmoving with respect to the earth, and (2) a local or moving reference frame, which is attached to the moving segment of an object and moves with the object. For the sake of consistency within this book and the works of others,[4] the definition of the local reference system within the body is (tx) = anterior or forward, (ty) = superior or upward, and (tz) = to the right.

KINEMATICS OF HUMAN GAIT

Center of Gravity

The center of gravity (CG) is that point on or near a body at which the entire weight of the body may be assumed to be concentrated. In normal standing, it is located in the midline, 1 inch anterior to the second sacral segment, or about 55 percent of the height of the total stature, from the base in adults. This position of the center of mass will shift with changes of the mass, such as changes in posture.

For the body as a whole to be stable, the line of gravity, which originates at the center of gravity and proceeds vertically downward, must fall within the base of support. In normal level walking, the CG describes a smooth, regular sinusoidal curve, or a series of arcs, in the plane of progression. This results in an overall mean linear displacement. The CG is displaced twice in the vertical direction during each gait cycle. The peaks of the oscillations appear at 25 and 75 percent of the cycle, corresponding to the midstance phase of each supporting limb. The lowest point the center of gravity attains corresponds to the point in time when both feet are in contact with the ground (double support).

There is also lateral displacement of the center of gravity in the horizontal plane. The peaks of lateral oscillation correspond to the stance phase of the ipsilateral limb. Therefore, maximum lateral displacement corresponds to maximum vertical displacement. If the displacement of the CG is traced as someone walks directly away from you, it would describe a crescent opening upward.

Truncal Rotation

As a person reaches forward with the left leg, the pelvis rotates in a clockwise manner as viewed from above. The trunk rotates in the opposite, counterclockwise, direction. This pattern of rotation reverses as the next step is taken, reaching forward with the right leg. This "simultaneous horizontal rotation" of the trunk and pelvis in opposite directions helps produce a smooth, efficient progression of the CG through a counterbalance mechanism. Motion of the pelvis and trunk is limited by rotational constraints of the thorax as a whole. In healthy males, at the self-selected walking velocity, the total amplitude of truncal rotation was measured at 6.8 ± 2.1°. When the gait velocity was increased, the truncal rotation increased to 8.9 ± 2.6°.[5]

Arm Swing

Causal observation of gait will readily confirm the presence of arm swing during walking. The arms swing in phase with the contralateral limb; as a person steps forward with the left leg, the right shoulder and elbow flex slightly. The total amplitude of motion is about 30° at both the shoulder and elbow.[5] This has implications in gait training. Many patients have a great deal of difficulty in coordinating arm swing with stepping, especially when attempting ambulation with a gait aid such as a cane or crutches. Correct arm swing will help generate correct trunk rotation, hence a more efficient gait pattern.

Hip Rotation

Kinematic analysis of the hip joint involves relative motion between the pelvis and femur with 3 DOF. Normally, there is 41° of motion in the sagittal plane, 9° of coronal plane motion, and 12° of transverse plane motion (Fig. 3-7).

In the sagittal plane at heel strike, the hip is at or near maximum flexion and beings to extend just after early stance. The hip extends through foot flat, and the joint is near 0° of flexion at about the time of heel-off. The hip continues to extend through heel rise and push off. Maximum extension is reached, and flexion begins just before toe-off. The hip will flex throughout swing phase, again reaching maximum flexion just before heel strike.

In the coronal plane, the hip is in neutral or slight abduction at the time of heel strike. Adduction occurs through foot flat and heel off, reaching maximum adduction at 80 percent of the stance phase period. There is a rather sharp inclination toward abduction, which peaks shortly after toe-off.

The hip is at or near neutral rotation in the transverse plane at heel strike. The hip immediately externally rotates in early stance, progressing to maximal internal rotation at the time of toe-off. The femur again rotates externally during the swing phase. Just before heel strike, the hip will rotate internally in preparation of weight acceptance.[6] The following generalization may be used to describe the motion at the hip during gait:

Stance phase: extension, adduction, and internal rotation
Swing phase: flexion, abduction, and external rotation

Knee Rotation

Rotation of the tibia relative to the femur takes place in three planes. Normally, there is 70° of rotation in the sagittal plane, 10 to 12° of frontal plane rotation, and 13° in the transverse plane[7,8] (Fig. 3-8).

In the sagittal plane, the knee is just short of full extension at heel strike. During early stance, the knee will flex to about 20°. As the body is progressing over the foot, from foot flat until heel-off, the knee is extending. Flexion occurs through toe-off, continues during early swing phase, and reaches maximum extension just before heel strike.

In the coronal plane, adduction of 5 to 10° occurs at heel strike and remains essentially stable through foot flat. During swing phase, the knee abducts, returning to the neutral position.

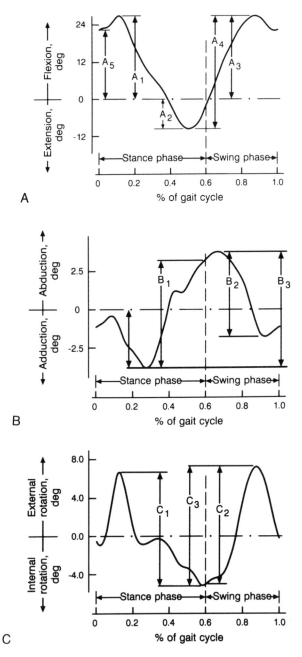

Fig. 3-7. (**A**) Continuous tracing of normal hip flexion/extension motion in a gait cycle. Important parameters are defined: A1, stance flexion; A2, stance extension; A3, swing flexion; A4, total sagittal motion; A5, hip flexion at heel strike. (**B**) Continuous tracing of normal hip abduction/adduction motion in a gait cycle. Important parameters are defined: B1, total coronal plane motion (B3 + B4); B2, stance coronal plane motion; B3, stance adduction; B4, swing abduction. (**C**) Continuous tracing of normal hip internal/external rotation in a gait cycle. Important parameters are defined: C1, stance rotation; C2, swing rotation; C3, total transverse plane motion. (From Chao et al.[6] By permission of Mayo Foundation.)

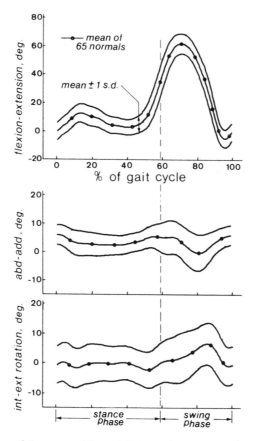

Fig. 3-8. Envelope of the general knee joint rotation patterns (mean and 1 SD) in 65 healthy subjects aged 32 to 65 years. (From Chao et al.,[7] with permission.)

In the transverse plane, the knee is externally rotated at heel strike. In early stance, as the knee flexes, it also rotates internally. As the knee extends at heel-off, the tibia rotates externally. During swing phase, external rotation continues until about midswing, when internal rotation starts.

In a study of the differences between level ground walking and treadmill ambulation, Strathy et al.[9] observed less knee extension at or near the time of heel contact. The changes resulted in less total sagittal plane knee motion, less swing phase sagittal motion, and altered knee position at heel contact. These changes resulted from altering the ground condition and have significant implications in the objective assessment of normal and pathologic gait.

Ankle and Foot Motion

Tibiotalar motion occurs primarily in the sagittal plane with the motions of plantar and dorsiflexion. When subtalar and midtarsal motion is included with the tibiotalar motion, 3 DOF is noted. At heel strike, the ankle angle is usually near the neutral position as in standing, but it may vary slightly due to ground conditions and footwear. At heel strike, there is initial plantar flexion to get the foot flat on the ground. From foot flat to heel-off, there is dorsiflexion (as the body translates over the foot), followed by rapid plantar flexion associated with push-off. During swing phase, dorsiflexion brings the ankle back to neutral, so the foot will clear the floor and be prepared for the next heel strike. Buck et al.[10] and Laughman et al.[11] found the motion used by a sample of normal subjects to range from 10° of dorsiflexion to 20° of plantar flexion (Fig. 3-9).

The subtalar joint is in supination at heel strike and quickly pronates to foot flat, while at heel-off, supination occurs again. The foot is a rigid lever in the supinated position (heel strike and push-off), and a mobile adaptor in the pronated position (foot flat).

The foot-floor contact pattern in the healthy subjects has shown to be quite consistent (Fig. 3-10). The heel makes the initial contact and usually stays on the floor for 55 percent of the stance phase. The area under the fifth matatarsal head makes contact with the floor from 15 to 85 percent of the stance phase. The first metatarsal head area closely follows the fifth, making contact at 20 percent, and

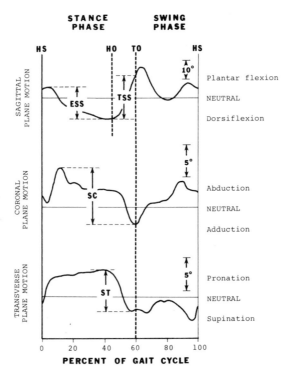

Fig. 3-9. Relative motion pattern of the foot to the ankle. ESS, early stance phase sagittal plane motion; TSS, terminal stance phase motion; SC, stance phase coronal plane motion; ST, stance phase transverse plane motion. (From Fogal et al,[23] with permission.)

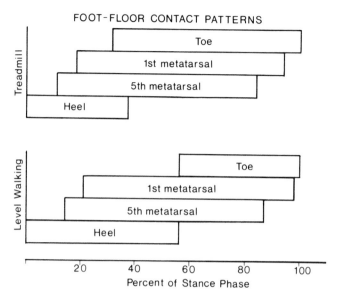

FOOT-FLOOR CONTACT PATTERNS

Fig. 3-10. Average contact times as measured with a foot-switch system, comparing different walking conditions. (From Strathy et al.,[9] with permission.)

finally leaving the floor at 95 percent of stance phase. The toe area makes contact with the floor at about the time the heel leaves the floor, or 55 percent of stance, and is the last part of the foot to leave the floor. Treadmill walking changes the duration of heel and toe contact. The heel has a shorter contact time (0 to 40 percent of stance phase), while the toe has a longer contact time (35 to 100 percent of the stance phase), with the subject walking on a treadmill.[9]

KINETICS OF HUMAN GAIT

Ground Reaction Force

With each step taken, a person applies a force to the ground. In accordance with *Newton's Third Law,* the ground generates a reaction force that is equal in magnitude and opposite in direction to the force applied by the foot. This ground reaction force (GRF) vector is easily determined with a force platform and can be decomposed into three orthogonal components represented by a vertical (compressive) component and fore-aft and mediolateral (sheer) components. Values can be identified from each of the three components that may be used for comparative purposes. A total of nine force parameters in percentage of body weight (F1 to F9) and their chronologic incidence of occurrence (T1 to T9) expressed in percentage of stance phase period have been defined[7] (Fig. 3-11).

Additional variables, such as heel-strike impulse,[12] foot-ground vertical impulse,[13] and foot center of pressure distribution,[14] can be determined from the

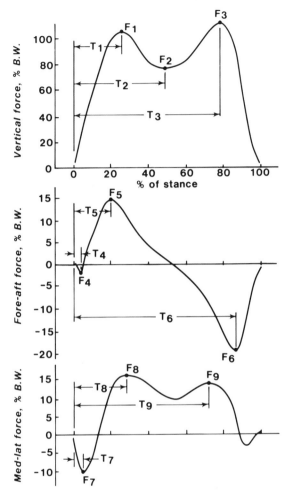

Fig. 3-11. Basic parameters used to describe the foot-floor reaction forces. The force directions are defined as the forces acting from the foot to the floor. (From Chao et al.,[7] with permission.)

data curves. These specialized definitions are suitable for the investigation of foot mechanics during gait.[7]

The vertical component of the GRF appears at the instant of heel strike and rapidly increases to a peak force of about 112 percent of body weight at 25 percent of stance phase. The slope of this line measures the rate of load acceptance of the limb. During foot flat, as the opposite limb propels the CG upward, the vertical force drops to about 93 percent of the body weight. Near heel-off, as the CG begins descending, the vertical force peaks again to about 110 to 115 percent of body weight at 80 percent of stance phase. After this final peak, the force drops off rapidly as the foot prepares to leave the ground.

The fore-aft component of the GRF has a brief initial backward or aft thrust at heel strike of about 2 percent body weight, followed immediately by a forward force (16 to 17 percent of body weight), which decelerates the body at midstance. The pattern then reverses itself, resulting in an aft force as the body is propelled forward, finally dropping to zero as the foot leaves the floor. This biphasic nature of the component of force indicates that although the body displaces forward in a smooth spiral pattern, abrupt, cyclic accelerations and decelerations are occurring.

The mediolateral component of the GRF is in the medial direction (8 percent of body weight) as the abducted leg is adducting at heel strike. This reverses to a lateral force of 8 percent as the center of gravity is supported entirely during single-limb stance. There is a second lateral peak as the CG is accelerated toward the contralateral limb, which is entering stance phase.

Joint Resultant Moments

Ignoring the gravity and inertial effects, the GRF vector tends to cause rotation about the joints of the lower extremity that must be controlled either by ligaments, by muscles, or both. This tendency to cause rotation is termed the moment of force. If the force vector is directed upward and is posterior to the center of rotation of the knee, for example, the knee will flex unless this external moment of force is resisted by an internal moment of force generated by the knee extensors. Generally, this moment is three-dimensional in nature but, during gait, the sagittal plane moment dominates and is usually more accurate to determine for practical applications.

Truncal Forces and Couples

In the anteroposterior (tx) axis during level walking, forces in the range of 10 to 29 percent of body weight are experienced by the pelvis. This force is the result of gravity acting on the upper body and of the forward lean of the body during gait. As the velocity of the gait increases, so does the forward lean and, consequentially, the force in the anteroposterior direction at the pelvis. The force pattern exhibited two relative peaks, occurring at the end of each stance phase.[15]

The couple about the tx axis tends to cause lateral bending of the trunk. During gait, peak-to-peak couples were noted to have a magnitude of 2 to 6 percent of the subject's body weight times height (recall that the unit of a couple is force × distance). This couple tends to flex the trunk laterally toward the right during late stance phase and swing phase on the right side, and visa versa. The maximum value of the couple occurred near toe off.[15]

The lateral force component (along the ty axis) has been calculated at 13 to 16 percent of body weight. The sign of the force is positive (directed toward the right) during right swing phase and negative (directed toward the left) during left swing phase. The couple about the ty axis extends the trunk *almost exclusively* with a magnitude of 1.1 to 2.7 percent of body weight $\times$ height at a gait velocity of 1 to 1.3 m/s. At a gait velocity of 1.9 to 2.35 m/s, the magnitude of this couple increases to 1.8 to 4.6 percent. This extension couple peaks just before each toe-off (corresponding closely to the peak forces along the tx axis).[15]

The force component acting on the pelvis along the tz axis in the negative (downward) direction is the vertical force component of the upper body. The amplitude of this force ranges from 34 to 93 percent body weight, acting to support the mass of the upper body. The peak forces occur about the time of heel strike, while the minima occur at mid- to late stance phase of each leg.[15]

The couple acting about the tx axis tends to twist the upper body to the right, starting at about one-third of the left swing phase. The direction of this couple reverses at one-third of the right swing phase. The inertial forces of the arms contribute significantly to this couple.[15]

The velocity of gait has a direct impact on the magnitude of the forces and couples at the pelvis. Generally, as the gait velocity increases, the amplitude of the force and couple patterns widens, (i.e., the magnitude of the forces and couples will increase in both the positive and negative directions).[15,16]

Resultant Moment About the Hip

In the normal gait pattern, the GRF vector passes anterior and medial to the hip joint throughout stance phase. However, in late stance, the vector passes posterior to the joint. Therefore, the moment of force during stance phase is controlled predominantly by the hip extensors in the sagittal plane and by the hip abductors in the frontal plane, until the GRF vector passes behind the joint and the hip flexors take over control.[4]

Resultant Moment About the Knee

The knee moment of force pattern is more complicated than the hip, exhibiting a biphasic pattern, with two distinct periods tending to flex the knee (30 percent and 90 percent of the stance phase) and two tending to extend the knee (13 percent and 71 percent of the stance phase).[4,17]

Resultant Moment About the Ankle

At heel strike, the moment of force tends to plantar flex the foot. The duration of this moment is rather short, until the foot is flat against the ground. From that instant until the foot leaves the ground, the GRF vector is anterior to the ankle, tending to cause dorsiflexion.

Joint Reaction Forces

The GRF results in external moments about the joints of the lower extremity. These external moments must be resisted by internal moments generated by the muscles and ligaments that cross the joints. The combination of external and internal moments produce internal forces within the joints often known as joint reaction forces.

The work of Paul indicates that the magnitude of the hip joint reaction force ranges from 1.7 to 9.2 times body weight in a group including healthy and pathologic subjects.[18] More recently, Rohrle et al.[19] reported the peak hip joint reaction forces, as a function of gait velocity, to vary from 2 to 5 times body weight at 0.7 m/s to 5 to 9 times body weight at 1.8 m/s.

Using the same techniques employed by Paul, Morrison[20] calculated the joint reaction force for the tibiofemoral joint. The average for a group of healthy adults was 3.03 times body weight, with a maximum of 4.0 times body weight. Morrison related the peak forces to contraction of the muscles crossing the joint (i.e., the hamstrings, quadriceps, and the gastrocnemius). Rohrle et al.[19] reported that the maximum resultant knee joint forces range from 2.5 to 5.5 times body weight at 0.7 m/s to 5 to 8.5 times body weight at 1.7 m/s.

Primary degenerative joint disease at the ankle is rare because, as believed by some, of the relatively smaller joint force and larger weightbearing surface area of the tibiotalor joint. This large surface area decreases the stress or pressure across the joint. The resultant force at this joint has been estimated to be as high as 5 times body weight occurring late in the stance phase.[21] Rohrle et al.[19] reported the maximum resultant ankle joint forces to range from 2.5 to 4 times body weight at 0.7 m/s to 3 to 4.5 times body weight at 1.7 m/s.

SUMMARY AND FUTURE PERSPECTIVES

The analysis of kinematic and kinetic parameters of human gait is difficult to perform accurately and consistently with the naked eye. While the naked eye is sensitive to even slight alterations in gait patterns, sophisticated instruments are needed in order to quantitate and record precisely the gait patterns of our patients. The question remains: How are these data to be used and are they cost effective?

As with any newly developed measurement technique, kinematic and kinetic analysis will ultimately find a niche in clinical practice. These techniques will overcome similar obstacles encountered 20 years ago by electrocardiogram (ECG) analysis, yet no one questions the clinical value of ECG today. Objective gait analysis will no doubt reach such status, provided it is regarded as a supplemental examination to reconfirm diagnosis and assist in treatment planning and assessment.

There seems to be a gap between the practical application of gait information developed and basic research efforts devoted to resolving the inherent problems in this branch of biomechanics. The main reason may have been a lack of communication among physicians, physiologists, physical therapists, and engineers. The absence of mutually acceptable definitions to specify joint motion and force during gait is an important contributing factor. In medical and biologic disciplines, the need for sophisticated theories may be limited but, when the mechanics of musculoskeletal systems are to be used for clinical or research purposes, a set of understandable and correct terminologies is indispensible.

Regardless of the methods used for motion measurement or force calculation in gait analysis, the experimental and computational procedures are too complex and costly for routine medical application. Efforts must be devoted in the future to simplify the method of analysis so that useful information, in legible form, can reach the hands of the physicians and physical therapists quickly. In the analysis of joint kinematics during gait, the translational component is usually small and often within the threshold of the experimental error involved. Under most circumstances, it may be necessary to ignore such motion for the sake of simplicity. In dynamic analysis of human gait, the joint constraint forces are of major concern to the related medical problems. A reliable and convenient relationship should be developed to correlate the joint forces with external measurements, to eliminate tedious computation in routine gait analysis. The degree of accuracy required in any analysis is dictated by the specific application. A proper trade-off must be carefully considered in the light of cost effectiveness before embarking on sophisticated development. Although many unsolved problems will remain an academic challenge for years to come, our present concern should be the use of available analysis and results in the areas of immediate demand.

Since direct validation of joint and muscle forces occurring during gait will be difficult, development of normative models is needed. Based on these models, various analytic methods used can be studied for benchmark comparison. In joint motion analysis, common standards must be established for convenient cross-checking of instrument reliability and data variation. It will be too costly for each institution to establish its own reference data base. The time is ripe to encourage sharing of models, analysis methodology, experimental devices, and reference data. To maintain the needed impetus and vitality of this exciting field, collaboration and communication must reach beyond the boundaries of various scientific and professional domains.

REFERENCES

1. Chao EYS: Jusitification of tri-axial odiometer for the measurement of joint rotation. J Biomech 13:989, 1980
2. Suntay WJ, Grood ES, Noyes FR, Butler DL: A coordinate system for describing joint position. Adv Bioeng ASME p. 59, 1978
3. Mital NK: Computation of rigid body rotation in 3-dimensional space from body-fixed acceleration measurements. Doctoral thesis, Graduate Division Wayne State University, Detroit, 1978
4. Winter DA: The Biomechanics and Motor Control of Human Gait. University of Waterloo Press, Waterloo, Ontario, Canada, 1987

5. Murray MP: Gait as a total pattern of movement. Am J Phys Med 46:290,1967
6. Chao EYS, Kaufman KR, Cahalan TD, Askew LJ: Comparison of objective gait analysis and clinical evaluation after total hip arthroplasty. p. 323 In Fitzgerald R (ed): Non-Cemented Total Hip Arthroplasty. Raven Press, New York, 1988
7. Chao EYS, Laughman RK, Schneider E, Stauffer RN: Normative data of knee joint motion and ground reaction forces in adult level walking. J Biomech 16:219, 1983
8. Laughman RK, Stauffer RN, Ilstrup DM, Dhao EYS: Functional evaluation of total knee replacement. J Orthop Res 2:307, 1984
9. Strathy GM, Chao EYS, Laughman RK: Changes in knee function associated with treadmill ambulation. J Biomech 16:517, 1983
10. Buck PG, Morrey BF, Chao EYS: The optimum position of arthrodesis of the ankle. A gait study of the knee and ankle. J Bone Joint Surg 69A: 1052, 1987
11. Laughman RK, Carr TA, Chao EYS, et al: Three-dimensional kinematics of the taped ankle before and after exercise. Am J Sports Med 8:425, 1980
12. Simon SR, Paul IL, Mansour J, et al: Peak dynamic force in human gait. J Biomech 14:817, 1982
13. Stott JRR, Hutton WC, Stokes IAF: Forces under the foot. J Bone Joint Surg 55B:335, 1973
14. Elftman HA: A cinematic study of the distribution of pressure in the human foot. Anat Res 59:481, 1934
15. Cappozzo A: Compressive loads in the lumbar vertebral column during normal level walking. J Orthop Res 1:292, 1984
16. Cappozzo A: The forces and couples in the human trunk during level walking. J Biomech 16:265, 1983
17. Andriacchi TP, Galante JO, Fermier RW: The influence of total knee-replacement design on walking and stair-climbing. J Bone Joint Surg 64A:1328, 1982
18. Paul JP: Loading on the head of the human femur. J Anat 105:187, 1969
19. Rohrle H, Scholten R, Sigolotto C, et al: Joint forces in the human pelvis-leg skeleton during walking. J Biomech 17:409, 1984
20. Morrison, JB: Function of the knee joint in various activities. Biomed Eng 3: 164, 1968
21. Stauffer RN, Chao EYS, Brewster RC: Force and motion analysis of the normal, diseased, and prosthetic ankle joint. Clin Orthop 127:189, 1977
22. Chao EYS, An KN: Perspectives in measurements and modeling of musculoskeletal joint dynamics p. 1. In Huiskes R, Van Campen D, DeWijn J (eds): Biomechanics: Principles and Applications. Martinus Nijhoff, The Hague, 1982
23. Fogal GR, Katoh Y, Rand JA, Chao EYS: Talonavicular arthrodesis for isolated arthrosis: 9.5-year results and gait analysis. Foot Ankle 3:105, 1982

4 | Energy Expenditure of Normal and Abnormal Ambulation

Robert Waters

Joy Yakura

The energy expenditure of ambulation in normal and disabled subjects has been measured to assess the physiologic penalties of disabled gait. The purpose of this chapter is to review the energy expenditure studies of normals and of patients with specific neurologic and orthopedic disabilities.

A number of investigators have measured the oxygen consumption of ambulation using different testing protocols under diverse laboratory conditions. Consequently, it is often difficult to compare the results. In order to facilitate comparisons of different patient disabilities, most of the data presented in this chapter are based on investigations using consistent procedures conducted in the Pathokinesiology Laboratory of Rancho Los Amigos Medical Center.

ENERGY SOURCES AND TRANSFER

The functional unit of energy for muscle contraction is adenosine triphosphate (ATP). Carbohydrates and fats are the principal food sources for generating ATP during sustained exercise. In aerobic oxidation (citric acid cycle), these substrates are oxidized through a series of enzymatic reactions leading to the production of ATP.

A second type of oxidative reaction is available that does not require oxygen. Anaerobic oxidation (glycolytic cycle) converts carbohydrates or fats to pyruvate and then to lactate. The utilization of either carbohydrates or fat is dependent on the type of muscular work (i.e., continuous, intermittent, brief or prolonged, intensity of work in relationship to muscle groups involved), the individual's training level, diet, and state of general health.

The amount of energy that can be produced by anaerobic means is limited. Approximately 19 times more energy is produced by the aerobic oxidation of carbohydrates than by anaerobic oxidation. Anaerobic oxidation is also limited by the individual's tolerance to acidosis resulting from the accumulation of lactate. From a practical standpoint, the anaerobic pathway provides muscle with an immediate supply of energy for short-term strenuous activity.

During continuous exercise there is an interplay between the aerobic and anaerobic metabolic pathways that depends on the exercise workload. During mild or moderate exercise, the oxygen supply to the cell and the capacity of aerobic energy-producing mechanisms are usually sufficient to satisfy ATP requirements. An individual can sustain exercise for a prolonged time without an easily definable point of exhaustion[1] and the serum lactate does not exceed resting values.

During more strenuous exercise, both anaerobic and aerobic oxidation processes occur, reflecting the additional anaerobic activity required to meet further ATP demands. The point of onset of anaerobic metabolism is heralded by a rise in the serum lactate, a drop in the blood pH, and a rise in the ratio of expired carbon dioxide to inspired oxygen.[2]

After several minutes of exercise at a constant submaximal workload, the rate of oxygen consumption reaches a level sufficient to meet the energy demands of the tissues. The cardiac output, heart rate, respiratory rate, and other parameters of physiologic workload also plateau and a steady-state condition is achieved. Measurement of the rate of oxygen consumption at this time reflects the energy expended during the activity.

Walking, Power, and Work Units

The terms *power* and *work* are used to describe energy expenditure. The power requirement (rate of O_2 consumption) is the milliliters of O_2 consumed per kilogram body weight per minute (ml/kg·min).

Physiologic work is the amount of energy required to perform a task. Physiologic work (O_2 cost) during level walking is the amount of oxygen consumed per kilogram body weight per unit distance traveled (ml/kg·m). The O_2 cost is determined by dividing the power requirement (rate of energy expenditure) by the speed of walking. By comparing the energy cost of pathologic gait to the corresponding value for normal walking, it is possible to determine the gait efficiency.

The rate of O_2 consumption relates to the level of physical effort and the O_2 cost determines the total energy required to perform the task of walking. In the interpretation of data, it is crucial to recognize that the velocity is in the denominator and the rate of O_2 consumption in the numerator of the energy cost calculation. Commonly there is a misinterpretation of the clinical significance of the O_2 cost due to the fact that the O_2 cost may be elevated, but the rate of O_2 uptake is below normal.

The following example illustrates the importance of understanding the difference in the parameters of power (rate of O_2 consumption) and work (O_2 cost). If a hemiplegic patient walks very slowly at 10 m/min (12.5 percent of normal velocity) and consumes oxygen at a rate of 7.3 ml/kg·min (halfway between the effort required for normal standing, 3.5 ml/kg·min, and normal walking, 12.1 ml/kg·m), the oxygen cost is 0.73 ml/kg·m. This is more than 500 percent greater than the normal value, 0.15 ml/kg·m. It is important to recognize that although the gait is extremely costly and inefficient, the rate of O_2 uptake is substantially less than during customary normal walking. The patient will not experience any physical stress, exertion, or fatigue. In this case the critical feature is the patient's slow speed, and the high energy cost is not clinically significant.

In the analysis of energy expenditure, the oxygen pulse and respiratory exchange ratio (RER) are commonly measured parameters. The oxygen pulse is the oxygen required per heartbeat (ml/kg·beat). The RER is the ratio of CO_2 production to O_2 consumption. Sustained strenuous exercise resulting in a RER greater than 0.90 is indicative of anaerobic activity.[1] A ratio greater than 1.00 is indicative of severe exercise. Since the metabolic contribution of anaerobic pathways is limited, as well as the individual's tolerance for acidosis, the endurance time progressively shortens and fatigue ensues earlier as the intensity of the work load rises. Other factors that influence RER in human testing conditions include hyperventilation and diet.

ENERGY CONSERVATION

Human locomotion involves smooth advancement of the body through space. While the goal of walking is progression in the forward direction, limb motion is based on the need to maintain a symmetric, low-amplitude displacement of the center of gravity of the head, arms, and trunk (HAT) in the vertical and lateral directions. This conserves both kinetic and potential energy and is the principle of biological *conservation of energy*.[3-5]

In both the stance and swing phases of gait, this energy transfer is apparent. At the end of the swing phase of gait, the HAT is posterior to the forward-extending leg. As the body progresses into the initial stance phase, the HAT begins to elevate over the leg following heel strike. Elevation of the HAT is generated by forward kinetic energy. As the HAT reaches maximal vertical elevation in the midstance phase, forward velocity of the HAT slows imperceptibly as forward kinetic energy is converted into potential energy of HAT elevation. This potential energy is reconverted into forward kinetic energy in late stance as the HAT passes ahead of the foot and descends, and forward velocity increases. This process is analogous to pole vaulting and enables energy transfer between successive steps as well as maintaining an approximately constant total mechanical energy level (sum of kinetic and potential energy).[3]

Another important energy-transfer mechanism occurs in the swing phase caused by the onset of hamstring muscle activity to decelerate the swinging limb preparatory to heel strike. At the outset of swing, forward velocity of the foot is zero and action of the hip muscles accelerates the foot and leg forward. During midswing the foot achieves a forward velocity more than twice the average walking speed.[6] The hamstrings fire in terminal swing to decelerate the limb preparatory to heel strike and forward velocity of the foot is again zero. Since the origin of the hamstrings is the ischium, the energy of the forward swinging leg is tranferred into a forward propulsive input acting on the pelvis.[3]

Muscle activity is responsible for producing limb movement. The design of the lower limbs and efficient use of two joint muscles enables muscles to fire with minimal change in length approaching isometric conditions of muscle efficiency.[3] Therefore, the shortening velocity of contracting muscle and the necessity for inefficient concentric activity is minimized.

Saunders et al.[5] described six determinants of normal gait that minimize energy expenditure. Pelvic rotation, pelvic tilt, and stance knee flexion minimize the vertical rise and fall of the trunk and, therefore, the need to perform lift work on the HAT against gravity. The fourth and fifth determinants involve interaction of the knee and ankle during stance to improve shock absorption and smooth out the points of inflection of vertical rise and fall of the HAT and the consequent vertical ground reaction force. The sixth determinant, lateral pelvic displacement, serves to minimize lateral shift of the body's center of gravity decreasing energy expenditure.

The above examples illustrate some of the numerous energy conserving characteristics of trunk and lower limb design and the complex interrelationships of muscle activity and movement in normal walking. Interruption of the normal gait cycle results in increased energy expenditure.[4,5] Nevertheless, in response to a gait disability, a patient will adapt by performing compensatory gait substitutions to minimize the additional energy expenditure.[4]

NORMAL WALKING

Range of Customary Walking Speeds

Most adults prefer to walk at speeds from 60 m/min up to 100 m/min.[7–9] In a study of adult pedestrians aged 20 to 60 years who were unaware they were observed, the mean velocity for males, 82 m/min, was significantly higher than for the females, 74 m/min.[8] Similar values were obtained during energy-expenditure studies performed around an outdoor circular track when subjects were instructed to select their natural comfortable walking speed (CWS)[9] (Table 4-1). Patients in the latter study were also tested at their customary slow and fast speeds. The customary slow, normal, and fast walking speeds, cadences, and stride lengths are listed in Table 4-2, indicating that the range of customary slow

Table 4-1. Gait Characteristics of Unobserved Adult Pedestrians and Adult Subjects Aged 20 to 60 Years Undergoing Energy Expenditure Testing at CWS

	Finley[a]			Waters[b]		
	M	F	T	M	F	T
Velocity (m/min)	82	74	78	82	78	80
Cadence (steps/min)	110	116	114	108	118	113
Stride (m)	1.48	1.31	1.38	1.51	1.32	1.42

[a] Data from Finley and Cody.[8]
[b] Data from Waters et al.[12]

and fast speeds in adults aged 20 to 59 years ranges from approximately 37 to 99 m/min.[9]

At speeds above 100 m/min there is a choice between walking or running. Thorstensson and Roberthson[10] studied adult males and found the transition speed between walking and running averaged 113 m/min with a tendency for longer-legged men to have a higher transition speed. Running becomes more efficient than walking at speeds above approximately 133 m/min.[7]

Controlled Speed versus Free-Velocity Walking

Although it is convenient to measure energy expenditure at a controlled velocity on a treadmill, the CWS is highly variable in different patient populations depending on the extent of disability. Consequent measurement of energy expenditure at predetermined controlled velocities may not reflect the true functional energy expenditure. Furthermore, patients with gait disabilities often have difficulty adjusting to walking on a treadmill. For these reasons, most investigators have found it preferable to perform testing on a track allowing patients to select their CWS.

An oxygen consumption study of normal adults using a modified Douglas Bag technique while walking around an outdoor track at their CWSs demonstrated no significant differences in mean velocity, stride length, or cadence as compared with Finley's measurements of unobserved adult pedestrians.[8,9] These findings support the conclusion that the gait of normal subjects tested in this manner is not altered by the experimental procedure.

Energy Expenditure at Customary Walking Speeds

At the CWS, the rate of oxygen consumption for young adults aged 20 to 59 years and senior subjects aged 60 to 80 years does not differ significantly, averaging 12.1 and 12.0 ml/kg·min.[9] The rate of O_2 uptake increases in younger subjects averaging 12.9 ml/kg·min in teens and 15.3 ml/kg·min in children (Table 4-3). Expressed as a percentage of the Vo_2max, the rate of oxygen consumption at the CWS requires approximately 32 percent of the Vo_2max of an untrained

Table 4-2. Gait Characteristics at Slow, Comfortable, and Fast Speeds

Group		Velocity (m/min)			Cadence (steps/min)			Stride (m)		
		SWS	CWS	FWS	SWS	CWS	FWS	SWS	CWS	FWS
Adults (20–59)	F	37	78	99[a]	68	118	137	0.89	1.32	1.24
	M	48	82	110[a]	76	108	125	1.03	1.51	1.67
	T	43	80	106	72	113	131	0.97	1.42	1.47

[a] Indicates significant ($p = 0.05$) difference between male and female subjects at slow walking speed (SWS), customary walking speed (CWS), and fast walking speed (FWS).
(From Waters and Yakura,[72] with permission.)

Table 4-3. Energy Expenditure at Comfortable and Fast Walking Speeds, the Influence of Age

Group	Speed (m/min)		O₂ Rate (ml/kg·min)		O₂ Cost (ml/kg·m)		Pulse (beats/min)		RER	
	CWS	FWS	CWS	FWS	CWS	FWS	CWS	FWS	CWS	FWS
Children (6–12)	70	88	15.3	19.6	0.22	0.22	114	127	0.84	0.87
Teens (13–19)	73[a]	99	12.9[a]	19.1	0.18	0.20	97	117	0.76	0.77
Adults (20–59)	80[a]	106[a]	12.1[a]	18.4[a]	0.15[a]	0.19	99	124[a]	0.81	0.92
Seniors (60–80)	74[a]	90[a]	12.0	15.4[a]	0.16[a]	0.17	103	119[a]	0.84	0.92

Speed values for O₂ Rate column headers: O₂ Rate (ml/kg·min), O₂ Cost (ml/kg·m), Pulse (beats/min)

[a] Indicates significant ($p = 0.05$) difference between preceding value in younger age group.
(From Waters and Yakura,[72] with permission.)

normal subject aged 20 to 30 years and nearly 48 percent of the Vo_2max of a senior subject 75 years of age.[11-13] The RER is less than 0.85 for normal subjects of all ages at their CWS,[9] indicating anaerobic metabolism is not required.

Senior subjects have a slightly lower rate of O_2 consumption at their CWS than do young adults; this may be a purposeful effort to keep the exercise within the aerobic range.[9] The fact that walking taxes less than 50 percent of the Vo_2max in normal subjects in all age groups and does not require anaerobic activity accounts for the perception that walking requires minimal effort in healthy individuals. It is significant that with advancing years older individuals have progressively smaller aerobic reserves (decline in Vo_2max) to accommodate to any added physiological penalties imposed by gait disorders that commonly occur due to aging.

Energy Expenditure at Customary Fast Walking Speeds

When asked to walk at a fast walking speed (FWS), the average rate of O_2 uptake for children, teens and young adults is approximately the same, averaging 19.6, 19.1, and 18.4 ml/kg·min[9,12,13] (Table 4-3). These values are significantly higher than for senior subjects at their CWS, 15.4 ml/kg·min. There is a corresponding decline in the average FWS in senior subjects. The decrease in the rate of energy expenditure in older subjects is similar to the decline observed of other physiologic parameters of performance, such as muscle strength. The decline of the CWS and FWS is associated with a decrease in the Vo_2max independent of age.[14]

The RER for children, teens, young adults, and seniors at their FWS average 0.87, 0.77, 0.92, and 0.92 respectively.[9] These findings indicate that normal adults customarily set their fast walking speed at approximately the threshold triggering anaerobic metabolism. Interestingly, long distance runners also select an exercise rate slightly above the anaerobic threshold.[2]

Rate of O_2 Consumption Versus Speed Relationship

In normal walking, the rate of O_2 consumption is dependent on walking speed, and there is a curvilinear rise at increasing velocities.[7,15-23] Different investigators have derived second-order equations to describe the energy-speed relationship:

$$O_2 \text{ rate } = 0.00110V^2 + 5.9 \quad \text{(Ralston[23])} \tag{1}$$
$$O_2 \text{ rate } = 0.00100V^2 + 6.2 \quad \text{(Corcoran and Gelmann[17])} \tag{2}$$
$$O_2 \text{ rate } = 0.00105V^2 + 7.1 \quad \text{(Molen and Roxendal[21])} \tag{3}$$

where the rate of oxygen consumption is the ml/kg·min of O_2 and V equals the velocity.

The curve of the energy-speed relationship is approximately linear within the customary range of walking speeds below 100 m/min.[9] Within this functional range of walking speeds, higher-order regressions do not improve data fit in comparison with a linear regression and yield the following equations for adult subjects aged 20 to 59 years[9]:

$$O_2 \text{ rate} = 0.129V + 2.60; \quad V \leq 100 \text{ m/min} \tag{4}$$
$$O_2 \text{ rate} = 0.213V - 4.06; \quad V \geq 100 \text{ m/min} \tag{5}$$

Comparison of Eqs. (1), (2), and (4) indicates that all generate nearly identical values for the customary range of normal walking speeds from 40 to 100 m/min (Fig. 4-1). All implicitly state that the rate of energy expenditure is proportional to body weight.

The regression equations for the energy-speed relationship of children, teens, and adults for speeds less than 100 m/min also differ significantly[9]:

Children: $O_2 \text{ rate} = 0.188V + 2.61$ (6)
Teens: $O_2 \text{ rate} = 0.147V + 2.68$ (7)
Adults: $O_2 \text{ rate} = 0.129V + 2.60$ (8)

The Y-intercept (Fig. 4-2) of the regression equations are essentially the same in all three groups and slightly below values for quiet standing (zero velocity).

The above equations were determined in the range of customary walking speeds and not at extremely slow velocities. Measurement of the rate of oxygen consumption at extremely slow speeds in adults resulted in an average of

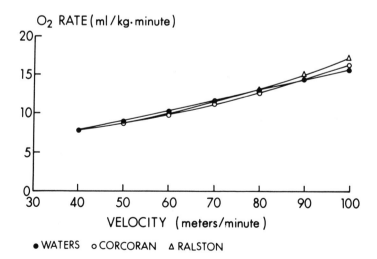

Fig. 4-1. Rate of O_2 consumption-speed relationship in three different studies. This relationship is approximately linear in the range of functional walking speeds between 40 and 100 m/min. (From Waters and Yakura[72], with permission.)

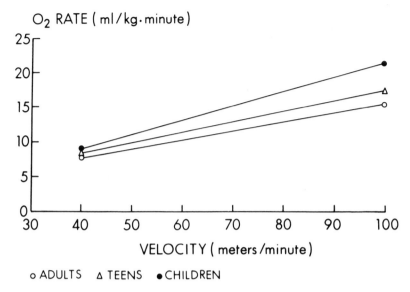

Fig. 4-2. Rate of O_2 consumption-speed relationship in children, teens, and adults. (From Waters and Yakura[72], with permission.)

5.7 ml/kg·min.[23] This value represents the power required to maintain the body in motion at a barely perceptible speed.

O_2 Cost Versus Speed Relationship

The oxygen cost per meter walked is obtained by dividing the rate of oxygen uptake by the velocity. The equation for O_2 cost at different speeds can be derived by dividing Eqs. (6)–(8) by the velocity yielding the following equations:

Children:	O_2 cost $= 0.188 + 2.61\ V^{-1}$	(9)
Teens:	O_2 cost $= 0.147 + 1.68\ V^{-1}$	(10)
Adults:	O_2 cost $= 0.129 + 2.60\ V^{-1}$	(11)

Adults are the most efficient walkers and children the least efficient (Fig. 4-3). The curves are relatively flat, indicating the efficiency of normal gait throughout the functional range of walking speeds.

Ralston demonstrated if the relationship between rate of O_2 consumption and speed is determined by a second-order equation, the equation relating O_2 cost to speed yields a curve that is concave upward with a minimal value of 80 m/min, which is approximately the same as the average speed of unobserved adult pedestrians, 78 m/min.[8,23] However, this mathematical result is the fortuitous choice of a second-order regression equation to characterize the data statistically; therefore, this finding is serendipitous.

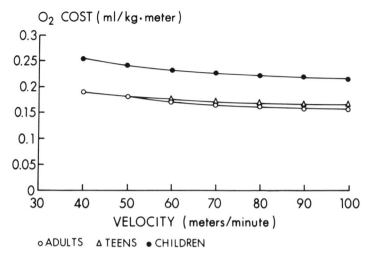

Fig. 4-3. O_2 cost-speed relationship in children, teens, and adults. (From Waters and Yakura[72], with permission.)

Range of Customary Walking Distances

Functional ambulation requires the individual to traverse a certain distance to perform a specific activity. The distance required to perform a walking task divided by the speed of ambulation determines the length of time ambulation must be sustained. Figure 4-4 lists the average distances for various daily living

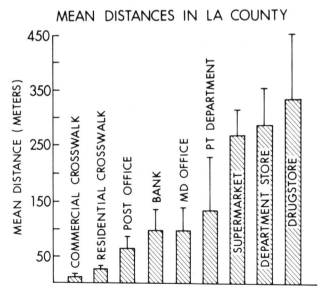

Fig. 4-4. Average walking distance necessary to perform routine activities of daily living in metropolitan Los Angeles. (From Waters and Yakura[72], with permission.)

activities measured in a cross section of different urban areas in Los Angeles, California.[24] Some activities necessitate a 300-m walking distance from available parking. Assuming automotive transport is available and the average speed is 80 m/min, it follows that most daily living activities require less than 5 minutes of walking.

Sex Differences

Several investigators have reported higher rates of oxygen consumption in males while walking.[17,18] Others have reported higher values in female subjects or no significant difference.[16,25] In a review of 225 normal subjects between the ages of 6 and 80 years, no significant differences due to sex were observed at the customary slow, normal, or fast speeds.[9,12,13] The heart rate was higher in females than in males in all age groups, consistent with other types of exercise in which higher heart rates are observed in females.

Effects of Loading During Walking

Loading the body with weights increases the rate of energy expenditure depending on the location of the loads. Loads placed peripherally on the foot have a much greater effect than loads placed over the trunk.[4] Placement of a 20-kg load on the trunk of a male subject did not result in a measurable increase in the rate of energy expenditure. By contrast, a 2-kg load placed on each foot increased the rate of O_2 uptake by 30 percent. This finding is predictible, since forward foot acceleration is much greater than trunk acceleration, requiring greater effort. These findings are of clinical significance for patients requiring lower extremity orthoses or prostheses and indicate the importance of minimizing weight.

SWING-THROUGH CRUTCH-ASSISTED GAIT

Swing-through crutch locomotion requires a high rate of physical effort in comparison with normal walking. The arms and shoulder girdle musculature must lift and then swing the entire body weight forward with each step. A linear relationship was observed between O_2 uptake and speed in normal subjects using upper extremity aids and weightbearing on both legs (four-point gait).[26] The energy-speed curve paralleled the normal walking curve and was 78 percent greater.

High rates of energy expenditure have been recorded with either three- or four-point swing-through gait patterns among unilateral above-knee (AK) amputees walking without a prosthesis, fracture patients, and paraplegics.[26-31] The results of studies in these different populations are summarized in Table 4-4. Unilateral amputees who were experienced crutch ambulators had the fastest

Table 4-4. Energy Expenditure of Swing-Through Crutch Walking

Group	Speed (m/min)	O$_2$ Rate (ml/kg·min)	O$_2$ Cost (ml/kg·m)	Pulse (beats/min)	RER
AK amputee[a]	65	12.8	—	129	0.95
Fracture[b]	50	15.7	0.32	153	1.08
Paraplegia[c]	29	16.3	0.88	140	—

[a] Data from Waters et al.[31]
[b] Data from Waters and Lunsford.[29]
[c] Data from Waters et al.[30]
AK, above-knee.

gait. The newly injured fracture patients with at least 2 weeks crutch experience with a three-point gait had a significantly slower speed and higher rate of energy expenditure and heart rate than that of the amputees, indicating that the effects of chronic crutch ambulation in the latter population resulted in significant upper-extremity conditioning and a training response.

Paraplegics with two paralyzed legs were the slowest ambulators, achieving a velocity less than one-half the value of the unilateral amputees, yet had the highest rate of O$_2$ uptake. The typical paraplegic using a swing-through gait requires bilateral knee-ankle-foot orthoses (KAFOs) to substitute for hip and knee instability; consequently, the arms must also contribute to stance-phase stability at either the hip or trunk, or both, in addition to swinging the body forward. Furthermore, paraplegics commonly have deficient trunk and hip flexors, concentrating the demand on the shoulder and arm musculature to swing the body forward.

The rate of energy expenditure for paraplegics was 16.3 ml/kg·min[30] (Table 4-4). The rate of O$_2$ uptake for normal subjects walking at the same speed as the paraplegics is 6.3 ml/kg·min (Eq. 4). Thus, the paraplegics consume O$_2$ at a rate 160 percent greater than normal. This level of effort is even relatively greater in consideration of the fact that the energy production capacity for paraplegics (Vo$_2$max) is lower in paraplegics than in able bodied subjects.[32,33] Fracture patients required a rate of energy expenditure 69 percent greater than normal value. Above-knee amputees who were experienced crutch ambulators had a rate 16 percent higher than that of normal subjects walking at the same speed.

Interestingly, the RER and heart rate for swing-through crutch ambulation in amputees, fracture patients, and paraplegics at their comfortable speeds are greater than corresponding values for normal subjects during fast walking (see Table 4-3). On this basis, it can be concluded that swing-through crutch ambulation is a strenuous exercise challenge. This accounts for the common clinical finding that patients who require a swing-through gait have a restricted sphere of ambulatory activities. Since the maximal aerobic capacity normally declines with age, older patients have more difficulty meeting the strenuous demands of crutch ambulation than do younger patients. If pulmonary, cardiac, or other disease processes further restrict oxygen delivery, the patient will have greater difficulty meeting the energy demand.

Conditioning programs to improve exercise capacity and locomotor performance in borderline patients may be indicated in patients whom a swing-through crutch-assisted gait pattern is required. A wheelchair may be a logical choice when it is necessary for a patient requiring a swing-through gait pattern to ambulate for a long distance.

CAST IMMOBILIZATION

The patient with lower-extremity trauma frequently is required to wear a cast. Several investigators have measured energy expenditure in normal subjects with unilateral weightbearing plaster casts applied to the leg to restrict joint motion.[34,35]

When normal subjects are allowed to select their CWS, the rate of O_2 consumption in short-leg, cylinder, or long-leg casts does not rise above the value for unrestricted normal walking.[35] Subjects adjust their gait velocity to keep their rate of energy expenditure within normal limits (Table 4-5). Immobilization of both ankle and knee in a long cast resulted in the slowest velocity. Ankle restriction in a short cast resulted in the least reduction in walking speed. Since the rate of O_2 uptake was the same in all three groups, the O_2 cost varied reciprocally with the gait velocity.

These results have important clinical implications for trauma patients. In the preceding section, it was shown that three-point crutch ambulation requires a high heart rate and rate of energy expenditure. Therefore, following lower extremity trauma, weightbearing should be allowed on the injured limb at the earliest possible time consistent with adequate healing to lessen energy expenditure. In this regard, it is often preferable to place an injured lower extremity in a cast and allow full or partial weightbearing, rather than not applying a cast necessitating a unilateral non-weightbearing three-point crutch-assisted gait.

HIP AND ANKLE FUSION

Measurement of energy expenditure following joint fusion provides a method of assessing the relative importance of specific joing movements to the gait cycle. Comparison of energy cost studies of lower-extremity joint fusions

Table 4-5. Energy Expenditure, Walking in Lower-Extremity Plaster Casts

Cast	Speed (m/min)	O_2 Rate (ml/kg·min)	O_2 Cost (ml/kg·m)	Pulse (beats/min)
Short-leg	70	13.0	0.19	92
Cylinder	64	12.7	0.20	93
Long-leg	56	13.0	0.24	92

(From Waters and Yakura,[72] with permission.)

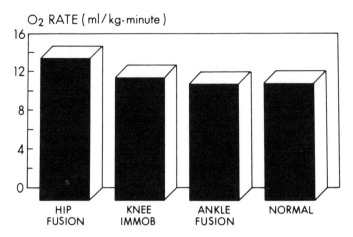

Fig. 4-5. Rate of O_2 consumption following hip or ankle arthrodesis and knee immobilization in a cylinder cast. There is a progressive increase in the rate of energy demand with the loss of joint motion at higher levels. (From Waters and Yakura[72], with permission.)

demonstrates a progressive rise in the energy expenditure with the loss of joint motion progressing from the ankle, to the knee, and to the hip (Figs. 4-5 and 4-6).

Ankle Fusion

During normal walking, ankle motion ranges from 15° of dorsiflexion in the midstance phase to 20° of plantar flexion in the terminal stance phase.[4] Altera-

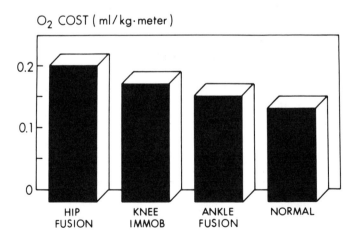

Fig. 4-6. O_2 cost following hip or ankle arthrodesis and knee immobilization in a cylinder cast. Note the progressive increase in O_2 cost when lower-extremity joint motion is lost at higher levels. (From Waters and Yakura[72], with permission.)

Table 4-6. Energy Expenditure Following Hip and Ankle Fusion

Group	Speed (m/min)	O$_2$ Rate (ml/kg·min)	O$_2$ Cost (ml/kg·m)	Pulse (beats/min)
Ankle fusion	67	12.0	0.17	93
Hip fusion	67	14.7	0.22	112

(From Waters and Yakura,[72] with permission.)

tions in the gait pattern created by ankle arthrodesis are difficult to identify by visual observation.[36]

Ankle-fusion patients select an average CWS, 67 m/min, which is 84 percent slower than normal[37] (Table 4-6). At their CWS, the average rate of O$_2$ uptake, 12.0 ml/kg·min was approximately the same as the mean for adult subjects, 12.1 ml/kg·min. Equation (4) shows that the average patient required a 3 percent greater rate of energy expenditure than for a normal subject walking at the same speed.

The oxygen cost averaged 0.166 ml/kg·m. By comparing this value with the mean for normal walking, 0.151 ml/kg·m, the physiologic efficiency of gait can be determined. Gait efficiency for ankle-fusion patients averaged 90 percent. The fact that gait efficiency is only slightly decreased is consistent with the finding that ankle fusion does not require major compensatory changes in the gait pattern.

Knee Immobilization

Since application of a cylinder cast provides excellent restriction of knee motion without interfering with ankle or hip motion, the results obtained following cylinder cast immobilization are probably comparable to those with knee fusion. Interestingly, the values for the rate of O$_2$ consumption, 12.7 ml/kg·min, and the O$_2$ cost per meter, 0.200 ml/kg·m following cylinder cast immobilization are greater than the values for ankle fusion and less than values for hip fusion patients.[38]

Often immobilization can lead to joint contracture. The significance of knee-flexion deformity was illustrated by a study in which the energy cost penalties associated with walking on a flexed knee were evaluated in normal subjects.[39] A specially designed hinged-knee orthosis restricted right knee extension to 15°, 30°, and 45° but allowed full flexion.

In normal walking, knee flexion deformities shorten the limb and lead to decreased lower-extremity shock absorption in stance, hence increased energy expenditure.[40] Progressively greater O$_2$ cost and rates of O$_2$ expenditure resulted when the amount of simulated knee-flexion contracture was increased (Table 4-7). These changes were associated with a decline in speed.

Table 4-7. Energy Expenditure of Flexed Knee Gait

Degrees	Speed (m/min)	O$_2$ Rate (ml/kg·min)	O$_2$ Cost (ml/kg·m)
0°	80	11.8	0.16
15°	77	12.8	0.17
30°	75	14.3	0.19
45°	67	14.5	0.22

(From Waters and Yakura,[72] with permission.)

Hip Fusion

In normal walking, pelvic rotation and tilt about the hip joint are important to energy conservation. The hip flexes 30° and internally rotates 7° during the swing phase, reaching full extension and 10° external rotation in the terminal stance phase.[4] Following hip fusion, excessive anterior pelvic tilt and lumbar lordosis are necessary to enable the femur on the fused limb to extend during the stance phase while the normal limb was advanced.[41] During the swing phase, less difficulty with advancing the fused limb is encountered due to the generally chosen position of fusion, 30° to 40° of flexion. Transverse pelvic rotation about the contralateral hip joint is increased to maintain stride length.

The mean CWS of the hip-fusion patients during energy expenditure testing is the same as the value for the ankle fusion patients, 67 m/min[37] (Table 4-6); however, the average rate of energy expenditure for hip fusion patients (14.7 ml/kg·min) was significantly greater than the preceding value for the ankle-fusion patients. This represents a 32 percent increase in comparison with normal values at the same walking speed according to Eq. (8). Inability to perform adequate gait substitutions to prevent this increase indicates the importance of hip motion in the normal gait cycle. Heart rate was also higher, indicating that hip-fusion patients expended more physiologic effort than did ankle fusion patients or normal subjects.

The O$_2$ cost averaged 0.223 ml/kg·m for patients with hip arthrodesis, which was significantly ($P < 0.05$) greater than the value following ankle arthrodesis (0.170 ml/kg·m). In comparison with normal walking, hip-fusion patients achieved a 53 percent gait efficiency.

It is of clinical interest to compare the energy expenditure of walking in patients with hip fusion with the results obtained following total hip arthroplasty. We have previously reported the energy expenditure in patients 1 year following unilateral total hip arthroplasty for osteoarthritis.[42] After walking for 5 minutes, the patient's rate of energy expenditure was significantly lower following total hip arthroplasty than following hip fusion (11.8 ml/kg·min versus 14.3 ml/kg·min). Favorable energy expenditure is an advantage of hip arthroplasty over hip fusion in the patient with unilateral disease.

AMPUTATION

Lower-extremity amputation with or without prosthetic replacement imposes energy penalties for ambulation. The patient must choose between walking without a prosthesis using crutches or using a prosthesis and using the remaining muscles to substitute for lost function and control the additional mass of the prosthesis.

There is a considerable body of literature on the energy expenditure of amputee gait. However, a direct comparison of the results of the different studies is difficult, since no distinction is made among age groups, use or nonuse of upper-extremity assistive devices, and adequacy of prosthetic fit and duration of experience is often not specified.

Unilateral Amputees

Different investigators have described linear or second-order equations to describe the energy-speed relationship in below-knee (BK) amputees.[43–46] Below-knee amputees expend a 20 percent higher rate of O_2 uptake that parallels the normal energy-speed relationship.[45] Other investigators have defined similar relationships for AK amputees indicating that values for the energy-speed relationship are greater for AK than for BK amputees.[43,47]

The combined results of two studies in which patients were tested at their CWSs under similar conditions illustrate the importance of the level of amputation.[31,48] The O_2 cost progressively increased at each higher amputation level, ranging from the BK to hemipelvectomy (HP) levels. Patients with higher level amputations had a less efficient gait and higher O_2 cost than those with lower level amputations.

The averaged rate of O_2 consumption for different level amputees was not dependent on level and was approximately the same as the value for normal subjects (Table 4-8). The CWS depended on the level of amputation and declined at each higher amputation level progressing from the BK, TK, AK, hip disarticulation (HD), and HP levels in the traumatic and surgical amputee groups. These values averaged 71 m/min, 61 m/min, 52 m/min, 47 m/min, and 40 m/min. Interestingly, in a group of vascular patients, Syme amputees had a faster velocity than that of BK amputees.[31]

These findings indicate the amputees purposefully adapted to the inefficient gait (higher O_2 cost) caused by progressively higher level amputations by selecting speeds so that the mean rate of O_2 uptake did not exceed the normal rate. Other investigators who have tested amputees at their CWS have also reported the rate of O_2 uptake was approximately the same as for normal subjects at their CWS.[44,49,50] Clearly, as more joints and muscles of the leg are lost due to higher-level amputations, the greater the loss of the normal locomotor mechanisms, hence the greater the energy cost and disability.[51]

Table 4-8. Energy Expenditure: Unilateral Amputees

Group	Speed (m/min)	O$_2$ Rate (ml/kg·min)	O$_2$ Cost (ml/kg·m)	Pulse (beats/min)
Vascular amputees[a]				
AK	36	10.8	0.28	126
BK	45	9.4	0.20	105
SYME	54	9.2	0.17	108
Surgical amputees[b]				
HP	40	11.5	0.29	97
HD	47	11.1	0.24	99
Traumatic amputees[a]				
AK	52	10.3	0.20	111
TK	61	13.4	0.20	109
BK	71	12.4	0.16	106

[a] Data from Waters et al.[31]
[b] Data from Nowrozzi and Salvanelli.[48]
AK, above-knee; BK, below-knee; TK, through knee; HP, hemipelvectomy; HD, hip disarticulation.

Traumatic Versus Vascular Amputees

A special problem confronting many older vascular amputees is their limited exercise ability. Physical work capacity and Vo$_2$max are reduced not only because of the effects of aging but as a result of commonly associated diseases such as arteriosclerotic heart and peripheral vascular disease. Diabetes, commonly present in the vascular amputee population, decreases capillary permeability, and therefore O$_2$ supply to the muscle, due to basement membrane thickening.

The data in Table 4-8 also permit comparison of the young traumatic amputees with the older vascular amputees at the BK level. The CWS and rate of O$_2$ uptake were significantly higher for the traumatic BK amputees than for the vascular BK amputees. It is probable the higher exercise capacity of the younger traumatic amputees permits selection of a higher CWS than for the older vascular counterpart.

Most older patients who have AK amputations for vascular disease are not successful long-term prosthetic ambulators. Only a small percentage of these patients are functional ambulators.[31,52] If able to walk, most have a very slow gait velocity and an elevated heart rate if crutch assistance is required.[31] By contrast, traumatic AK amputees usually have an adequate gait and can walk without crutches.[31,53] It may be concluded that every effort must be made to protect dysvascular limbs early so that AK amputation does not become necessary. If amputation is required every effort should be made to amputate below the knee.

Prosthesis Versus Crutches

Crutch walking without a prosthesis with a three-point gait pattern in unilateral amputees may be a primary or secondary means of transportation when an adequate prosthesis is unavailable or inadequate. A direct comparison of walking in unilateral amputees with and without a prosthesis using a three-point crutch-assisted gait pattern revealed that all, with the single exception of vascular AK amputees, had a lower rate of energy expenditure, heart rate, and O_2 cost when using a prosthesis.[31] This difference was insignificant in the vascular AK group and probably relates to the fact that, even with a prosthesis, most of these patients relied on crutches for some support increasing the energy demand and heart rate. Traugh et al.[54] also compared energy expenditure with and without a prosthesis in middle-aged and elderly AK patients and reported similar findings.

It may be concluded a well-fitted prosthesis that results in a satisfactory gait not requiring crutches significantly reduces the physiologic energy demand. Since crutch walking requires more exertion than walking with a prosthesis, crutch walking without a prosthesis should not be considered an absolute requirement for prosthetic prescription and training.

Bilateral Amputees

Few energy expenditure studies have been performed on bilateral amputees.[55] Table 4-9 summarizes data on both traumatic and vascular patients with bilateral amputation. This limited information indicates that the bilateral amputee expends greater effort than the unilateral amputee. Of interest, vascular patients with the Syme/Syme combination walked faster and had a lower O_2 cost than did vascular patients with the BK/BK combination. This parallels the findings among the unilateral amputees demonstrating performance relates to

Table 4-9. Energy Expenditure: Bilateral Amputees

Group	Speed (m/min)	O_2 Rate (ml/kg·min)	O_2 Cost (ml/kg·m)	Pulse (beats/min)
Traumatic				
BK/BK[a]	67	13.6	0.20	112
AK/AK[a]	54	17.6	0.33	104
Vascular				
Syme/Syme[a]	62	12.8	0.21	99
BK/BK[a]	40	11.6	0.31	113
Stubbies[b]	46	9.9	0.22	86

[a] Data from Waters et al.[31]
[b] Data from Wainapel et al.[56]
AK, above-knee; BK, below-knee.

amputation level. Traumatic BK/BK amputees walked faster and at a lower energy cost than did their vascular BK/BK counterparts (Table 4-9).

Gonzalez et al.[49] pointed out that considering approximately 24 to 35 percent of diabetic amputees lose the remaining leg within 3 years. It is important to preserve the knee joint even if the stump is short because, should a unilateral BK amputee undergo another BK amputation, 24 percent less energy would still be expended than with a unilateral AK amputation. Bilateral vascular amputees rarely achieve a functional ambulation status if one amputation is at the AK level.

Finally, of special interest, Wainapel[56] measured energy expenditure in a 21-year-old bilateral through knee (TK/TK) patient who walked on stubby prostheses with a walker. The patient walked faster at a slightly greater rate of O_2 consumption than with conventional prostheses and crutches. While walking on stubbies is cosmetically unacceptable for most patients (except for gait training or limited walking in the home), the data from this single patient illustrates that it can result in a functional gait.

Cardiovascular Efficiency

The status of physical fitness can be assessed by examining the oxygen pulse. Comparison of the mean rate of O_2 uptake and heart rate in different amputee groups walking without crutches indicates a lower than normal O_2 pulse. This suggests amputees may lead a less active life-style, resulting in a lower level of physical conditioning.[55] This conclusion is supported by the result of Vo_2max measurements during one-legged and two-legged exercise in normal subjects and AK amputees.[50]

ARTHRITIS

Few energy-expenditure studies have been performed on arthritis patients.[42,57,58] In a study of 24 patients with unilateral osteoarthritis of the hip tested before and after total hip replacement (THR), Brown et al.[42] found that the energy cost was significantly reduced after operation, reflecting an improved gait velocity. In a follow-up study of 60 patients, energy expenditure was measured after Girdlestone resection arthroplasty of the hip and both before and after total knee arthoplasty (TKA).[58] Both osteoarthritis and rheumatoid arthritis patients were tested.

Arthritis of the Hip

Pain resulting from arthritis of the hip results in an antalgic gait pattern. The patient leans excessively in the lateral plane over the involved hip to keep the center of gravity of the trunk over the hip joint. This pattern lowers the demand on the hip abductor muscles and lessens the compressive forces across the hip joint. When this gait pattern is no longer sufficient to ameliorate pain, patients require upper-extremity gait-assistive devices to lessen the load across the hip.

In a group of patients with unilateral osteoarthritis of the hip tested prior to the total hip arthroplasty (THA), walking speed averaged 41 m/min and the rate of O_2 uptake 10.3 ml/kg·min.[42] One year following surgery, speed increased to 55 m/min and the rate of O_2 uptake was not significantly changed. Since the speed improved without a corresponding increase in the O_2 rate, the efficiency of gait also improved and the O_2 cost declined from 0.28 to 0.20 ml/kg·m (Table 4-10).

It is useful to compare the results of THA procedure to the previously discussed results following hip fusion (see Table 4-6). Hip fusion is often performed in young patients as an alternative to THA. Hip fusion resulted in a faster gait but required a 32 percent greater rate of O_2 uptake than THA and was slightly less efficient (0.22 versus 0.20 ml/kg·m).

Girdlestone hip resection arthroplasty is commonly performed as a salvage procedure following failed THA or following hip sepsis. Following this procedure, speed averaged 46 m/min, O_2 rate 12.2 ml/kg·min, and O_2 cost 0.39 ml/kg·m.[55] The heart rate averaged 118 beats/min, reflecting reliance of the majority of these patients on crutches for partial weight support. These findings imply that the functional energetic impairment of the patient following Girdlestone resection arthroplasty as a salvage procedure is approximately the same as that for the typical patient with unilateral osteoarthritis of the hip prior to any surgery. In other words, the functional outcome of a failed THR arthroplasty, which results in removal of prosthesis, is probably no worse than the disability caused by the patient's primary pathology.

Arthritis of the Knee

Evaluation of patients with osteoarthritis of the knee prior to total knee arthroplasty revealed approximately the same speed, rate of O_2 uptake, and O_2 cost as that of patients with osteoarthritis of the hip tested prior to total hip arthroplasty.[55] These results indicate that the energetic impairment caused by

Table 4-10. Energy Expenditure: Arthritis of the Hip

Group	Speed (m/min)	O_2 Rate (ml/kg·min)	O_2 Cost (ml/kg·m)	Pulse (beats/min)
Preoperative THR[a]	41	10.3	0.28	106
Postoperative THR[a]	55	11.1	0.20	108
Girdlestone[b]	46	12.2	0.39	118
Fusion[c]	67	14.7	0.22	112

[a] Data from Brown et al.[42]
[b] Data from Waters et al.[58]
[c] Data from Waters et al.[37]

Table 4-11. Energy Expenditure: Arthritis of the Knee

Group	Speed (m/min)	O$_2$ Rate (ml/kg·min)	O$_2$ Cost (ml/kg·m)	Pulse (beats/min)
Osteoarthritis	46	10.1	0.23	112
Rheumatoid arthritis	33	10.3	0.40	115

(From Waters and Yakura,[72] with permission.)

severe arthritis of the knee is generally the same as by arthritis of the hip (Table 4-11).

A study of patients with rheumatoid arthritis revealed the functional benefit of total joint replacement in patients with systemic illness.[55] Although the rheumatoid patients had involvement of other lower extremity joints, severe degeneration of the knee joint was the primary problem. After surgery a significant improvement in gait velocity without an increase in the rate of O$_2$ uptake was noted to result in a significant improvement in the O$_2$ cost and walking efficiency (Table 4-12). These results suggest that the same magnitude of improvement from surgery can be obtained from surgery in a rheumatoid patient as in an osteoarthritis patient if the primary pathology is restricted to a single joint.

Influence of Upper Extremity Assistive Devices

The use of crutches, canes, or walkers by arthritis patients reflects the severity of the patient's pathology and functional performance (Table 4-13). The type of device prescribed depends on the magnitude of pain. Forces across a joint are progressively unloaded by prescription of a cane, one crutch, two crutches, or a walker.

In a group of rheumatoid arthritis patients, those patients using a walker had the highest O$_2$ cost and slowest gait.[55] Speed progressively increased in the groups of patients requiring two crutches, one crutch, cane(s), or no assistive devices. Conversely, O$_2$ cost was highest in patients requiring a walker and least in those patients requiring no upper-extremity assistive devices.

Since the use of gait-assistive devices is associated with a slow walking speed and higher O$_2$ cost, the question arises as to whether the device is responsible for the additional energy demand rather than the patient's disability. McBeath et al.[26] tested patients with hip impairment with and without walking aids (one crutch, two crutches, or a cane). Most of the patients were able to walk faster with their assistive device. The effect on energy expenditure was variable.

Table 4-12. Rheumatoid Arthritis of the Knee: Pre- and Postoperative Total Knee Arthroplasty

Group	Speed (m/min)	O$_2$ Rate (ml/kg·min)	O$_2$ Cost (ml/kg·m)	Pulse (beats/min)
Preoperative	33	10.3	0.40	115
Postoperative	58	11.4	0.71	111

(From Waters and Yakura,[72] with permission.)

Table 4-13. Rheumatoid Arthritis of the Knee: Preoperative Evaluation: Influence Upper-Extremity Assistive Devices

Device	Speed (m/min)	O_2 Rate (ml/kg·min)	O_2 Cost (ml/kg·m)	Pulse (beats/min)
Walker	21	7.2	0.63	124
Crutches	26	10.6	0.50	124
Crutch	31	10.9	0.37	102
Cane(s)	32	9.8	0.36	97
No assistive device	45	11.0	0.26	115

(From Waters and Yakura,[72] with permission.)

McBeath et al. concluded that when hip impairment exists, assistive devices enable upper-extremity power to compensate for the hip impairment and permit an increase in speed with an inconsistent effect on energy expenditure.

Deconditioning

The heart rate in arthritis patients tested prior to surgery is higher than in normal subjects.[55] Two factors—the patient's level of physical fitness and the necessity of using upper-extremity assistive devices to aid walking—account for the elevated heart rate.

The heart rate was highest in patients using crutches or a walker, reflecting the greater arm work required by these devices. The use of upper-extremity assistive devices, however, does not account for the elevated cardiac response in all patients. In arthritis patients not using upper-extremity devices, higher than normal heart rates and lower than normal rates of O_2 uptake were recorded, indicating a lower O_2 pulse. This leads to the conclusion that pain limits ambulatory activities and leads to a more sedentary and deconditioning lifestyle.

PARAPLEGIA

Increased energy expenditure of paraplegic gait has been closely linked to the type of orthoses, gait pattern, and upper-extremity assistive device(s) used during gait.[59] A recent study of 36 spinal cord injury patients (34 patients utilized a reciprocal gait) has demonstrated that the lower-extremity strength or, conversely, the severity of paralysis, determines gait performance.[59]

Effects of Lower-Extremity Strength on Energy Expenditure

Lower-extremity strength was calculated by the ambulatory motor index (AMI) representing the sum of manual muscle scores for bilateral hip flexors, extensors, abductors, knee flexors, and extensors and expressed as a percentage of the total possible score.[59] The AMI was significantly correlated with the rate of O_2 consumption, velocity, O_2 cost, percentage increase of O_2 consumption as compared with normals walking at the same speed (O_2 rate increase), and upper-extremity load on assistive devices.

Furthermore, when patients were grouped according to assistive device (cane, crutch, or walker), general level of lesion (quadriparetic, paraparetic), and orthoses (two KAFOs, one KAFO, or no orthoses), the differences among the groups in terms of energy cost parameters were attributable to differences in lower-extremity strength scores (AMI). Those patients with an AMI greater than 60 percent of normal demonstrated gait performance characteristics and energy expenditure values that approximated normal values, consistent with community ambulation. Those patients having an AMI of less than 40 percent of normal had a slow speed and high-energy expenditure, consistent with restricted ambulatory capabilities.

Gait Pattern

Paraplegics with quadriceps weakness requiring bilateral KAFOs generally walk with a four-point, swing-through crutch-assisted gait. This type of a gait pattern requires a high rate of energy expenditure and energy cost.[30,60–62]

A 38 percent increase in the rate of O_2 consumption and a 560 percent increase in the O_2 cost was recorded in complete paraplegics using bilateral KAFOs with a swing-through crutch-assisted gait[30] (Table 4-14). Further studies comparing the standard KAFO design with a rigid ankle with the Scott-Craig brace (fixed in dorsiflexion, extended sole to the metatarsal heads, and a crossbar across the ankle to provide mediolateral stability) found no differences between braces in the energy cost of standing.[60,61] Furthermore, there was no significant difference between standard braces and Scott-Craig braces when ambulating with a walker, negotiating turns, or walking up and/or down steps or down ramps.

Although the rate of energy expenditure and heart rate in reciprocal gait is significantly below that required for swing-through gait pattern, the reciprocal gait pattern still severely restricts the paraplegic's ability to walk. The AMI of reciprocal walkers determined energy expenditure.[59] Compared with normal subjects walking at their CWS, the O_2 cost can be 500 percent greater, the rate of O_2 expenditure in reciprocal gait is 20 percent greater, and the speed is 67 percent slower[30] (Table 4-15). No differences in the speed or rate of energy expenditure were found between patients with one or two free knees (AFO/AFO versus AFO/KAFO).

Table 4-14. Paraplegic Swing-Through Gait Versus Wheelchair Propulsion

Group	Speed (m/min)	O_2 Rate (ml/kg·min)	O_2 Cost (ml/kg·m)	Pulse (beats/min)
Wheelchair (N = 124)	72	11.5	0.16	123
Walking (N = 20)	29	16.3	0.64	140

(From Waters and Yakura,[72] with permission.)

Table 4-15. Paraplegic Reciprocal Gait

Group	Speed (m/min)	O₂ Rate (ml/kg·min)	O₂ Cost (ml/kg·m)	Pulse (beats/min)
KAFO/KAFO	18	16.5	1.02	168
KAFO/AFO	26	13.0	0.58	132
AFO/AFO	26	13.8	0.73	131

(From Waters and Yakura,[72] with permission.)
AFO, ankle-foot orthosis; KAFO, knee-ankle-foot orthosis.

MYELODYSPLASIA

The child with myelodysplasia has a pattern of motor paralysis that parallels that observed following traumatic spinal cord injury (SCI) in the absence of brain dysfunction secondary to hydrocephalus or Arnold-Chiari malformation. Following a preliminary report on 15 children with myelodysplasia, we have tested 22 children averaging 12.1 years of age[63] (Waters RL: unpublished data). Patients with clinically significant neurologic impairment above the level of their spinal lesion impairing use of the upper extremities or clinically significant spine or hip instability/dislocation were excluded.

Categorization of subjects by their orthotic requirement (KAFO, AFO) permitted classification of the children according to their functional neurologic lesion. They were subdivided into the following four groups. The thoracolumbar group required two KAFOs due to bilaterally inadequate quadriceps strength; the high lumbar group required only one KAFO and having one free knee with functionally intact quadriceps strength; the low lumbar group had two AFOs and less than fair hip extensor and abductor strength; and the sacral group consisted of children with two free knees and bilateral fair or greater hip abductor and extensor strength.

Six of eight patients requiring bilateral KAFOs preferred walking with a swing-through gait. Three of six patients requiring only one KAFO and having one free knee (with or without an AFO on the opposite limb) preferred walking with a reciprocal gait and crutches. Nine of 14 patients using only AFOs chose a reciprocal gait pattern.

Patients were tested using their preferred mode of walking. Those patients requiring crutch assistance were asked to walk with both a swing-through and reciprocal gait pattern.

Swing-Through Gait

Oxygen cost was highest, but the speed of walking slowest in the thoracolumbar group (Table 4-16). The average heart rates were elevated (>143 beats/min) beyond the values for normal walking (106 beats/min) in the high lumbar, low lumbar, and sacral groups, indicating intense physical exertion. Only the one patient with a sacral lesion had energy expenditure values approaching normal.

Table 4-16. Myelodysplasia: Swing-Through Gait

Group	Speed (m/min)	O₂ Rate (ml/kg·min)	O₂ Cost (ml/kg·m)	Pulse (beats/min)
Sacral (N = 1)	47	13.8	0.29	120
Low lumbar 0-KAFO (N = 5)	41	15.6	0.41	147
High lumbar 1-KAFO (N = 3)	46	18.7	0.41	143
Thoracolumbar 2-KAFO (N = 6)	22	14.9	0.77	149

(Data from Waters RL: unpublished data.)
KAFO, knee-ankle-foot orthosis.

Reciprocal Gait

The findings for children using a reciprocal gait pattern paralleled the results obtained for swing-through gait. Patients in the thoracolumbar group had the highest O_2 cost, greatest O_2 consumption rate, and slowest speed (Table 4-17). With the cumulative addition of hip flexion, knee extension, and antigravity hip support in lower-level patient groups, gait performance progressively improved providing a faster and more efficient gait at a lower O_2 cost and rate of O_2 consumption.

Swing-Through Gait Versus Reciprocal Gait

A direct comparison of energy expenditure during both swing-through and reciprocal walking was obtained in 10 children: thoracolumbar (two patients); high lumbar (two patients); low lumbar (five patients); and sacral (one patient). The mean values of the indices reflecting physiologic effort (rate of O_2 uptake

Table 4-17. Myelodysplasia: Reciprocal Gait

	Speed (m/min)	O₂ Rate (ml/kg·min)	O₂ Cost (ml/kg·m)	Pulse (beats/min)
Sacral (N = 1)	48	13.0	0.28	117
Lumbar 0-KAFO (N = 8)	38	16.6	0.49	145
Lumbar 1-KAFO (N = 5)	29	17.5	0.77	146
Thoracic 2-KAFO (N = 6)	19	18.1	1.35	146

(Data from Waters RL: unpublished data.)
KAFO, knee-ankle-foot orthosis.

and heart rate) were slightly higher during swing-through crutch-assisted gait; however, gait velocity was faster during swing-through gait. As a consequence, swing-through walking proved the more efficient gait (0.68 ml/kg·m versus 0.40 ml/kg·m). Not surprisingly, seven of 10 children preferred the swing-through mode of crutch use for most activities. It may be concluded that attempts to train children who prefer a swing-through gait to a reciprocal gait are probably unwarranted.

These findings are in contrast to the experience in adult SCI patients indicating the intense physiological energy expenditure of a swing-through gait infrequently provides a functionally useful ambulation. The difference probably relates to the higher ratio of upper arm strength to gross body weight in children as compared with adults. Also, myelodysplastic children have proportionately smaller and lighter lower limbs because of the effects of paralysis during the growth years. Nevertheless, as the child ages, approaches maturity, and gains weight, sustaining walking activity is difficult, and increased reliance is placed on the wheelchair. These factors, coupled with the normal decline in the maximal exercise capacity with aging, account for the reason that many severely paralyzed patients choose wheeling rather than walking in later years.

HEMIPLEGIA (STROKE)

Energy expenditure of hemiplegic gait is variable depending on the extent of neurologic dysfunction and spasticity. The hemiplegic population generally consists of older persons with a high prevalence of cardiovascular disease who are often further deconditioned by the effects of acute illness and bed rest before active rehabilitation. Exercise capacity is therefore typically reduced.

Spasticity and primitive patterns of motion characterize hemiplegic gait.[64] Bard[65,66] demonstrated the energy cost of walking correlated with the degree of spasticity. Step length is decreased due to the inability to extend the knee and flex the hip and ankle simultaneously in late swing.[6] Gait analysis in a typical group of hemiplegics indicated only 33 percent of the step cycle of the involved extremity is spent during the swing phase, and 80 percent of the step cycle of the uninvolved leg is spent during stance as compared with the normal swing to stance ratio of 40 percent and 60 percent, respectively.[67]

Because of the marked reduction in the speed of walking, the rate of O_2 consumption in hemiplegic walking is less than the rate for normal subjects walking at their CWS despite the inefficiency of the gait pattern and high energy cost.[65,66,68-70] It can be concluded that hemiplegic gait is not physiologically stressful for the typical patient, and the primary gait disability is the slow speed.

Hash[70] measured energy expenditure in hemiplegic subjects both walking and using one hand and one leg to propel a wheelchair and found the rate of O_2 consumption and O_2 cost were comparable to normal walking (Table 4-18). During wheeling, the speed of locomotion was greater and the rate of O_2 uptake and the O_2 cost less than during walking.

Table 4-18. Hemiplegia

Group	Speed (m/min)	O₂ Rate (ml/kg·min)	O₂ Cost (ml/kg·m)	Pulse (beats/min)
Wheelchair	37	10.0	0.27	107
Walking	30	11.5	0.54	109

(From Waters and Yakura,[72] with permission.)

SPASTIC DIPLEGIA (CEREBRAL PALSY)

The child with spastic diplegia has spasticity and a pervasive loss of motor control throughout both lower limbs that depend on the degree of involvement. Campbell and Ball[71] evaluated 35 spastic diplegic children aged 5 to 17 years. All had spasticity and varying degrees of impaired motor control. Upright balance reactions were present in six subjects, delayed or absent in 17 subjects, and absent in 12. Six children wore bilateral AFOs and six wore unilateral AFOs. Walking aids were used by 14 children: three used forearm crutches, five used quad canes, and six used walkers.

The average walking speed averaged 40 m/min, 57 percent of normal velocity (Table 4-19). The mean rate of energy expenditure was higher than normal exemplified by an elevated heart rate, 145 beats/min, and rate of oxygen uptake, 18.6 ml/kg·min. As a group, these children had an inefficient gait averaging 0.72 ml/kg·m.

In normal children, the rate of energy expenditure required for walking per kilogram of body weight decreases as the child grows older.[12] The opposite trend occurred in children with spastic diplegia. The rate of energy expenditure increased as the children approached maturity.[71] This observation has clinical significance for the spastic child who complains of fatigue or the need for rest. The older child may prefer to walk less or rely on a wheelchair because walking requires greater physical exertion than at a younger age. This is because of increased body weight and size, and the inability of the child with impaired motor control, spasticity, and impaired balance reactions to transport the added weight efficiently.

Most children with gait disabilities that do not require the use of upper-extremity assistive devices purposefully slow the speed to keep the rate of O₂ consumption from rising above normal limits. Elevated rates of O₂ consumption were consistently recorded in spastic diplegics even when upper-extremity assistive devices were not required. These children customarily maintain the hip and knee in flexion throughout the gait cycle requiring greater than normal hip and knee extensor muscle effort for joint stabilization even at reduced speeds.

Table 4-19. Cerebral Palsy

Group	Speed (m/min)	O₂ Rate (ml/kg·min)	O₂ Cost (ml/kg·m)	Pulse (beats/min)
Spastic diplegia	40	18.6	0.72	145

(From Waters and Yakura,[72] with permission.)

Another reason for the elevated rate of O_2 consumption relates to the inability of the child to perform the necessary compensatory gait substitutions. The hemiplegic patient spends approximately 80 percent of the gait cycle on the uninvolved limb and during the period of single limb support is able to maintain the hip and knee in a relatively extended position.[68] Compensatory maneuvers are performed with the intact limb. As a consequence of bilateral limb impairment, the child with spastic diplegia cannot compensate to keep the rate of energy expenditure from rising above the mean for normal children at their CWS.

REFERENCES

1. Astrand PO, Rodahl K: Textbook of Work Physiology, 2nd Ed. McGraw-Hill, New York, 1977
2. McArdle WD, Katch FI, Katch VL: Exercise Physiology. Lea & Febiger, Philadelphia, 1986
3. Elftman H: Biomechanics of muscle with particular application to studies of gait. J Bone Joint Surg 48A:363, 1966
4. Inman VT, Ralston HJ, Todd F: Human Walking. Waverly Press, Baltimore, 1981
5. Saunders JB, Inman VT, Eberhart HD: Major determinants in normal and pathological gait. J Bone Joint Surg 35A:543, 1953
6. Perry JP: Mechanics of walking in hemiplegia. Clin Orthop North Am 63:23, 1969
7. Falls HB, Humphrey LA: Energy cost of running and walking in young women. Med Sci Sports 8:9, 1976
8. Finley FR, Cody KA: Locomotive characteristics of urban pedestrians. Arch Phys Med Rehabil 51:423, 1970
9. Waters RL, Lunsford BR, Perry J, Byrd R: Energy-speed relationship of walking: Standard tables. J Orthop Res 6:215, 1988
10. Thorstensson A, Roberthson HR: Adaptations to changing speed in human locomotion: Speed of transition between walking and running. Acta Physiol Scand 131:211, 1987
11. Astrand A, Astrand I, Hallback I, Kilbom A: Reduction in maximal oxygen uptake with age. J Appl Physiol 35:649, 1973
12. Waters RL, Hislop HJ, Perry J, et al: Comparative cost of walking in young and old adults. J Orthop Res 1:73, 1983
13. Waters RL, Hislop HJ, Thomas L, Campbell J: Energy cost of walking in normal children and teenagers. Med Child Neurol 25:184, 1983
14. Cunningham DA, Rechnitzer PA, Pearce ME, Donner AP: Determinants of self-selected walking pace across ages 19 to 66. J Gerontol 37:560, 1982
15. Bobbert AC: Energy expenditure in level and grade walking. J Appl Physiol 15: 1015, 1961
16. Booyens J, Keatinge WR: The expenditure of energy by men and women walking. J Physiol (Lond) 138:165, 1957
17. Corcoran PJ, Gelmann B: Oxygen uptake in normal and handicapped subjects in relation to the speed of walking beside a velocity-controlled cart. Arch Phys Med Rehabil 51:78, 1970
18. Cotes JE, Meade F: The energy expenditure and mechanical energy demand in walking. Ergon 3(2):97, 1960

19. Dill DB: Oxygen use in horizontal and grade walking and running on the treadmill. J Appl Physiol 20:165, 1957
20. Erickson L, Simonson E, Talor HC, et al: Energy cost of horizontal and grade walking on motor-driven treadmill. Am J Physiol 145:391, 1946
21. Molen NH, Roxendal RH: Energy expenditure in normal test subjects walking on a motor driven treadmill. Proc Kon Ned Akad Wetensch Senes 70:192, 1967
22. Passmore R, Durnin JUGA: Human energy expenditure. Physiol Rev 35:801, 1953
23. Ralston HJ: Energy-speed relation and optimal speed during level walking. Int Z Angew Physiol Einschl Arbeitsphysiol 17:277, 1958
24. Lerner-Frankeil M, Vargas S, et al: Functional community ambulation: What are your criteria. Clin Man Phys Ther 6:12, 1986
25. Mahadeva K, Passmore R, Woolf B: Individual variations in the metabolic cost of standardized exercises: The effects of food, age, sex, and race. J Physiol (Lond) 121:225, 1953
26. McBeath AA, Bahrke M, Balke B: Efficiency of assisted ambulation determined by oxygen consumption measurement. J Bone Joint Surg 56A:994, 1974
27. Imms FJ, MacDonald IC, Prestidge SP: Energy expenditure during walking in patients recovering from fractures of the leg. Scand J Rehabil Med 8:1, 1976
28. Patterson R, Fisher SV: Cardiovascular stress of crutch walking. Arch Phys Med Rehabil 62:257, 1967
29. Waters RL, Campbell J, Perry J: Energy cost of three-point crutch ambulation in fracture patients. J Orthop Trauma 1:170, 1987
30. Waters RL, Lunsford BR: Energy cost of paraplegic ambulation. J Bone Joint Surg 67A:1245, 1985
31. Waters RL, Perry J, Antonelli D, Hislop H: The energy cost of walking of amputees—Influence of level of amputation. J Bone Joint Surg 58A:42, 1976
32. Hjeltnes N: Oxygen uptake and cardiac output in graded arm exercise in paraplegics with low level spinal lesions. Scand J Rehabil Med 9:107, 1977
33. Wolf E, Magora A: Orthostatic and ergometric evaluation of cord-injured patients. Scand J Rehabil Med 8:93, 1976
34. Ralston HJ: Effects of immobilization of various body segments on the energy cost of human locomotion. In Proceedings of the I.E.A. Conference, Dortmund, 1964. Ergonomics (suppl) p. 53, 1965
35. Waters RL, Campbell J, Thomas L, et al: Energy cost of walking in lower extremity plaster casts. J Bone Joint Surg 64A:896, 1982
36. Mazur JM, Schwartz E, Simon SR: Ankle arthrodesis: Long-term followup with gait analysis. J Bone Joint Surg 61A:964, 1979
37. Waters RL, Barnes G, Husserl T, et al: Energy expenditure following hip and ankle arthrodesis. J Bone Joint Surg 70A:1032, 1988
38. Waters RL, Hislop HJ, Perry J, Antonelli D: Energetics: Application to the study and management of locomotor disabilities. Orthop Clin North Am 9:351, 1978
39. Reuter K, Pierre M: Energy cost and gait characteristics of flexed knee ambulation. (unpublished)
40. Perry J, Antonelli D, Ford, W: Analysis of knee joint forces during flexed knee stance. J Bone Joint Surg 57A:961, 1975
41. Gore DR, Murray MP, Sepic SB, Gardner GM: Walking patterns of men with unilateral surgical hip fusion. J Bone Joint Surg 57A:759, 1975
42. Brown M, Hislop HJ, Waters RL, Porell D: Walking efficiency before and after total hip replacement. Phys Ther 60:1259, 1980
43. Ganguli S, Datta SR, Chatterjee BB, Roy BN: Metabolic cost of walking at different speeds with patellar tendon-bearing prosthesis. J Appl Physiol 36:440, 1974

44. Huang CT, Jackson JR, Moore NB, et al: Amputation: Energy cost of ambulation. Arch Phys Med Rehabil 60:18, 1979

45. Molen NH: Energy/speed relation of below-knee amputees walking on a motor-driven treadmill. Int Z Angew Physiol 31:173, 1973

46. Pagliarulo MA, Waters R, Hislop HJ: Energy cost of walking of below-knee amputees have no vascular disease. Phys Ther 59:538, 1979

47. James U: Oxygen uptake and heart rate during prosthetic walking in healthy male unilateral above-knee amputees. Scand J Rehabil Med 5:71, 1973

48. Nowrozzi F, Salvanelli ML: Energy expenditure in hip disarticulation and hemipelvectomy amputees. Arch Phys Med Rehabil 64:300, 1983

49. Gonzalez EG, Corcoran PJ, Reyes, RL: Energy expenditure in below-knee amputees: Correlation with stump length. Arch Phys Med Rehabil 55:111, 1974

50. James U, Nordgren B: Physical work capacity measured by bike ergometry (one leg) and prosthetic treadmill walking in healthy active unilateral above knee amputees. Scand J Rehabil Med 5:81, 1973

51. Eberhart HD, Elftman H, Inman VT: Locomotor mechanism of amputee. p. 472. In Klopsteg PE, Wilson PD (eds): Human Limbs and Their Substitutes. McGraw-Hill, New York, 1954

52. Steinberg FU, Garcia WJ, Roettger RF, Shelton DJ: Rehabilitation of the geriatric amputee. J Am Gerontol Soc 22:62, 1974

53. James U, Oberg K: Prosthetic gait pattern in unilateral above-knee amputees. Scand J Rehabil Med 5:35, 1973

54. Traugh GH, Corcoran PF, Reyes RL: Energy expenditure of ambulation in patients with above-knee amputations. Arch Phys Med Rehabil 56:67, 1975

55. Waters RL, Perry J, Chambers R: Energy expenditure of amputee gait. p. 250. In Lower Extremity Amputation. WB Saunders, Philadelphia, 1989

56. Wainapel SF, March H, Steve L: Stubby prostheses: An alternative to conventional prosthetic devices. Arch Phys Med Rehabil 66:264, 1985

57. Pugh L: The oxygen uptake and energy cost of walking before and after unilateral hip replacement with some observations on the use of crutches. J Bone Joint Surg 55B:742, 1973

58. Waters RL, Perry J, Conaty P, et al: The energy cost of walking with arthritis of the hip and knee. Clin Orthop 214:278, 1987

59. Waters RL, Yakura JS, Adkins RH, Barnes G: Determinants of gait performance following spinal injury. Arch Phys Med Rehabil 70:589, 1989

60. Merkel K, Miller N, Merritt J: Energy expenditure in patients with low-, mid-, or high-thoracic paraplegia using Scott-Craig knee-ankle-foot orthoses. Mayo Clin Proc 60:165, 1985

61. Miller HE, Merritt JL, Merkel KD, Westbrook PR: Paraplegic energy expenditure during negotiation of architectural barriers. Arch Phys Med Rehabil 65:778, 1984

62. Huang CR, Kuhlemeier KV, Moore NB, Fine PR: Energy cost of ambulation in paraplegic patients using craig-scott braces. Arch Phys Med Rehabil 60:595, 1979

63. Williams LO, Anderson AD, Campbell J, et al: Energy cost of walking and of wheelchair propulsion by children with myelodysplasia: Comparison with normal children. Dev Med Child Neurol 25:617, 1983

64. Olney SJ, Monga TN, Costigan PA: Mechanical energy of walking of stroke patients. Arch Phys Med Rehabil 67:92, 1986

65. Bard G, Ralston H: Measurement of energy expenditure during ambulation, with special reference to evaluation of assistive devices. Arch Phys Med Rehabil 40:415, 1959

66. Bard G: Energy expenditure of hemiplegic subjects during walking. Arch Phys Med Rehabil 44:368, 1963
67. Peat M, Hyman I: Electromyographic temporal analysis of gait: hemiplegic locomotion. Arch Phys Med Rehabil 57:421, 1976
68. Corcoran P, Jebsen R, Brengelmann G, Simons B: Effects of plastic and metal leg braces on speed and energy cost of hemiparetic ambulation. Arch Phys Med Rehabil 51:69, 1970
69. Dasco J, Luczak A, Hass A, Rusk H: Bracing and rehabilitation training: Effect on the energy expenditure of the elderly hemiplegic. Postgrad Med 34:42, 1963
70. Hash D: Energetics of wheelchair propulsion and walking in stroke patients. p. 372. In Energetics: Application to the Study and Management of Locomotor Disabilities. Orthop Clin North Am 9:351, 1978
71. Campbell J, Ball J: Energetics of walking in cerebral palsy. p. 374. In Energetics: Application to the Study and Management of Locomotor Disabilities. Orthop Clin North Am 9:351, 1978
72. Waters RL, Yakura JS: The energy expenditure of normal and pathological gait. Critical Rev in Phys Rehab Med 1:183, 1989

5 | Electromyographic Patterns in Normal Adult Locomotion

Richard Shiavi

Investigations of muscular synergy patterns in locomotion have had a variety of purposes, and the results have been presented in different degrees of detail. Some were focused on muscles acting on a particular joint, while others considered selected muscle groups of the lower extremity. Partial summaries appear in several of the major books and papers written on the kinesiology of gait. Included are the works of Eberhart et al.,[1] Basmajian,[2] Perry,[3] and Inman et al.[4] Inman's book contains an excellent pictorial representation of general muscle function, differentiating eccentric and concentric action. An example of the classic results is shown in Figure 5-1.

Population variabilities in electromyographic (EMG) patterns have been noted[5,6]; more recently, attention has been directed toward this fact.[7-9] Paul[10] and, more recently, Shiavi[11] have compiled the results of several reported investigations and indicated some significant inconsistencies on the phasings of particular muscles or groups. These apparent disagreements may be attributed either to differences in investigatory protocol or to actual interindividual dynamic variations.[12] For instance, EMG patterns can change with walking speed.[5,13-16] The preference of the investigator or the size and depth of the muscles or groups also influenced whether surface or intramuscular electrodes were used to record EMG activity. The investigatory paradigms differed generally, and the results were presented in terms of the action of either groups or specific muscles. Some investigators state that muscles in a group had patterns similar enough to average their patterns, whereas others have stated the opposite. For instance, compare the statements of Battye and Joseph[17] and Grieve

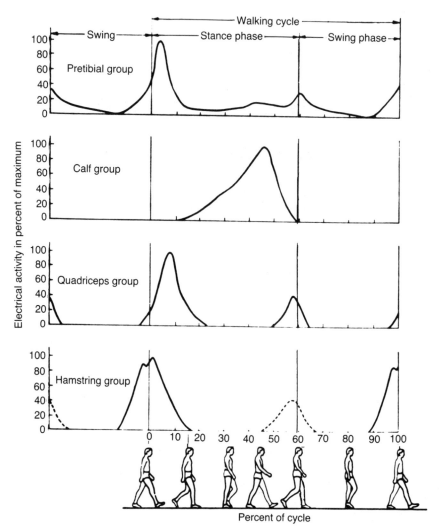

Fig. 5-1. Electromyographic envelopes of major muscle groups. (**Figure continues.**)

and Cavanagh[18] on the EMG patterns of thigh musculature. At the other extreme, such investigators as Basmajian[2] and Inman et al.[4] state that regions within a specific muscle are functionally different. The principal differences in experimental protocol are whether

1. Subjects walked freely or in cadence with a metronome.
2. Subjects walked at their free speed or other speed.
3. Subjects wore shoes or were barefooted.
4. Subjects walked on a floor, metal plate, or treadmill.
5. EMG were recorded with surface, wire, or needle electrodes.

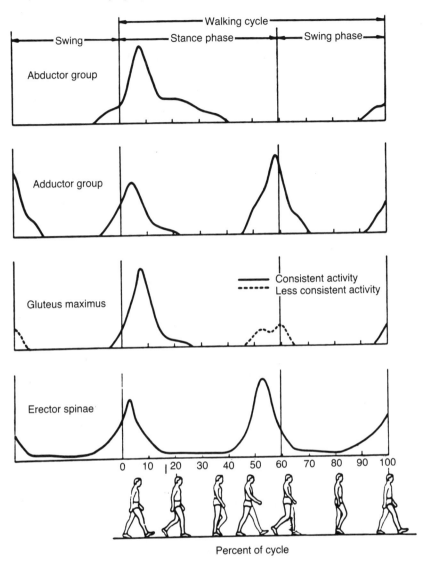

Fig. 5-1. (*Continued*). (From Eberhart et al.,[1] with permission.)

Another factor that complicates the assimilation of the results of all the investigations has been the different methods used to analyze and represent EMG activity. This has also hindered the creation of a common data base for all investigators. Investigators have used a variety of representations, which include (1) raw data, (2) on-off patterns, (3) full wave rectified and integrated values in 5% stride segments, and (4) the linear envelope.

A recent standards report contains a plea for standardization of research results.[19,20] This report and subsequent publications cogently argue that the best method is the ensemble average of the time-normalized linear envelope.[13,21,22] Another significant question is the type of amplitude normalization to reduce intersubject variability. Again, publications show that normalization by the stride average reduces the variability the most.[8,9,23]

The significance of the results is also influenced by the number of subjects in any particular investigation. In most investigations, less than 14 subjects were studied and often not all the experimental conditions were mentioned. A summary of the various investigatory methods used is tabulated in the review article by Shiavi.[11]

This material in this chapter is presented as an attempt to coalesce most of the known results into an informational base on locomotor EMG in normal adults. It is not intended to be a kinesiology review, although some of the current concepts, including the methodology for forming the time-normalized linear envelope, are mentioned to provide a more relevant understanding.

MUSCULAR SYNERGY PATTERNS

The EMG patterns are presented modularly, according to anatomic regions of the body. The discussions will be initiated with a presentation either of the results of a particular investigator, usually often-quoted, or of a consensus of consistent results. Again, Figure 5-1 tabulates the classically accepted synergy patterns for muscle groups and is referenced. Figures are indispensable for this review. They are primarily selected or adapted from publications that focus on many individual muscles in a particular functional group (e.g., adductors). Other investigators who have contributed to the knowledge of their function are listed in the references. The adapted figures are general estimates of consistent results from the referenced publications. Because of the varieties of representation mentioned above, no attempt was made to average any patterns quantitatively. However, all the pattern variations are discussed.

Intrinsic Muscles of the Foot

The intrinsic muscles of the foot have been studied by several investigators.[2,24–26] Mann and Inman[27] have studied the most, six, simultaneously; their results are shown in Figure 5-2. All the EMG results are presented in measured form. All except Sheffield et al.[25] used wire electrodes, and all their subjects walked at free speed; the actual speeds were not reported. The number of subjects ranged between 10 and 20.

These muscles are primarily active during late midstance and unloading periods. In persons with pronated (flat) feet, the activity of the abductor hallucis, flexor hallucis, and flexor digitorum brevis muscles began earlier in the stride, sometimes at foot strike. The only inconsistent result is that the extensor digitorum brevis can be active throughout the stride in some individuals.[25] This may be due to the surface electrode measurement or the slow speed of walking; a stride time of 2.0 seconds was used. It is concluded that the intrinsic muscles stabilize the foot and enable it to act as a functional unit.

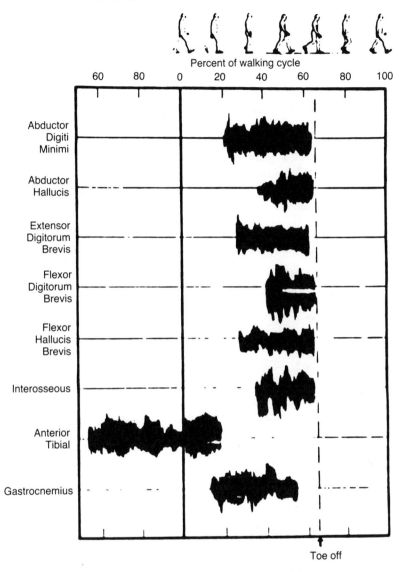

Fig. 5-2. Electromyographic activity of intrinsic muscles of the foot. (From Mann and Inman,[27] with permission.)

Ankle Dorsiflexors

Figure 5-3 presents a synopsis of the activity and function of the pretibial muscles, which have been well documented.[1,5,17,24–26,28–31] Only Sheffield[25] and Rozin et al.,[29] in addition to the University of California (UC) group, studied all three simultaneously. Interestingly, they used intramuscular electrodes and 10

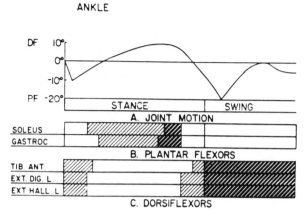

Fig. 5-3. On-off patterns of EMG activity of ankle plantar flexors (**B**) and ankle dorsiflexors (**C**). A normal ankle joint angle trajectory is also shown (**A**). (From Perry,[3] with permission.)

or fewer subjects. In general, the pretibial muscles are active from the unloading stage through swing and the loading stage. Their activity in midswing is highly variable and can be nonexistent in some persons (see Fig. 5-1). The stance-swing transition period controls floor clearance by causing rapid dorsiflexion of the foot, and the swing-stance transition controls the deceleration of plantar flexion at foot strike. The concentric contraction activity during the latter part of the loading stage shows that these muscles, especially the tibialis anterior, contribute to ankle stabilization. The tibialis anterior, being also an invertor, is contributing to the transfer of weight to the lateral border of the foot.

Many other investigators have studied the tibialis anterior on-off and envelope patterns. Their studies confirm the high degree of interindividual variability during midswing and show additional variability during midstance.[10,28,30] Basmajian[2] indicates that the midstance activity exists in those with pronated feet. It appears that the biphasic EMG pattern tends to occur more often at faster walking speeds.[13]

Ankle Plantar Flexors

The function of the plantar flexors has been investigated quite extensively. In fact, the plantar flexors have been studied under almost all variations of the experimental paradigms.[1,5,17,24–26,28–32] The triceps surae received the most attention, whereas the toe flexors received the least. Only Sutherland[6] studied all of them simultaneously (Fig. 5-4 presents his results). The plantar flexors represent a consensus of on-off patterns for free speed walking.

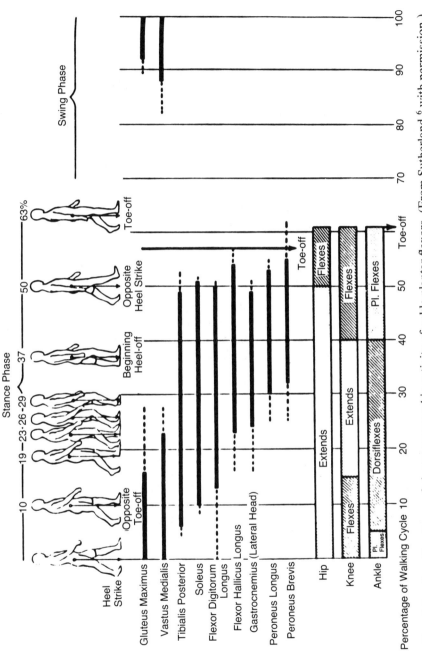

Fig. 5-4. On-off patterns of electromyographic activity of ankle plantar flexors. (From Sutherland,[6] with permission.)

Triceps Surae

All the plantar flexor muscles are single joint muscles, with the exception of the gastrocnemius. They are mainly stance phase muscles and, interestingly, all contract eccentrically until late midstance (40 percent of gait cycle) when they have a switch in function. The triceps surae are mainly concerned with control of forward momentum. During midstance, they decelerate tibial-talar rotation and permit forward momentum to extend the knee joint. At the end of midstance, the concentric contraction phase begins, and they impart forward momentum (push-off).[6] Activity usually ceases during the unloading period.[1,2,10]

More recent investigations show that the triceps surae, more often the soleus, are sometimes active during the swing-stance transition period,[28,29] especially at faster walking speeds.[5,13,33] The activity is still monophasic. The eccentric contraction of the gastrocnemius during the deceleration stage at faster speeds contributes to deceleration of the tibia.

Toe Flexors

The function of the long toe flexors seems to be primarily to stabilize the toes during metatarsal contact, since their size would imply that there is little contribution to plantar flexor moment. Their timing has been investigated with intramuscular electrodes only at free speed and is consistent.

Peronei and Tibialis Posterior

The peronei and tibialis posterior are antagonists that primarily control inversion-eversion of the foot.[34] During walking, they control weight distribution on the lateral border of the foot during stance and orientation of the foot during swing.[24,32] The tibialis posterior is fairly consistent in its activity, whereas the peronei, although usually synchronous, are definitely variable.[30,32] The peronei in many persons are active during swing phase and transition periods regardless of electrode type and walking speed.

Anterior Thigh Musculature

A typical estimate of the patterns of activity of the muscles located in the anterior thigh during free speed walking is shown in Figure 5-5.[2,5,10,17,28–31,33,35] The quadriceps, except for the vastus intermedius, have undergone intense investigation. The other muscles have not, probably either because of their relative unimportance for essential function or because of the difficulty of measurement. There is considerable variation, both intra- and interindividually.

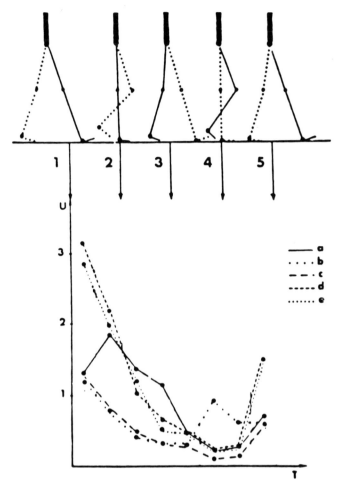

Fig. 5-5. Patterns of activity of anterior thigh musculature. (From Rideau and Duval,[35] with permission.)

Quadriceps

The quadriceps are consistently active during the swing-stance transition period. There is much variability during the remainder of the stride, no matter which type of electrodes are used. The activity of the vastus intermedius is synchronized with the other vasti.[36] The predominant variation is the activity during the stance-swing transition period, as depicted in Figure 5-1. The collation of the results of many investigations show the following general trends:

1. At free speed, approximately 67 percent of the rectus femoris patterns have a stance-wing transition period, while 45 percent of the vasti have one.

2. The frequency of occurrence of this period correlates with walking speed.

3. The major phase of activity of the quadriceps tends to elongate into midstance as walking speed increases in approximately 40 percent of the patterns.

Interestingly, Brandell's results are the only ones showing the vastus medialis having predominantly midstance activity. His subjects walked on a treadmill.[33]

The first phase provides knee stability for load bearing and ironically ceases activity when knee extension commences. The second phase of activity occurs primarily during the loading stage of the opposite extremity. It may help to fix the knee during gastrocnemius contraction and is associated with acceleration of the leg at the onset of swing.

Sartorius

The sartorius can be biphasically active during loading and early swing.[35] Only Basmajian[2] does not report a loading period action. The early swing activity elongates into the unloading period with faster walking speeds.[31] This latter activity contributes to hip flexion.

Posterior Thigh Muscles

The hamstring muscles comprise the posterior thigh muscle group. The hamstrings have been studied under a variety of conditions, separately, as medial and lateral groups, with surface or wire electrodes, as so forth. Figure 5-6 is an adaptation of the work of several investigators[1,2,5,10,17,28,30,31] and shows the most consistent activities.

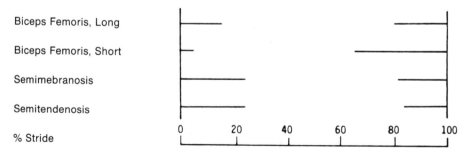

Fig. 5-6. On-off patterns of consistent electromyographic activity of posterior knee musculature.

All heads of the hamstrings are active within the swing-stance transition period. However, at slower speeds of walking, the late swing portion changes with walking speed. As speed increases from slow to fast, the swing phase activity elongates from terminal swing period into initial swing period.[30,37] An inconsistent second phase during the stance-swing transition period (see Fig. 5-1) has been found by most investigators in approximately 40 percent of subjects. A level of activity of the medial hamstrings during the most of midstance has also been reported by Paul.[10] His subjects walked only in the fast speed range, 1.4 to 2.1 m/s. However, Milner et al.[5] did not find this activity at speeds of 2.28 m/s.

In the consistent phase, the muscles undergo a switch in function. The well-known deceleration of the lower extremity is accomplished in late swing with eccentric contraction. At heel strike, the muscles contract concentrically, causing hip extension and forward propulsion during the loading and initial midstance stages. The inconsistent second phase is also an eccentric contraction, occurring while the hip joint is flexing. This action serves to assist knee flexion and leg clearance.

Popliteus

The activity of the popliteus has been reported by Perry.[3] It is active during midstance and seems to contribute to deceleration of knee joint extension.

Hip Joint Musculature

Hip Extensor

The gluteus maximus is the primary single-joint hip extensor. It is consistently active during the swing-stance transition period and contributes initially to hip joint stabilization and then to hip extension.[1,2,10,17,31] (Fig. 5-7). An inconsistent second phase of smaller magnitude during the stance-swing transition period also exists.[1,2,17] (see Fig. 5-1). Given that hip flexion is occurring, this second phase would contribute to pelvic stabilization.

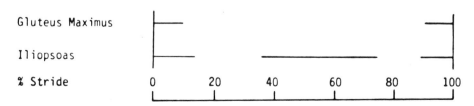

Fig. 5-7. On-off patterns of consistent electromyographic activity of single joint hip extensor/flexors.

Hip Flexor

The iliopsoas is the primary single-joint hip-flexor muscle. Its activity from terminal midstance through midswing is a consistent finding. From a small study, it appears that the duration is shorter in women.[17] However, several investigators have claimed that another phase of activity exists during the swing-stance transition period. Since these latter investigators used surface electrodes in the femoral triangle, this second phase could be the result of cross-talk.[10,17] Figure 5-7 summarizes these findings.[1,2,10,17,31]

The iliopsoas actually shows a switch in function during its acknowledged range of activity. During stance, it lengthens and must be assisting hip stabilization. During swing, it flexes the hip and becomes quiescent when the hip joint angle becomes constant. If the questionable phase of activity is accurate, the precise function is difficult to discern because of the multitude of hip muscles that are active during that time.

Abductor Group

Figures 5-1 and 5-8 show a consensus of patterns for the abductor muscles.[1,2,10,17,30,31] The results of studies of the gluteus medius using surface electrodes are merged into the group pattern. The gluteus medius and the gluteus minimus are active in all subjects from loading through midstance and cease activity prior to loading of the opposite extremity. As walking speed increases this phase for the gluteus medius extends into late swing in a a greater percentage of people.[30] This activity stabilizes the pelvis in the frontal plane during stance. A second phase exists in approximately 40 percent of people during the stance-swing transition period.[2,30] This causes a slight abduction to promote leg clearance. Only Battye and Joseph report a few observations of isolated gluteus medius activity during midswing.[17] The gluteus minimus also has a second phase of activity, but it occurs during midswing.[2] The tensor fasciae latae has biphasic activity in synergy with the other abductors. The function is generally the same and may also control the rotation of the femur.[2]

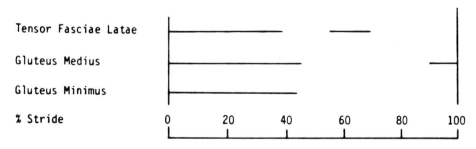

Fig. 5-8.   On-off patterns of consistent electromyographic activity of abductors.

Adductor Group

A few earlier articles report the activity of the adductor group, adductors and gracilis.[1,2,17,31,35,38] A synopsis is presented in Figure 5-9. The three reports on the gracilis are perplexing, although all used wire electrodes. Paul[10] shows it to be monophasically active through most of swing and loading, whereas Basmajian[2] reports it to be more like the adductor longus pattern in Figure 5-9. The UC group reported both types of activity.[31] This duality remains unexplained.

The adductors can be biphasically active close to or during the transition periods. Both phases correspond to the times when the direction of transverse rotation of the pelvis is changing.[1] The stance-swing transition phase is also thought to contribute to lateral rotation of the femur. The adductor magnus is functionally two muscles. The upper portion is a true adductor, whereas the lower portion functions as a hamstring muscle.[2] It essentially has the biphasic activity shown and reflects the group activity. The exception is the treadmill study by Green and Morris[38]; their results do not show any stance-swing transition activity. Only Basmajian[2] reports on the adductor brevis. Its pattern varies with the speed of walking; at free speed, the pattern is biphasic. The variations are not documented.

Trunk Musculature

There has been very little investigation into the activity of the trunk musculature during level walking. Figure 5-10 summarizes the currently known EMG patterns.[39]

Abdominal

The abdominal muscles (rectus abdominus, external oblique, internal oblique) are quite variable in their activity.[39,40] The latter two are continuously active at free speed and have superimposed phases at faster speed as shown.

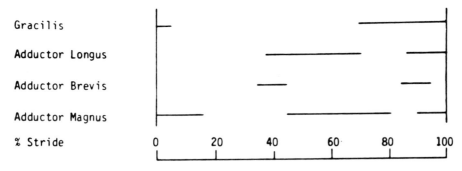

Fig. 5-9. On-off patterns of consistent electromyographic activity of adductors.

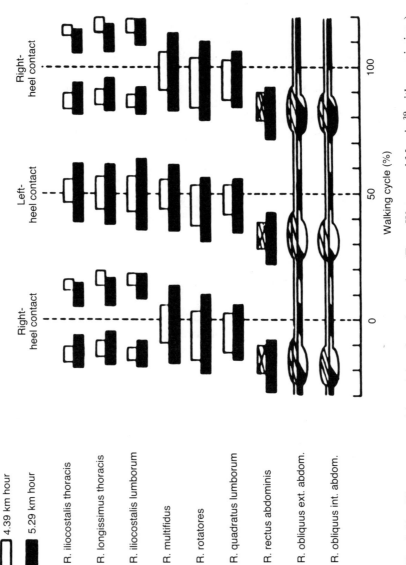

Fig. 5-10. Electromyographic activity of trunk muscles. (From Waters and Morris,[39] with permission.)

The rectus abdominus is active in only 50 percent of subjects at free speed (stance duration = 1.2 second) and always phasically active at faster speeds (stance duration = 1.0 second). This seems to be consistent with Sheffield who reports no activity; however, his subjects were walking slowly with a stance time equaling 2 seconds.

Paraspinal

Even though the paradigms were diverse (e.g., floor and treadmill, wire and surface electrodes), the results are similar.[1,17,31,39,41] The paraspinal muscles are active during the transitions periods at free and fast speeds. The only inconsistency is that the erector spinae is not always active during the swing-stance transition at free speed.[39] A major difference is that the wire electrode recordings showed two bursts of EMG during the stance-swing transition, whereas the surface recordings showed continuous activity. Stance times were equal for free speed.

The transitional stage activities coincide with the time when the pelvic and thoracic rotations are changing direction and the weight support is being shifted. Note that the phases differ in timing by 50 percent; that is, the first phase of the ipsilateral extremity has the same timing as the second phase of the contralateral extremity. Since all these muscles exist bilaterally, they are contracting bilaterally, one concentrically and the other eccentrically, performing a stable balancing of the torso and pelvis and elevating the pelvis in preparation for swing phase.

PATTERN VARIABILITY

There are two general sources of pattern variability, one inherent in the measurement process and the other a reflection of the adaptability of the motor control process. The former is handled using normalization procedures, and the latter is a phenomenon to be investigated. The adaptability is demonstrated by studies showing changes in EMG patterns from stride to stride within the same individual, differences in patterns among individuals walking at the same speed, and changes in patterns as walking speed increases. A comprehensive discussion of these topics would be very lengthy; the reader interested in these topics is encouraged to consult the references cited in this brief summary of the current knowledge.

Normalization

The major cause of the variability in pattern is the amplitude of the linear envelope of the recorded EMG. This is because of such factors as the variations in size of the surfaces of the recording electrodes used for different studies and differences in skin resistance across a subject population. Several investigations have addressed this issue using variability indices.[8,9,23] Yang and Winter[23] investigated four parameters of the linear envelope for reducing the pattern variability across subject populations: subject pattern average, subject pattern maximum, percentage of maximum voluntary contraction, and EMG magnitude per unit isometric torque. Pattern average was found to reduce the population variability the most.

It is anticipated that time-base normalization may also be required. Consider Figure 5-11, which shows the ensemble averages of the tibialis anterior muscle EMG pattern for 25 normal adults sorted by walking speed, which means that stride times are also different. If the stride is segmented such that the stance and swing phases have equal normalized durations, the pattern alignment would be better, resulting in reduced variation. This is a rational procedure, since functional regions of gait become aligned. Perry et al.[42] suggested and used this when studying on-off patterns in hemiplegic gait. The UC group also presented their data in this manner.[31] Definitive analyses need to be undertaken to find the optimal normalization procedures.

Intraindividual Variability

Many gait investigations have acknowledged a stride-to-stride variability in EMG patterns. This is why individual EMG profiles are used. The profile is defined as the ensemble average and standard deviation of a set of linear envelopes. Figure 5-12 shows such a profile for a normal subject.[43] It is to be hoped that the results from one measurement session are representative of an individual's performance. The variabilities among successive strides and successive trials are low. However, the standard deviations doubles for measurements repeated over separate days.[43,44] Even with amplitude normalization, measurements using wire electrodes produce variabilities 30 percent larger than those using surface electrodes.[44]

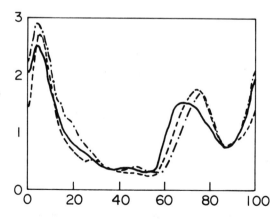

Fig. 5-11. Ensemble averages of electromyographic envelopes from tibialis anterior muscle for three speed ranges: slow $(-\cdot-\cdot)$, free $(- -)$, fast $(—)$.

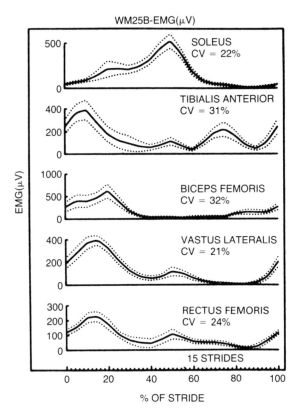

Fig. 5-12.   Ensemble averages (middle curves) and 1 SD band (outer curves) of electromyographic envelopes from 15 strides in a normal subject walking at free speed. (From Winter and Yack,[43] with permission.)

Population Variability

As was surmised from the descriptions of the periods of activity of the various skeletal muscles, there can be much interindividual variability. Some persons display monophasic activity in the hamstring or other muscle group, while others exhibit biphasic activity, as illustrated in Figure 5-1.[7-9,43,45] Other possible variations include differences in timing of peaks of activity and differences in the ratios of the magnitudes of the peak activities in biphasic patterns. The magnitude of the variability seems to be a function of anatomic location. The distal muscles are the most consistent, whereas the two joint muscles about the knee and hip are the most variable. The single joint muscles about the knee and hip have moderate variability.[43]

Walking speed is another factor. An individual's pattern can change as walking speed is increased from very slow to fast. At very slow walking speeds, a population can exhibit a great variety of patterns, whereas as they walk faster, individuals tend to exhibit the same pattern. Figure 5-13 plots a variability index as a function of walking speed for several muscles illustrating this phenomenon.[8,9,46]

DATA ACQUISITION AND LINEAR ENVELOPE FORMATION

Data Acquisition

Electromyograms are measured using standard bipolar surface or wire electrodes with differential amplification. The total amplification factor, gain, should be adjustable from 1,000 to at least 10,000. The entire system can be either a telemetry or hard-wired system with the capability of measuring a minimum of four EMG channels simultaneously. Most of the power in a EMG signal lies within a frequency band from 20 to 200 Hz for surface measurements and from 20 to 400 Hz for intramuscular measurements. Bandpass filters with a passband from 35 to 400 or 500 Hz are used to eliminate noise and motion artifacts. The EMG signals are acquired by a computer via an analog-to-digital (A/D) converter. The measurement, sampling, rate is 1,000 samples per second

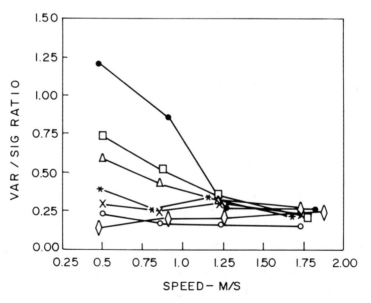

Fig. 5-13. The variation-to-signal ratio (VAR/SIG) plotted with respect to average walking speed in each category. Muscle symbols: ○, tibialis anterior; ◇, soleus; X, gastrocnemius; △, rectus femoris; □, medial hamstring; ●, vastus lateralis; *, gluteus medius.

for each channel. The resulting data are stored in computer files for further processing.

Since the major concern is the behavior of muscular activity over the stride, some technique must be used to demarcate the beginning and end of stance phase. This is typically accomplished either with foot switches or with a video technique.

Linear Envelope Formation

After data acquisition, additional computer software is used to form the linear envelope and ensemble average gait pattern from the sampled data file in several stages. The linear envelope is formed from the interference EMG signal through the operations of rectification and envelope detection. These operations are graphically depicted in Figure 5-14.[19] The linear envelopes are formed in software by taking the absolute value of the EMG and passing it through a digital recursive filter that implements a third-order Paynter finite-time integrator.[25,26] The time constant of the integrator varies from 25 ms to 200 ms, depending on the smoothness desired.[44]

The average linear envelope for an EMG channel, the EMG profile, is calculated in a three-step process. First, the foot-contact measurements are scanned and the beginning and end times of each stride determined. Each stride has a different duration, individual linear envelopes have different durations, as shown in Figure 5-15. The second step to ensure that the linear envelope in each stride has an equal number of points; 256 points is a sufficient number. This is accomplished through a process called interpolation. Finally, all the interpolated linear envelopes from a given channel are averaged together in an ensemble manner.[25,26] The ensemble standard deviation is also calculated during the averaging step. The profiles are then stored. Typical profiles are plotted in Figures 5-11 and 5-12.

OVERVIEW

The investigations of the EMG patterns produced during normal adult locomotion have been under investigation for several decades. Many of the initial questions (e.g., Is there a "typical" normal pattern? or Can an individual use different patterns?) have recently been addressed more comprehensively with the aid of computerized data processing. The motor system is capable of adapting to different conditions by changing the balance of muscular activities. The next important question is: How can this information be used effectively for evaluating locomotor disorders? All this information must be compiled into a useful data base for a comprehensive understanding of the variations in EMG gait patterns and for providing a normative data base to evaluate locomotor deficits.[47,48] For the immediate future, it appears that the quantitative form of individual patterns in the data base must be the EMG profile.

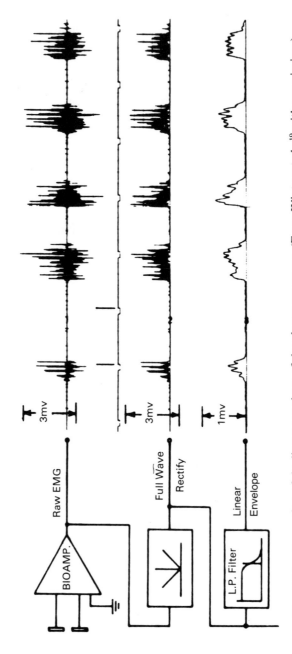

Fig. 5-14. Formation of the linear envelope of the electromyogram. (From Winter et al.,[19] with permission.)

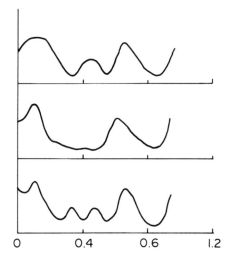

Fig. 5-15. Three consecutive strides of the linear envelope of an electromyogram from the rectus femoris muscle. (From Shiavi and Green,[26] with permission.)

REFERENCES

1. Eberhart H, Inman V, Bresler B: The principal elements in human locomotion. In Klopsteg P, Wilson P (eds): Human Limbs and Their Substitutes. Hafner Publishing Company, p. 464
2. Basmajian JV: Muscles Alive. Williams & Wilkins, Baltimore, 1978
3. Perry J: Kinesiology of lower extremity bracing. Clin Orthop 102:18, 1974
4. Inman V, Ralston H, Todd F: Human Walking. William & Wilkins, Baltimore, 1981
5. Milner M, Basmajian J, Quanbury A: Multifactorial analysis of walking by electromyography and computer. Am J Phys Med 50:235, 1971
6. Sutherland DH: An electromyographic study of the plantar flexors of the ankle in normal walking on the level. J Bone Joint Surg 48A:66, 1966
7. Arsenault B, Winter D, Marteniuk R: Is there a "normal" profile of EMG activity in gait? Med Biol Eng Comput 24:337, 1986
8. Shiavi R, Bourne J, Holland A: Automated extraction of activity features in linear envelopes of locomotor electromyographic patterns. IEEE Trans Biomed Eng 33:594, 1987
9. Shiavi R, Bugle H, Limbird T: Electromyographic gait assessment. Part 1. Adult EMG profiles and walking speed. J Rehabil Res & Dev 24(2):13, 1987
10. Paul J: Comparison of EMG signals from leg muscles with the corresponding force actions calculated from walkpath measurements. p. 16. In Human Locomotor Engineering. Institute of Mechanical Engineering, London, 1974
11. Shiavi R: Electromyographic patterns in adult locomotion—A comprehensive review. J Rehabil Res Dev 22(3):85, 1985
12. Pedotti A: A study of motor coordination and neuromuscular activities in human locomotion. Biol Cybern 26:53, 1977
13. Shiavi R, Griffin P: Changes in electromyographic gait patterns of calf muscles with walking speed. IEEE Trans Biomed Eng 30:73, 1983

14. Murray M, Mollinger L, Gardner G, Sepic S: Kinematic and EMG patterns during slow, free, and fast walking. J Orthop Res 2:272, 1984

15. Nilsson J, Thortensson A, Halbertsma J: Changes in leg movements and muscle activity with speed of locomotion and modes of progression in humans. Acta Physiol Scand 123:457, 1985

16. Shiavi R, Green N, McFadyen B, et al: Normative Childhood EMG Gait Patterns. J Orthop Res 5:283, 1987

17. Battye C, Joseph J: An investigation by telemetering of the activity of some muscles in walking. Med Biol Eng 4:125, 1966

18. Grieve DW, Cavanagh PR: The validity of quantitative statements about surface electromyograms recorded during locomotion. Scand J Rehabil Med 3:19, 1974

19. Winter D, Rau G, Kadefors R, et al: Units, terms, and standards in the reporting of EMG research. Report of Ad Hoc Committee of the International Society of Electrophysiological Kinesiology, August 1980

20. Sutherland D: Events measurements in normal and pathological gait. Gait Analysis Workshop, Rehabilitative Engineering Research and Development Service, Veterans Administration, Long Beach, CA, September 1979. Bull Prosthet Res 18:281, 1981

21. Boden F, Brussatis F, Wunderlich T, Mertin B: A kinesiologic electromyography system for the computer-controlled analog and digital recording and processing of muscle action potentials of walking subjects. Med Prog Technol 8:129, 1981

22. Winter D: Pathologic gait diagnosis with computer-averaged electromyographic profiles. Arch Phys Med Rehabil 65:393, 1984

23. Yang J, Winter D: Electromyographic amplitude normalization methods—Improving their sensitivity as diagnostic tools in gait analysis. Arch Phys Med Rehabil 65:517, 1984

24. Gray E, Basmajian J: Electromyography and cinematography of leg and foot ("normal" and "flat") during walking. Anat Rec 161:1, 1968

25. Sheffield F, Gersten J, Mastellone A: Electromyographic study of the muscles of the foot in normal walking. Am J Phys Med 35:223, 1956

26. Shiavi R, Green N: Ensemble averaging of locomotor electromyographic patterns using interpolation. Med Biol Eng Comput 21:573, 1983

27. Mann R, Inman V: Phasic activity of intrinsic muscles of the foot. J Bone Joint Surg 406A:469, 1964

28. Dubo H, Peat M, Winter D, et al: Electromyographic temporal analysis of gait: Normal human locomotion. Arch Phys Med Rehabil 57:415, 1976

29. Rozin R, Robin G, Magora A, et al: Investigation of fait. 2. Gait analysis of normal individuals. Electromyography 12:183, 1971

30. Shiavi R, Champion S, Freemon F, Griffin P: Variability of electromyographic patterns for level surface walking through a range of self-selected speeds. Bull Pros Res 18:5, 1981

31. University of California, Berkeley: The pattern of muscular activity in the lower of extremity during walking. Advisory Committee on Artificial Limbs—National Research Council; Prosthetic Devices Research Project, Institute of Engineering Research Report Series 11 Issue 25, September 1953

32. Walmsley R: Electromyographic study of the phasic activity of peroneus longus and brevis. Arch Phys Med 58:65, 1977

33. Brandell B: Functional roles of the calf and vastus muscles in locomotion. Am J Phys Med 56:59, 1977

34. Matsusaka N: Control of the medial-lateral balance in walking. Acta Orthop Scand 57:555, 1986
35. Rideau X, Duval A: Function of the anterior thigh muscles. Anat Clin 1:29, 1978
36. Adler N, Kent B: Electromyography of the vastus medialis in normal subjects during gait. Presented at the Fourth Congress of International Society of Electrophysiological Kinesiology, Boston, 1979, p. 222
37. Lyons K, Perry J, Gronley J, et al: Timing and relative intensity of hip extensor and abductor muscle action during level and stair ambulation. Phys Ther 63:1597, 1983
38. Green D, Morris J: Role of adductor longus and adductor magnus in postural movements and in ambulation. Am J Phys Med 49:223, 1970
39. Waters R, Morris J: Electrical activity of muscles of the trunk during walking. J Anat 111:191, 1972
40. Sheffield F: Electromyographic study of the abdominal muscles in walking and other movements. Am J Phys Med 41:142, 1962
41. Dofferhof A, Vink P: The stabilizing function of the mm. iliocostalis and the mm. multifidi during walking. J Anat 140:329, 1985
42. Perry J, Waters R, Perrin T: Electromyographic analysis of equinovarus following stroke. Clin Orthop 131:47, 1978
43. Winter D, Yack H: EMG profiles during normal walking: Stride-to-stride and inter-subject variability. EEG Clin Neurophysiol 67:402, 1987
44. Kadaba M, Wooten M, Gainey J, Cochran G: Repeatability of phasic activity—Performance of surface and intramuscular wire electrodes in gait analysis. J Orthop Res 3:350, 1985
45. Shiavi R, Griffin P: Representing and clustering electromyographic gait patterns with multivariate techniques. Med Biol Eng Comput 19:605, 1981
46. Yang J, Winter D: Surface EMG profiles during different walking cadences in humans. EEG Clin Neurophysiol 60:485, 1985
47. Guth V, Abink F, Theysohn H: Electromyographic investigations on gait. Electromyograph Clin Neurophysiol 19:305, 1979
48. Sutherland D: The value of normative data in gait analysis. p. 89. Gait Research Workshop, U.S. Department of Health, Education and Welfare (NIH 78-119), Washington, DC, 1978

6 Early Motor Development and Control: Foundations for Independent Walking

Elizabeth L. Leonard

The human infant comes into this world kicking. Over the next 12 months, a remarkably short period within the life span, these seemingly undifferentiated, random, and purposeless movements are transformed to permit development of bipedal gait. The ontogeny of human motor function is central to understanding motor development and its disorders. Surprisingly, despite great interest in motor function by physical therapists, relatively little is known about the determinants and underlying dynamics of motor abilities. Renewed interest in early motor development has come from many disciplines: motor science, neurobiology, and psychology. Experimental approaches to normal and abnormal motor development and their significance for remediation through physical therapy are discussed in this review of locomotor development during the first year of life.

ONTOGENY, MATURATION, AND MOTOR DEVELOPMENT

Ontogenic theories of motor development postulate that motor development occurs in an invariant, hierarchically ordered sequence that is principally dependent on cortical maturation. Motor milestones are thought to mirror central nervous system (CNS) maturation. Cardinal postulates of motor development, based primarily on the work of Gesell,[1,2] have remained prominent in contemporary physical therapy. A maturational model is firmly rooted within child development and has occupied a central theoretical position for more than 50 years.

Recent developmental studies[3-8] questioned whether a maturational model accounts adequately for the complexities of human motor development and addressed how other processes compose and underlie motor behavior. The importance of maturation within motor ontogeny is acknowledged. These studies, however, establish perception, cognition, and experience as additional determinants of motor behavior. The traditional formulation of maturation posits no role for learning or experience. Current motor development research suggests that a maturational model is reductionistic and fails to account for the complexities of the infant's biology and its relation to the environment. Connolly[9] stated that the conceptualization of motor development as a mere unfolding is an oversimplification. Explanations of motor development, not exclusively linked to maturational theory, support a role for maturation within human ontogeny and acknowledge how processes like epigenesis affect canalization of motor development. Development is nonlinear and consists of spurts, plateaus, and regressions that produce quantitative and qualitative changes in motor behavior.[10]

Interval synchrony defines the emergence of new behaviors across different developmental domains within a relative time frame.[11,12] Basal ages, possibly fixed by maturation, set a lower limit for the emergence of specific motor abilities. For example, independent sitting is not seen in a child under 6 months of age, and independent ambulation seldom emerges before 9 months of age.

Maturation has had heuristic value for diagnosing developmental deviance. Developmental diagnosis[13] is predicated on the notion that stage-related changes in behavior mirror growth of the CNS. Maturation is conceptualized as a process that is uniform, invariant, and marked by the passage of time. Maturation thus serves as an anchor by which one can mark development. But maturation is not only a sequence of motor behaviors chronologically yoked to age. Maturation is dynamic and complex; it is influenced by constitutional, environmental, and experiential factors through the processes of interaction and covariance.[9] To conceive of motor development solely as a predetermined sequence tied to chronologic age is to deprive ourselves of the richness of human ontogeny. Changes in motor behavior require explanations that transcend maturation as a unitary cause.

VARIABILITY AND INDIVIDUAL DIFFERENCES IN MOTOR DEVELOPMENT

Physical therapists have emphasized uniformity in development rather than variability. A model of motor development must apply universally and account for intraindividual and interindividual variability. A maturational model of motor development fails to account adequately for individual differences and cultural variability. Alternative pathways to the same motor end point exist. Although most children crawl before they walk, crawling is not a necessary condition for ambulation. Variability in the path to bipedalism includes behaviors such as scooting and hitching. Culture and environment impact on the expression, rate, and sequence with which motor behaviors develop.[6,7,14]

To assume that an infant must pass through the prone progression sequences described by Gesell[1,2] and McGraw[15,16] enforces arbitrary constraints on locomotor development. Some would have you believe that these sequences are necessary conditions for developing higher cortical function necessary for reading.[17] The relationship between sensorimotor experience and higher cortical abilities is largely unknown. To assume that recapitulation of these motor sequences is the route to advancing mental function is unjustified. The role of individual differences in human motor development should not be underestimated. Acknowledging variability in the rate and sequence with which children attain milestones is important in recognizing breadth and diversity within human motor ontogeny.

THE ROLE OF REFLEXES IN LOCOMOTOR DEVELOPMENT

Despite great significance accorded assessment of reflexes within child development there is not uniform agreement as to their significance within human ontogeny. Much effort has been expended in determining whether the presence or absence of particular reflexes at given points in time signifies motoric normality or deviance. Touwen[18] provided a comprehensive review of the subject and illustrated two salient points. First, he stated that these responses were called reflexes because the infant is considered to respond on a reflexive basis in contrast to being able to execute controlled movement volitionally. Second, these responses were termed primitive to indicate a low level of differentiation.

The motor competencies of the human neonate have been described as reflexive. Neonatal stepping and placing are topologically similar to motor patterns used for locomotion. These stereotypical responses remain in the infant's movement repertoire until approximately the end of the third postnatal month when they traditionally are thought to disappear. Their disappearance has been attributed to inhibition by maturing higher cortical centers. Reappearance of these neuromotor patterns in pediatric and adult brain injury is said to occur because of cortical disinhibition.

The development of motor abilities from innate reflexive motor patterns to the development of skilled motor behavior under voluntary, higher-order control continues to be investigated.[5-7] Zelazo and colleagues proposed that the so called primitive reflexes, are instead innate motor patterns that are modified by instrumental learning. Reflexes are transformed from automatically elicited motor behaviors to responses that are volitionally controlled through practice and experience. Zelazo's[4,5] reflexive-to-instrumental control model proposes that transitions in motor behavior are concordant with changes in central processing. Moreover, he states that cognitive maturation and information processing capacity may be limiting factors in the onset of unaided walking.

At about 1 year of age, qualitative changes in motor function appear in developmental synchrony with centrally mediated changes in information processing ability. Profound changes in motor, cognitive, and linguistic development occur at this time.[19,20] Babies take their first independent steps, utter their first words, and begin to use objects in goal directed activity. Zelazo[5,6] proposes that the basis for these changes lies in a fundamental transformation in the rapidity with which infants can form associations and retrieve stored information. This transformation in information processing ability is particularly significant for motor development. Changes in central processing capacity permit the integration of spatial, perceptual, and coordinative abilities that enable the transition from quadripedal bipedal locomotion. Age-related changes in motor and cognitive behavior reported by Zelazo[19] and Zelazo and Leonard[20] are so pronounced that they constitute a developmental metamorphosis.

It is likely that there are other developmental epochs during which interval synchrony accounts for qualitative changes in development. Prechtl and Hopkins[21] studied spontaneous movement in infants aged 3 to 18 weeks and reported a major motor reorganization between 2 to 3 months characterized by a shift from gross movement to voluntary control. This change was concordant with the onset of social smiling. The concordance of social smiling and a reorganization in motor behavior is probably not coincidental. About age three months is one point during infancy when motor behaviors are known to change as evidenced by the diminution of neonatal stepping, placing, and the Moro response.

It is unlikely that this change in motor activity is independent of change in other developmental domains. The concordance between smiling and the onset of voluntary motor activity constitutes interval synchrony. Zelazo[22-24] noted that the onset of smiling and vocalizing were basic constituents of early cognitive activity. The relationship between the onset of smiling, vocalization, and emergent voluntary motor activity may be dictated by a common change in central processing ability at age 3 months as it is in the year-old infant.

CULTURAL VARIABILITY AND
THE ACQUISITION OF
MOTOR BEHAVIOR

Cross-cultural investigations demonstrated that the cephalocaudal motor progression recognized by European and American societies as invariant may not be universal.[14,25,26] Phenotypic variability in motor development of African infants is present and not explained by maturational theory. Variability in the sequence with which children acquire motor milestones can occur because of the effects of environment and culture.[3-6] Furthermore, nonsequential development of motor abilities does not support the hierarchical invariance described by motor development theory.

Super[25] studied motor development in Kenyan Kipsigis babies who were precocious relative to Western norms regarding onset of ambulation. Kipsigis infants were advanced in sitting, standing and walking but were behind Western infants in development of rolling and crawling. Kipsigis mothers believed that their infants had to be instructed in how to sit and walk, but not to crawl or roll over, and thus trained their infants in the desired behaviors. Super illustrated that motor precocity probably was not due to differences in genotype but was specific to behaviors that were trained. Konner[26] studied San infants in the Kalahari Desert in Botswana. San infants maintained the stepping response during infancy and had an earlier onset of sitting relative to Western norms. In both instances functionally valued motor behaviors were shaped by childrearing conditions influenced by a particular culture.

Variability in the rate and sequence of motor development is not limited to African infants. Caesar[27] described postural development in Dutch neonates and noted that head control was strongly influenced by maternal handling during caretaking. Solomon and Solomon[28] studied motor development in year-old Mexican infants living in the Yucatan who displayed advanced fine motor skills in contrast to slower developing gross motor abilities. Yucatan parents rarely allowed their children to be on the floor which restricted opportunities for crawling or creeping. Conversely, these infants were carried about with their hands free and had increased opportunities to develop prehensile skills. Finnish investigators Lagerspetz et al.[29] demonstrated that the onset of creeping was accelerated with practice and concluded that motor development was not solely dependent on maturation.

Individual and cultural variability in the rate and sequence of motor development is not well recognized within physical therapy. Therapists are generally taught that motor development proceeds in an invariant cephalocaudal sequence. Variations from this pattern constitute abnormality. Moreover, repetition of this cephalocaudal sequence forms the foundation for motor remediation procedures used to correct motor deviance in infants with neuromotor pathology.[30-33] There have been no exceptions to this approach. The research reviewed illustrated clearly that variation occurred in the sequence of motor development. Furthermore, acceleration of motor behaviors occurred with training although there may be limits determined by maturation.

THE TRANSITION FROM INNATE MOTOR PATTERNS TO VOLUNTARY CONTROL

Traditionally neonatal reflexes are believed to be suppressed by encephalization which is thought to be necessary for development of mature motor behavior. It has also been assumed that neonatal stepping and later walking are unrelated. In this model failure of primitive reflexes to disappear connotes neuromotor pathology. Surprisingly, there have been few studies of developmental transitions of infant movement. The control mechanisms that underlie the change from innate motor patterns to development of voluntary motor behavior are largely unexplored. Development of higher order control, in relation to infant motor behavior, has not been investigated extensively. This is noteworthy given the role that encephalization plays in motor development theory.

Cioni et al.[34] described the interindividual and intraindividual variability of the motor repertoire of the newborn. These investigators could not confirm the commonly accepted predominance of a flexion posture in neonates. Their study suggested that (1) preference for a flexion posture may not predominate neonatal development, and (2) the sequence of motor development may not take place as previously thought.

Principles that underlie transitions from innate to voluntary control of motor behavior are particularly relevant for physical therapy. Zelazo et al.[3] investigated whether as little as 8 minutes of daily practice in neonatal stepping could lead to an increase in stepping. Stepping rates of exercised infants increased from a mean base rate of 12 steps/min to 30 steps/min, whereas rates of control infants declined. Qualitative changes in the walking pattern also occurred. The amplitude of the flexion phase of the gait cycle increased, as did cadence and velocity.

Several important points emerge from this research. First, daily practice of neonatal stepping prevented its disappearance. Second, the increase in stepping over the training period suggested that instrumental learning occurred. Third, infants appeared to gain the capacity to harness congenital neuromotor patterns (reflexes) by gaining control of the initiation, modulation, and termination of the response.

Zelazo[4–6] and Leonard[7,35] and co-workers argued that innate motor patterns are retained within a hierarchy of motor behavior and are modified during the development from a subcortically activated stereotypical response to one that is governed by higher-order control. These workers proposed that innate motor patterns constitute a substrate for later voluntary motor behavior. Activation and transformation of these elemental motor patterns to sophisticated and controlled motor behavior occurs gradually during infancy and early childhood. These transformations argue for continuity in motor function from prenatal development through maturity such that early and later forms of walking are isomorphic. Furthermore, instrumental control of innate motor patterns is acquired through practice and experience, as stereotypical movement is modified to produce mature, skilled motor function. Innate motor patterns are transformed during infancy to form the scaffolding for development of skilled movement. The belief that primitive reflexes are phylogenetically old motor patterns and that innate and later forms of the same motor behavior are unrelated does not appear to be valid.

Neonatal stepping differs from later walking on several dimensions. First, neonatal stepping, appears to be driven by a stretch over the hip joint as the infant is tilted forward to initiate gait.[36] Second, infants require external support to remain upright. Third, infant gait is digitigrade rather than plantigrade.

There appear to be fundamental similarities in the gait cycle that argue that the two constitute an isomorphic response. Forssberg[37-40] employed electromyography (EMG) and kinematics to show transitions from neonatal to mature stepping. Stepping was transformed from a reflexive to an acquired form through modification of the innate condition rather than through creation of a new form. The possibility that neonatal stepping was transformed to form the foundation for mature locomotion had been proposed previously by Zelazo,[4] who issued a challenge that the reflexive-to-instrumental control model be refuted or validated using electromyography.

The capacity of infants to activate innate motor patterns, inhibit reflex activity, and transform innate patterns into voluntary motor acts stands in direct contrast to prevailing beliefs within physical therapy that embrace the necessity for therapeutic activity to inhibit primitive reflex behaviors.[30,31] This is a critical distinction since the concept of reflex dominance implies that the infant is unable to modulate innate reflexive responses. The concept of reflex dominance does not appear to be valid.

The notion that innate neuromotor patterns and later voluntary behaviors are linked has perinatal research support. Milani-Comparetti[41] recorded the progressive development of prenatal motor patterns using real-time ultrasound and demonstrated fetal-infant continuity in motor function. Milani-Comparetti observed fetuses practicing pushing against the wall of the uterus to prepare for parturition. Several motor behaviors were graphed during gestation. Development of these behaviors peaked at 40 weeks gestation coinciding with the birth of the infant and then began to decline. Innate motor patterns appear to be species-specific behaviors that are ecologically valid for development of motor behavior.

CONTINUITY IN MOTOR DEVELOPMENT

The course of locomotor development appears to follow a U-shaped trajectory.[35] Neonatal walking decays by the third postnatal month to a period of locomotor inactivity from 2 to 5 months.[39-40] Supported locomotion develops between 6 to 9 months with the onset of independent ambulation emerging from 9 months onward. U-shaped trajectories are not unique to locomotor behavior. They are present in other development functions including grasping[42] and auditory orientation and localization of infants to sound.[43]

Clearly, differences in neonatal walking and independent bipedal locomotion exist. Zelazo,[4] Zelazo et al.,[6] Forssberg,[37-40] and recently Thelen and Cooke[44-46] argued that neonatal and later forms of locomotion are more related than disparate. Does the development of locomotion represent a U-shaped developmental function or is continuity of locomotor responses from neonatal to unsupported locomotion possible?

Zelazo[3,4] provided experimental support for the instrumental adaptation of neonatal stepping and demonstrated that practice and reinforcement resulted in an increase in stepping over time. He argued that instrumental learning accounted for the increase in stepping and modulation of locomotor control.

Forssberg[37-40] described similarities and differences in various stages of locomotor development from neonatal stepping to independent ambulation. Neonatal activity was characterized by marked hip flexion, a digitigrade strike pattern, the need for external support to initiate the gait cycle and maintain postural control, coactivation of antagonist muscles, and phase coupling of joint motion. There was rhythmic movement during stepping, but it had an irregular quality often accompanied by crossed extension. During the inactive phase, no rhythmic locomotor activity could be induced. Forssberg noted that some infants may never enter an inactive phase and maintained stepping from the neonatal period. A stage of supported locomotion ensued after the inactive period. During supported locomotion, the gait was infant initiated; that is, no afferent input was required to induce stepping.

Independent walking was characterized by a more vertical posture with decreased flexion of the hip and knee, an increase in step length, and desynchronization of the hip, knee, and ankle joints. After the onset of independent locomotion, no changes in the EMG pattern occurred for several weeks. The foot was still placed with full sole contact preceding ankle dorsiflexion. Transformation of this pattern occurred relative rapidly prior to age 3 and then more slowly until age 5 years, when an adult pattern was complete.

Differences between newborn stepping and mature locomotion were also described by Thelen and Cooke.[36,44,45] Kinematic analysis of infant stepping demonstrated that knee flexion lead hip flexion at the beginning of the swing cycle. There was tight synchronization of the hip, knee, and ankle joints with co-contraction of agonist-antagonist muscles. During mature locomotion hip and knee flexion were coupled but there was a phase reversal at the ankle. This reciprocol innervation rather than coactivation allowed development of a heel strike. Although newborn and later patterns were not identical, the differences observed didn't preclude continuity. Thus, infant stepping, supported locomotion, and independent locomotion have elements that are quite different from mature locomotor patterns, but possess constituent components that share several collective features and have a developmental progression.

Forssberg[39] postulated a neural control theory to account for changes in locomotor ontogeny. Innate, possibly spinal controlled, neuronal networks generate locomotor patterns. While these patterns change with maturation, the same neural circuitry is believed to be used for newborn and mature locomotion. A species-specific central control mechanism operates to transform an initial digitigrade pattern into an efficient bipedal plantigrade pattern.

Spinal mechanisms are initially activated by an external force that stimulates stepping. This circuitry is maintained throughout development despite an apparent discontinuity in locomotor behavior. Zelazo[4] previously postulated that original patterns were not lost, but were suppressed possibly because of disuse. The maintenance of the neonatal gait EMG pattern after the inactive locomotor phase argues against two different locomotor mechanisms, that is, an innate and acquired form.

Regulation of posture and balance appears to be dependent on higher-order motor control developing during midinfancy. It is hypothesized that spinally activated stepping may link up with higher order control mechanisms toward the end of the first year. Spinally activated and cortically driven systems may converge to permit development of independent locomotion. Zelazo[5] suggested that information processing and maturational constraints may set a lower limit on the onset of unaided walking.

Supraspinal control may be governed by multiple mechanisms.[39,40] A locomotor driving system is hypothesized to control the locomotor pattern generator by initiating and regulating spinal locomotor activity. An adaptive control system is postulated that modifies stereotypical locomotor behavior to meet environmental conditions. Forssberg hypothesized that development of independent locomotion is dependent on maturation of the equilibrium system and not solely reliant on changes in the locomotor pattern. The locomotor pattern generator is present in the newborn and remains throughout development. Changes in locomotion appear to take place because of more rostral influences on the spinal locomotor generator. Approximately 30 to 50 weeks following the onset of independent ambulation, ankle dorsiflexion begins to precede heel contact—a pattern that is continually refined over the next 36 months. Infants do not appear to drive locomotion volitionally until balance is adequately developed to maintain antigravity postural control.[40]

Thelen[46] provided presumptive evidence for a central motor program that generates spatial and temporally patterned movement. Thelen found that kicking and stepping shared the same topography. She also found evidence of interlimb coordination that argued for phase-related coupling of leg movement during infancy.

Clark and Phillips[47] studied step-cycle organization during infant locomotion. The step cycles of babies with 3, 6, and 9 months walking experience were compared with step cycles of adults. Infants with 3 months walking experience displayed a step-cycle pattern similar to that of adult walkers, including the presence of all four Phillippson phases, which occurred in approximately the same proportion as that of adults. Moreover, infant walkers adapted to differences in walking speeds in a manner analogous to that of adults. Absolute and relative timing patterns across walking speeds were similar between infants and adults, suggesting that shortly after the onset of ambulation, the infant possesses the essential pattern of coordination required for mature independent locomotion.

Clark et al.[48] analyzed interlimb coordination during the first 6 months of locomotion. Newly walking infants, that is, babies who are just able to take three independent steps, were studied during ambulation with and without support. In addition, infants with 0.5, 1, 3, and 6 months walking experience were analyzed and compared with adults. Temporal phasing and distance phasing were measured. For each measure, the mean and variability were analyzed to determine whether this pattern displayed the phase relationships that characterize mature walking. Clark et al. found no differences in the mean temporal phasing between groups and an inverse relationship between walking age and temporal variability. As walking experience increased, there was a decrease in the temporal phasing that approached adult values by the age of 3 months. Differences were found in the mean distance phasing only for supported walkers. Variability was present between groups that approached adult values after 3 months ambulation.

Clark et al. concluded that a coordinative structure for interlimb coordination was present early in infancy. The variability of interlimb coordination was improved by providing external support to newly walking infants who were less facile in integrating the demands of upright posture. Clark et al. suggested that coordination patterns employed by the newly walking infant were not dictated by a central nervous system encoded pattern, but rather reflected an emergent capacity for dynamic organization.

Two important points derive from this research. First, the data established that a pattern for interlimb coordination is present at the onset of unaided walking. Second, although not addressed from a cognitive perspective, these data appear to support a role for instrumental learning in the postural and biomechanical adaptation of newly walking infants. Variability in temporal and distance phasing improved with physical support in newly walking infants. This supports the contention that new walkers are unable to integrate the perceptual, cognitive, and motoric components required to produce coordinated movement.

Antigravity postural control, equilibrium, and coordination of movement require considerable intersensory integration of not only motor components but also vision and a motivational drive to ambulate. An increased capacity for central processing might be a necessary condition for the integration of these abilities to enable independent bipedal locomotion.[5] Independent perceptual, neurologic, and biomechanical developmental research converge on age 3 months and show qualitative changes in motor organization providing strong support for interval synchrony. Furthermore, the explanation proposed by Clark et al. that the "pattern of coordination first used by the upright infant is not prescribed by the central nervous system, but is one that emerges because it affords the most dynamic stability" supports a role for higher functions governing this response. Neural substrates particular to the locomotor system appear to play a role in the development of walking as acknowledged by Clark et al., but undoubtedly other factors also operative within the developing nervous system.

ORGANIZATION OF EARLY MOTOR BEHAVIOR

Research in early motor development supports a prefunctional organization of the infant's nervous system for movement. Movements are organized and constrained by coordinative structures that become progressively differentiated with age. Forssberg[39] and Thelen et al.[49] suggest that the infant's capacity for rhythmic movement may be influenced by subcortical mechanisms that control pattern generation. These neuromotor patterns are innate and appear to be activated initially by proprioceptive inputs that induce movement. These mechanisms may be responsible for movement associated with the behaviors classically termed *primitive reflexes.*

The term *primitive reflex* is a misnomer, since these motor responses do not fit the neurophysiological definition of a motor reflex. Katona[50] distinguished between movements that he termed *primitive reflexes* and *elementary neuromotor patterns.* Elementary neuromotor patterns illustrate a species-specific human motor capacity for organized movement and a high degree of stereotypy. These patterns are elicited under specific releasing conditions in all infants, as well as nonviable fetuses and represent primordial complex movements. They herald the later appearance of crawling, creeping, sitting, and walking. Elementary neuromotor patterns are believed to be represented at a higher level of CNS integration minimally requiring the basal ganglia. Once stimulated, elementary neuromotor patterns can generate cyclical movement. Conversely, primitive reflexes are short singular reactions that require stimulation to activate each response. Innate neuromotor patterns are organized, provide a substrate from which controlled movement develops, and enable the execution of rhythmic, temporally, and spatially patterned movement.

Motor development is dependent on the infant's biology, behavior and environment and may be less reliant on neurological maturation then previously believed. Fogel and Thelen[8] stated that behavior does not preceed uniformly across different domains of development prompted by a single cause. Rather, asynchronous changes are produced from various component actions that account for developmental change. Dynamic systems theory postulates that de novo forms of motor behavior can be generated from innate coordinative structures depending on the task at hand and environmental demands. For example, the desire to look around may provide an initial condition for prone lying infants to elevate the head and view the world around them. Zelazo[4] suggested that perceptual inputs produced by the assumption of a vertical posture might pique the infant's interest in distal events and provide the motivation to take his first independent steps. Furthermore, Zelazo[19] and Zelazo and Leonard[20] argued that motor and mental development may proceed in tandem but need not and can develop independently in children with motoric dysfunction.

CLINICAL IMPLICATIONS FOR PHYSICAL THERAPY

How might this new knowledge about the ontogeny of motor behavior be used to help children with motoric impairment? While interest in early motor development has burgeoned in the last decade, little attention has focused on applications of this research to children with motoric dysfunction. Heriza[51] stated the need for applied research with motor impaired infants; however, few studies speak to this issue.

A method of comprehensive neurohabilitation for brain injured infants has been described by Katona.[50,52,53] This method is based on a comprehensive neurological investigation of brain activity using electrophysiology (EEG, EMG, BAER) computed axial tomography, and behavioral evaluation. Motor habilitation is accomplished by placing infants in positions activating innate motor patterns. Hypotonia, spasticity, and dyskinesia are treated with exercises that facilitate walking, crawling, and sitting.

An exercise profile is developed for the neurologic deficits exhibited by the infant. Daily exercises are taught to parents. Progress in motor development is monitored regularly by a child neurologist, physical therapist, and pediatrician. Katona reported on a sample of 886 infants who were enrolled at less than 4 months of age (N = 547), at 4 to 6 months of age (N = 156), or at 6 to 8 months of age (N = 183) and on a group of 75 children who were recommended for treatment but were untreated because of medical or social factors. Developmental outcome was assessed after 18 months and overall development was found to be better in treated infants. Developmental dysfunction increased linearly as a function of age of treatment initiation. According to Katona, activation of elementary neuromotor patterns is a prime component for motor habilitation of infants with neurologic deficits and can be shaped and facilitated by early training.

Exercise of neonatal stepping, with the specific intent of strengthening walking in infants at risk of cerebral palsy, represents a considerable departure from neurodevelopmental treatment. In a pilot investigation, Leonard and Zelazo[54] studied whether daily practice of neonatal walking would increase stepping in 4-month-old infants who had had neonatal neurologic signs and were considered at risk of cerebral palsy. Eleven infants (four experimentally treated and seven conventionally treated) participated in this study. Infants in the experimental group received training in stepping, standing, and placing for 12 min/day for 10 weeks. Mean stepping, standing, and placing responses were recorded weekly for experimental infants and at baseline and at week 10 for controls. Infants were recruited at 20 ± 6 weeks of age. As neonates, these infants displayed two or more abnormalities, including disorders in posture, muscle tone, or the quality of movement. Parents of infants receiving treatment provided daily exercise. Weekly measurements were recorded during 10 weeks of intervention. The mean number of stepping and placing responses to occur over two 1-minute test sessions and the mean duration of standing until the knees buckled during two trials were the principal dependent measures.

These data are illustrated in Figure 6-1. Experimental infants displayed statistically significant higher rates of stepping and standing after 10 weeks of training relative to the conventionally treated controls. Placing approached statistical significance. The mean number of steps and the duration of standing increased almost fourfold from the beginning to the end of treatment. These results implied that the newborn stepping pattern developed into an instrumental behavior for infants at risk of neuromotor disabilities as it did for infants with normal neuromotor status.[3]

The specificity of practice on the development of two innate neuromotor patterns—stepping and sitting—was investigated by Zelazo et al.[55] as an experi-

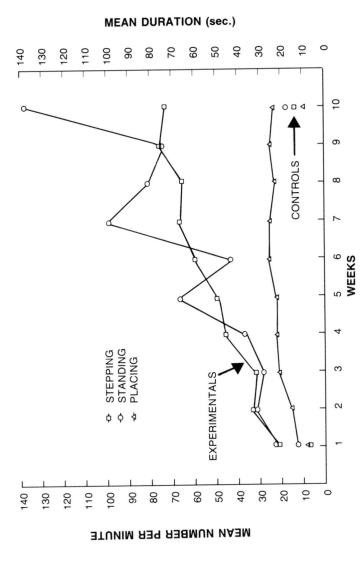

Fig. 6-1. Mean number of placing and stepping responses and mean duration of standing for high-risk infants receiving exercise and their matched controls. (From Zelazo et al.,[6] with permission.)

mental test of Super's observation that infant motor precocity is specific to the behaviors trained. Thirty-six week-old male infants were assigned to one of five groups. There were three experimental groups who received 6 minutes of daily exercise of stepping or sitting or both stepping and sitting. Weekly and 14-week control infants received no exercise. The elicitation of stepping is as previously described in the literature. Infants were held under the axillae from the rear and inclined forward to activate the stepping pattern.

Elicitation of elementary sitting requires special mention because it is a neuromotor pattern that is not generally known within North America. Neonatal sitting has been described by Katona.[52] Infants are held posteriorly by the thighs and buttocks and their backs are allowed to rest on the chest of the examiner. Once secure, the examiner withdraws the support on the infant's back. Infants straighten their back, center and elevate their head, and sit upright. Dependent variables were the mean number of steps per minute taken by the infant during 2 minutes of stepping and the mean number of seconds that the infant sat upright before losing his balance.

Infants who received practice in stepping alone or in combination with sitting, stepped more than infants who received no exercise or sitting exercise only. No statistically significant differences in stepping occurred between infants who received stimulation of the sitting pattern alone or no treatment controls. There was a similar effect of practice on sitting. Both groups receiving sitting exercises sat upright longer than did infants who were unexercised or infants who received only stepping practice. Stimulation of stepping without sitting did not influence the duration of sitting. The authors concluded that practice in stepping and sitting was specific to the patterns trained.

It should be noted that in comparison with conventional physical therapy, the intervention was brief for these cited studies. Facilitation and training of innate motor patterns required only a few minutes of daily practice. Brief periods of daily practice can have meaningful facilitative effects if performed regularly.

FACILITATING MOTOR DEVELOPMENT IN A NEUROLOGICALLY IMPAIRED INFANT

Leonard and Zelazo[7] argued that this paradigm has profound implications for habilitating motor impairment in children at risk of cerebral palsy. A single case study using the sitting and stepping procedures with a premature infant illustrates the application of this paradigm for facilitating motor development in infants with neurologic impairments. (Leonard EL, Zelazo PR, Tarby TJ: unpublished data). A 1,247-g female infant was born at 27 weeks gestation following a pregnancy complicated by intermittent spotting and placenta previa. The infant was asphyxiated, required endotracheal intubation, and subsequent high-frequency jet ventilation. The postnatal course was complicated. A large symptomatic patent ductus arteriosis required ligation. The infant developed extensive cystic periventricular leukomalacia with moderate ventricular dilation.

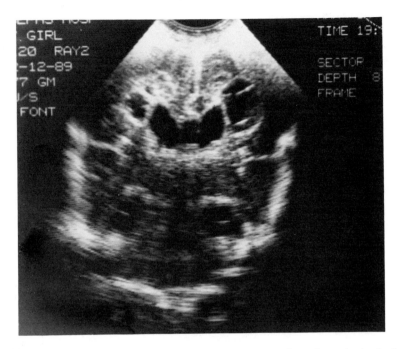

Fig. 6-2. Cranial ultrasound of preterm infant showing cystic periventricular leukoma-lacia.

Stepping and sitting procedures were initiated at a chronologic age of 4 months and at a corrected age of 3 weeks (Fig. 6-3). She received 3 minutes of stepping and 3 minutes of sitting practice twice daily using procedures described above. Weekly measurements were taken that included the mean number of steps for two 1-minute trials and the mean sitting time for two trials. The infant received 14 weeks of treatment but did not receive any exercise during weeks 7 and 8 because she required eye surgery for retinopathy of prematurity.

Early signs of cerebral palsy became evident. Arching was noted, the infant started easily, and there were twitchlike, myoclonic movements of the upper extremities. Deep tendon reflexes were brisk, but there was no clonus. Resistance to movement when the legs were manipulated (passive tone) was normal.

Despite early signs of cerebral palsy there were clear advances in motor behavior. Figure 6-3 illustrates the progression of stepping and sitting over the weeks of training. Initially the infant would drag her legs as she moved forward. Over time, the legs were lifted high and advanced to initiate a step. Stepping increased from a mean base rate of 11.5 to 23.5 steps/min. Stepping was best performed when the infant was crying—a highly aroused state.

Sitting also changed noticeably. The back became straighter, the head was elevated and held midline, and postural correction was observed when the infant's weight shifted over her base of support. The duration of sitting increased from a mean of 27.5 to 132.5 seconds.

Whether these procedures can significantly ameliorate disability imposed

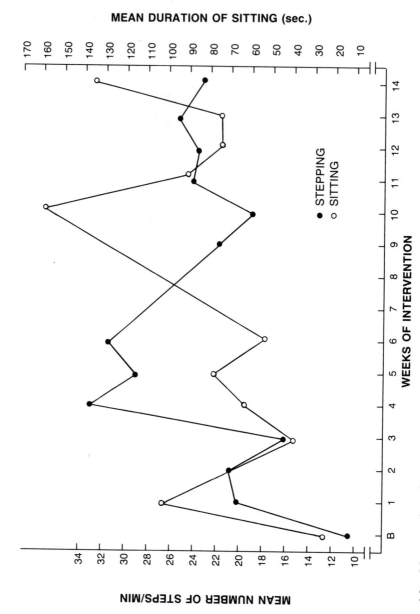

MEAN DURATION OF SITTING (sec.)

WEEKS OF INTERVENTION

MEAN NUMBER OF STEPS/MIN

● STEPPING
○ SITTING

Fig. 6-3. Mean number of steps per minute and mean duration of sitting from baseline through 14 weeks of intervention.

by cerebral palsy remains to be clarified by future research. A prospective study with random assignment of infants to different treatment conditions will be essential to determine whether stimulating innate motor patterns is therapeutically efficacious in facilitating motor development in infants with cerebral palsy. Experimental investigations that employed neurodevelopmental therapy as a procedure to facilitate motor development have recently appeared in the literature.[56,57] Additional studies are critically needed to determine how physical therapy can best help infants with cerebral palsy and related motor disabilities.[58]

SUMMARY AND CONCLUDING REMARKS

Recent studies of early motor development raise many questions about the validity of maturational theory, cephalocaudal development, and the role primitive reflexes play in motor development. Cross-cultural studies suggest that the presumed invariance in the temporal sequence with which motor behaviors emerge may not be universal and is strongly influenced by culture and experience.

Reflexes may not play as significant a role in motor development as previously believed. Primitive reflexes are generally thought to represent phylogenetic artifacts encoded as part of our evolutionary history. Instead, studies reviewed here suggest that these innate motor patterns form the foundation from which skilled movement develops.

The traditional view of discontinuity between neonatal and later emergent motor behaviors must be questioned. In a facilitating environment, the stereotypical motor repertoire present from birth becomes progressively refined through practice, instrumental learning and experience. Studies using EMG and kinematic procedures have demonstrated a transformation from reflexive to voluntary controlled motor behavior.

Cognitive development appears to pace and constrain the rate at which new motor behaviors appear. Maturation may set a basal limit on the emergence of new motor behaviors. Zelazo[5] has shown that changes in information-processing ability may dictate when specific motor behaviors emerge. A qualitative change in information processing ability may underlie the necessary integrative capacity needed for independent locomotion. The ability to assume an upright posture and the development of bipedalism require integration of perceptual, cognitive, and motor components. Ambulation is a complex skill requiring a drive to move forward in addition to neuromuscular maturation and coordination of neural and muscular elements.

Physical therapists interested in exploring applications of new theory to the development of therapeutic remediation programs have fertile ground for new research. Not since the 1950s, when the neurophysiologic approaches to therapeutic exercise were developed, have sound new paradigms for treating motor disorders been so available. New treatment paradigms should be a stimulus for further investigation. The validation or refutation of these new theories and the creation of new therapeutic approaches to improve the quality of life for children with neuromotor disorders will provide a major challenge for the next decade.

ACKNOWLEDGMENTS

I would like to thank Andrew Schwartz, Theodore Tarby, and Philip R. Zelazo for their helpful comments on an earlier draft of this chapter. I am indebted to Philip R. Zelazo for recognizing the relationship between early motor and cognitive development and their significance for habilitating infant motor dysfunction. I accept responsibility for the views expressed.

REFERENCES

1. Gesell A: The First Five Years of Life. Harper and Brothers, New York, 1940
2. Gesell A: The Embryology of Behavior. Harper and Brothers, New York, 1945
3. Zelazo PR, Zelazo NA, Kolb S: Walking in the newborn. Science 176:314, 1972
4. Zelazo PR: From reflexive to instrumental behavior. p. 87. In Lipsett L (ed): Developmental Psychobiology: The Significance of Infancy. Lawrence Erlbaum Associates, Hillsdale, NJ, 1976
5. Zelazo PR: The development of walking: New findings and old assumptions. J Motor Behav 15:99, 1983
6. Zelazo PR, Weiss MJ, Leonard EL: The development of unaided walking: The acquisition of higher order control. p. 139. In Zelazo P, Barr R (eds): Challenges to Developmental Paradigms. Lawrence Erlbaum Associates, Hillsdale, NJ, 1989
7. Leonard EL, Zelazo PR: From reflexive to instrumental control: A developmental model of motor learning. Presented at the American Physical Therapy Association/Canadian Physical Therapy Association Joint Congress, Las Vegas, Nevada, June, 1988
8. Fogel A, Thelen E: Development of early expressive and communicative action: Reinterupting the evidence from a dynamic systems perspective. Dev Psychol 23:747, 1987
9. Connolly KJ: Maturation and the Ontogeny of Motor Skills. In Connolly KJ, Prechtl HF (ed): Maturation and Development: Biological and Psychological Perspectives. William Heinemann Medical Books, London, 1981
10. Bever T: (ed): Regressions in Development: Basic Phenomena and Theoretical Alternatives. Lawrence Erlbaum Associates, Hillsdale, NJ, 1982
11. Fisher KW, Bullock D: Patterns of Data: Sequence, Synchrony, and Constraint in Cognitive Development. p. 12. In Fisher KW, (ed): Cognitive Development. New Directions in Child Development, Jossey-Bass, San Francisco, 1981
12. Fisher KW: Developmental levels as periods of discontinuity. p. 21. In Fisher KW (ed): Levels and Transitions in Children's Development. New Directions for Child Development. Jossey-Bass, San Francisco, 1983
13. Gesell A, Amatruda C: Developmental Diagnosis. 2nd Ed. Harper & Row, New York, 1947
14. Cintas HM: Cross cultural variation in infant motor development. Phys Occup Ther Pediatr 8(4):1, 1988
15. McGraw MB: From reflex to muscular control in the assumption of an erect posture and ambulation in the human infant. Child Dev 3:291, 1932
16. McGraw MB: Neuromuscular development of the human infant as exemplified in achievement of erect locomotion. J Pediatr 17:747, 1940

17. Delacato CH: Neurological Organization and Reading. Charles C Thomas, Springfield, IL, 1966
18. Touwen BC: Primitive reflexes: Conceptual or semantic problem. In Prechtl HF (ed): Continuity of Neuro Functions from Prenatal to Postnatal Life. Spastics International Medical Publications, Oxford, Blackwell Scientific Publications, Ltd., 1984
19. Zelazo P: The year-old infant: A period of major cognitive change. p. 47. In Bever T (ed): Regressions in Development: Basic Phenomena and Theoretical Alternatives. Lawrence Erlbaum Associates, Hillsdale, NJ, 1982
20. Zelazo PR, Leonard EL: The dawn of active thought. p. 37. In Fisher K (ed): Levels and Transitions in Children's Development. New Directions for Child Development. Jossey-Bass, San Francisco, 1983
21. Prechtl HF, Hopkins B: Developmental transformations of spontaneous movements in early infancy. Early Hum Dev 14:233, 1986
22. Zelazo PR: Smiling to social stimuli: Eliciting and conditioning effects. Dev Psychol 4(1):32, 1971
23. Zelazo PR: Smiling and vocalizing: A cognitive emphasis. Merrill-Palmer Q 18(4):349, 1972
24. Zelazo PR, Komer MJ: Infant smiling to non-social stimuli and the recognition hypothesis. Child Dev 42:1327, 1971
25. Super C: Environmental effects on motor development: The case of African infant precocity. Dev Med Child Neurol 18:561, 1976
26. Konner M: Maternal care infant behavior and development among the Kalahari Desert San. In Lee RB, DeVore I (eds): Kalahari Hunter Gatherers. Harvard University Press, Cambridge, MA, 1977
27. Caesar P: Postural Behavior in Newborn Infants. Acco, Leuven, Belgium, 1976
28. Solomon G, Solomon H: Motor development in Yucatecan infants. Dev Med Child Neurol 17:41, 1975
29. Lagerspetz K, Nygard M, Strandvick C: The effects of training in crawling on the motor and mental development of infants. Scand J Psychol 12:192, 1971
30. Bobath B: The very early treatment of cerebral palsy. Dev Med Child Neurol 93:73, 1967
31. Bobath B: Abnormal Postrual Reflex Activity Caused by Brain Lesions. 2nd Ed. London, William Heinemann Medical Books Ltd, 1971
32. Knott M, Voss D: Proprioceptive Neuromuscular Facilitation. 2nd Ed. Harper & Row, New York, 1974
33. Rood M: The use of sensory receptors to activate, facilitate, and inhibit motor response, automatic and somatic in developmental sequence. In Satteby A (ed): Study Course VI, Third International Congress of the World Federation of Occupational Therapy: WC Brown, Dubuque, 1962
34. Cioni G, Ferrari F, Prechtl HF: Posture and spontaneous motility in full-term infants. Early Hum Dev 18:207, 1989
35. Leonard EL: Neonatal neuromotor abnormalities: Effect on infant mental test performance. Doctoral dissertation, Tufts University, 1986
36. Thelen E: Treadmill-elicited stepping in seven-month old infants. Child Dev 57:1498, 1986
37. Forssberg H: Ontogeny of human locomotor control. I. Infant stepping, supported locomotion, and transition to independent locomotion. Exp Brain Res 57:480, 1985
38. Forssberg H, Wallberg H: Infant locomotion: A preliminary movement and electromyographic study. p. 32. In Berg K, Eriksson B (eds): Children and Exercise. Vol. IX. University Park Press, Baltimore, 1980

39. Forssberg H: A developmental model of human locomotion. p. 485. In Grillner S, Stein P, Stuart D, Forssberg H, Herman R (eds): Neuro Biology of Vertebrae Locomotion. London, Macmillan, 1986

40. Forssberg H: Development and integration of human locomotor functions. In Goldberger ME, Gorio A, Murray M (eds): Development and Plasticity of the Mammalian Spinal Cord. Fidia Research Series. Vol. III. Liviana Press, Padova, 1986

41. Milani-Comparetti A: The neurophysiologic and clinical implication of studies on fetal motor behavior. Semin Perinatol 5:183, 1981

42. Twitchell T: Reflex mechanisms and the development of prehension. In Connolly K (ed): Mechanisms of Motor Skill Development. Academic Press, Orlando, FL, 1970

43. Muir D, Abraham W, Forbes B, et al: The ontogenesis of an auditory localization response from birth to four months of age. Can J Psychol 33:326, 1979

44. Thelen E, Cooke DW: Relationship between newborn stepping and later walking: A new interpretation. Dev Med Child Neurol 29:380, 1987

45. Cooke DW, Thelen E: Newborn stepping: A review of puzzling infant coordination. Dev Med Child Neurol 29:394, 1987

46. Thelen E: Developmental origins of motor coordination: Leg movements in human infants. Dev Psychobiol 18:1, 1985

47. Clark J, Phillips S: The step cycle organization of infant walkers. J Motor Behav 19:421, 1987

48. Clark JE, Whitall J, Phillips SJ: Human interlimb coordination: The first six months of independent walking. Dev Psychobiol 21:445, 1988

49. Thelen E, Bradshaw G, Ward JA: Spontaneous kicking in month old infants: Manifestation of a human central locomotor program. Behav Neural Biol 32:45, 1981

50. Katona F: Clinical neuro-developmental diagnosis and treatment. p. 167. In Zelazo P, Barr R (eds): Challenges to Developmental Paradigms. Lawrence Erlbaum Associates, Hillsdale, NJ, 1989

51. Heriza C: Organization of leg movements in preterm infants. Phys Ther 68:1340, 1988

52. Katona F: Developmental clinical neurology and neurohabilitation in the secondary prevention of pre- and perinatal injuries of the brain. In Early Identification of Infants with Developmental Disabilities. Grune & Stratton, Orlando, FL, 1988

53. Katona F: An orienting diagnostic system in neonatal and infantile neurology. Acta Paediatr Hung 24:299, 1983

54. Leonard EL, Zelazo PR: Exercise of the reflexive stepping pattern with high risk infants. Poster presented at the International Conference on Infant Studies, Washington, DC, 1988

55. Zelazo NA, Zelazo PR, Cohen K, Zelazo PD: Specificity of practice on elementary neuromotor patterns. Unpublished manuscript.

56. Piper MC, Kunos VI, Willis DM, et al: Early physical therapy effects on the high risk infant: A randomized control trial. Pediatrics 78:216, 1986

57. Palmer F, Shapiro B, Wachtel, et al: The effects of physical therapy on cerebral palsy. N Engl J Med 318:803, 1988

58. Campbell SK: Editorial. Phys Occup Ther Pediat 9(2):1, 1989

7 | Assistive Devices

Elisabeth C. Olsson
Gary L. Smidt

Assistive devices or ambulatory aids are commonly recommended to relieve clinical problems of pain, fatigue, equilibrium, joint stability, muscular weakness, excessive structural loading, and cosmesis. Assistive devices function to increase balance or safety, to relieve weight from a weak or painful leg, and sometimes for cosmetic purposes. The reason for using an assistive device is often of a neuromuscular or musculoskeletal nature. It can be used either temporarily (i.e., after a surgical intervention or during fracture healing) or permanently (i.e., after a spinal cord injury).

Prescription, adjustment, information, and training with the device are generally handled by physical therapists, but also by physicians, occupational therapists, and nurses. In studies involving home calls to elderly patients, assistive devices have been reported to be underprovided, underused, and undermaintained. Distributions without length adjustment or information to the user have also been reported.

The scientific literature on assistive devices has dealt with the unloading of the affected leg,[1-8] loads on the upper extremity,[9-11] methods to control weight-bearing,[12-14] and energy consumption[5,14]; very little has been written on design improvement.[9]

TYPES OF ASSISTIVE DEVICES

The type of assistive device chosen depends on the patient's disability, general condition (pain, fatigue, and weakness), and age. There are three main categories of walking aids: canes, crutches, and walkers. In order to meet different patient needs, a great variety of shapes and designs exist within each category.

For the severely disabled (i.e., an amputee or a spinal cord injury patient), gait training begins on the parallel bars. Because the bars stand firmly on the floor, they provide stability and security that no other assistive device does, making it possible for patients to pull themselves forward against the bars. This is not possible with other walking aids, with which the hands must instead press downward on the assistive device.

CANES OR WALKING STICKS

Canes formerly served several purposes and therefore appeared in many shapes. Ornamented canes with a silver hand piece or those decorated with flowers and ribbons are now scarce and canes with a sword inside or with a secret place for poison are found only in museums.

Canes are prescribed to provide stability, which is accomplished by the increase of the base of support, when the cane is used in the hand opposite the involved leg. The standard wooden cane, which has to be cut to fit the patient, has basically looked the same for hundreds of years. It has a straight or half-circle hand piece and the rubber tip or suction ferrule is not standard. Canes made of aluminum tubing are lightweight and adjustable and have a grip-shaped hand piece that does not necessarily fit every patient's hand. No matter which assistive device it belongs to, the hand piece is the source of many problems connected to the use of walking aids. The more load on the hand, the more uncomfortable the hand piece, which is why one often sees home-made polstering of the hand piece. This problem becomes even more pronounced in patients with rheumatoid arthritis, for whom poor incongruity between the handle and grip often causes an intolerable increase in pain. An individually molded hand piece that is also adjustable to fit the available range of wrist extension on an adapted lightweight cane has demonstrated its importance in helping these patients maintain independent ambulation.[9] Canes should not be prescribed when cane loads above 20 percent body weight (BW) are wanted. Preoperative studies on patients with osteoarthritis and severe weightbearing hip pain have shown that cane loads will cause instability as the cane will rotate around its own axis leading to a tendency to support the cane towards the side of the body for increased stability.[15]

Quad Canes, Walk Canes, and Trestles

Quad canes and trestles provide a broader base of support, as they offer four points of floor contact. Unless all four legs of the cane are in contact with the ground, the cane will rock and not be able to load. The pressure on the handle must be centered over the cane's base of support, forcing the patient to take shorter steps and consequently walk more slowly. A disadvantage is that broad-based canes are difficult to use on stairs.

CRUTCHES

Crutches give more stability than canes. They are used to improve balance and to relieve weightbearing either fully or partially on the lower extremity.

Forearm or Elbow Crutches

Forearm, elbow, Canadian, or Lofstrand crutches are the most functional assistive devices for unloading and balancing. The downward pressure on the handle creates a counterpressure of the cuff on the forearm, giving stability to the work of the triceps and latissimus muscles and a possibility to transfer body weight to the floor. When long-term use of crutches is needed, forearm crutches are indicated. A disadvantage is that long-term use for a patient who puts a lot of weight on the crutches will cause strain on hands, wrists, and elbows. Hand pieces wrapped with all sorts of padding to soften or enlarge the grip are a common sight. Forearm crutches are the most functional type of crutch, as they are easier to handle on stairs and when getting in and out of a car.

Axillary or Underarm Crutches

Axillary and orthocrutches are less expensive and provide greater lateral stability than do forearm crutches. They should only be prescribed for short-term use, because of the tendency of some patients to lean on the axillary bar, which may cause nervous and vascular damage in the shoulder region. However, for patients with high levels of myelomeningocele or those with rheumatoid arthritis, who cannot use forearm crutches, the use of axillary crutches might be considered.

Shelf or Gutter Crutches

Shelf or gutter crutches, also referred to as trough crutches, transfer bodyweight through the forearm, which rests in the gutter to the upright cane. Velcro straps fix the forearm to the trough. They are used when weightbearing on wrists and hands is contraindicated and intended for patients with arthritis or arm fractures.

WALKERS AND WALKING FRAMES

Walkers provide the greatest stability of all assistive devices mentioned, as they have the broadest base of support. They are most commonly used by elderly patients. A great variety of walkers exist. They can be provided with two front wheels, making it easier for those who cannot lift the walking aid forward.

Reciprocal walkers with hinged side pieces are made for the same reason but provide less stability. Walkers are cumbersome and difficult to maneuver but provide a sense of security for the fearful patient, and are most commonly used indoors.

ADJUSTMENT OF WALKING AIDS

Length Adjustment

For a person standing with arms hanging and shoulders relaxed, the upper part of the hand piece should correspond to the styloid process. An adjustable cane is necessary for measuring the proper length of the assistive device. However, this static measurement is not enough. The therapist must also inspect the way in which the patient makes use of the cane. An assistive device used for unloading should be put closer to the body, hence shorter than one used for balance, when the purpose is to broaden the base of support. A fast walker may need a longer cane. If the cane is too long, the elbow will come into too much flexion, which will either increase the moment around the elbow joint or push up the shoulder.

If the cane is too short, the hip, knee, or ankle of the involved leg must flex more than usually to clear the foot from the floor during the swing phase and during cane support the vertical trajectory of the head will describe a descent instead of an elevation. A change in heel height may also call for a length adjustment.

Forearm crutches should be adjustable for length between both handle and floor and handle and elbow. The cuff should be placed within the proximal third of the forearm. A crutch that is adjustable at eight points to try out individual rheumatoid patient needs has recently been developed.[9]

Adjustment of Axillary Crutches

For adjustment of the hand piece, the same rule applies as to canes. For a patient standing erect with shoulders relaxed, a space of two to three fingers must be allowed between the pad and the axilla or the patient will place too much weight on the pads. Incorrectly adapted or improper use of axillary crutches can cause nerve damage; both brachial plexus neuropathy and carpal tunnel syndrome have been reported. The distal end of the crutch should come to a point 2 inches lateral and 6 inches anterior to the foot.[16]

Adjustment of a Shelf Crutch

With the patient standing erect and the forearm comfortably placed in the gutter, the hand piece should be raised slightly, so that the patient can press down to elevate the body.

WALKING PATTERNS

The approach to using one or two assistive devices depends on the disease, strength, and skill of the patient. Methods differ in the sequence of crutch and foot steps.

Method for Clinical Reporting

For accurate depiction and standardization, an approach for labeling and describing assisted gait patterns has been proposed by Smidt and Mommens.[17] (Figures 7-1 to 7-6 are based on this system.[17])

Specific terms are needed for describing assisted gait using ambulatory aids. The term *point* refers to the number of floor contacts on a line perpendicular to the direction of walking that occurs simultaneously during any part of stance phase for the lead foot. When the lead foot is clearly slower than the assistive device in making floor contact, the term *delayed* should be used. *Laterality* describes the associated placement on the walking surface of the side of the upper extremity holding the assistive device and the side of placement for the lead foot in the cycle. For example, laterality in the case of *ipsilateral left* indicates that both the assistive device held on the left and the left foot are concurrently in contact with the walking surface during a portion of the cycle. For completeness, the specific type of assistive device is identified. The recommended sequence for presenting descriptors for types of assisted gait is (1) delayed (when appropriate), (2) number of points, (3) laterality (when appropriate), and (4) type of assistive device. Common forms of assisted gait are illustrated in Figures 7-1 to 7-6, which show three of the descriptors (assistive device not included) and the numerical order of walking surface contact. The type of assistive device might be a crutch or a cane and, in the example of five-point gait, a walker.

A final term, designated a *count,* identifies the number of separate floor-contact events that occurs in one walking cycle. Unassisted gait has two counts. Several assisted-gait patterns also have two counts: two-point, three-point, five-point, swing-to, and swing-through. Three counts are involved in the delayed two-point, three-point, and five-point gait patterns. The four-point contralateral assisted gait with two devices requires a four-count involved walking cycle.

To illustrate further the use of this system, a delayed two-point contralateral cane crutch gait (right hand-left foot) is shown in Figure 7-1. The first event in the cycle is forward movement and floor placement of the crutch on the right side. The second event is the forward movement and floor placement of the left foot in line horizontally with the crutch tip on the floor. The one crutch and left foot constitute the two-point count. Also the laterality is identified as right hand-left foot. The term *delayed* is included because the left foot floor contact was a distinct event that followed the floor placement of the crutch. *Contralateral* as opposed to *ipsilateral* is included to differentiate from the situation in which the patient's lead foot and assistive device are on the same side. Finally, the third event is the forward movement and floor placement of the right foot.

The system also permits classification of various assisted gaits from most to least external assistance provided:

1. Four-point crutch gait
2. Delayed five-point gait with walker
3. Delayed three-point gait with two crutches
4. Five-point gait with walker
5. Three-point gait with two crutches
6. Delayed three-point gait with two canes
7. Three-point gait with two canes
8. Delayed two-point gait with one crutch
9. Delayed two-point gait with cane
10. Two-point gait with one crutch
11. Two-point gait with cane
12. Walk with assistive device

CANE ON OPPOSITE SIDE: CONTRALATERAL CANE USE

If a cane is used to improve balance, it should be used on the side contralateral to the weakest leg in order to broaden the base of support. If the assistive device is used to unload a hip, it should also be used in the hand opposite the involved leg (Fig. 7-1). A cane or a crutch on the opposite side carries not only some of the superincumbent body weight but also, through the long lever arm to the hip joint, reduces the force required by the abductors to balance the pelvis in the frontal plane.[1]

Instrumented canes have been used to study the amount of body weight placed by patients with unilateral lower extremity disability on a cane in the opposite hand. Several investigators have found that cane users seldom place more than 15 to 20 percent body weight on a cane.[4,7] In an unpublished study by Olsson,[15] in which healthy and well-motivated people were asked to unload as much as possible on a cane in the opposite hand, 37 percent body weight could be placed on the cane. Considering the effort and instability demonstrated by these people, canes should not be used if more than 15 to 20 percent body weight will be borne on it.

Free walking speed will decrease with the use of a cane even if the person has no locomotor problem.

CANE ON SAME SIDE: IPSILATERAL CANE USE

When an assistive device is used on the same side as the involved leg, the cane and the leg move together and the cane functions as a brace. This way of

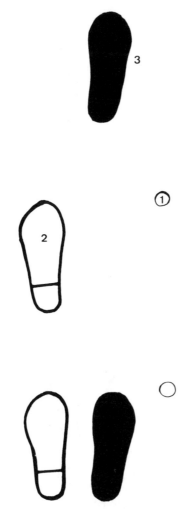

Fig. 7-1. Delayed two-point contralateral gait, right hand-left foot. (From Smidt and Mommens[17], with permission.)

walking creates an increased lateral shift and also restricts the reciprocal upper-/lower-extremity movement pattern. It also makes the base of support smaller compared with using the cane on the opposite side (Fig. 7-2). Edwards[3] suggested that an ipsilateral cane should be used when limited hip or knee motion was desired.

A cane on the same side can take as much load as a cane on the opposite side, but it has a much less favorable level arm, requiring considerably more pressure on the hand to relieve hip pressure to the same degree as if the cane were held on the opposite side.[15]

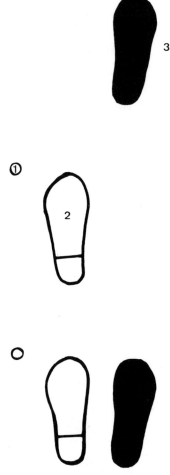

Fig. 7-2. Delayed two-point ipsilateral gait, left hand-left foot. (From Smidt and Mommens[17], with permission.)

THREE-POINT GAIT

Three-point gait indicates that the two walking aids are put forward, followed by the affected and then the unaffected leg (Fig. 7-3). Delayed three-point gait, stressing the sequence of assistive devices making floor contact before the affected leg, is the only way of walking when unloading of a lower extremity is prescribed.[15]

Partial weightbearing is often prescribed for the treatment of many orthopedic conditions without specifying the amount of weight to be relieved. As soon as the physician is able to specify the percentage body weight that the involved leg can tolerate, therapists must find a method to control this, as none of the suggestions to control weightbearing in the clinic has gained widespread use—

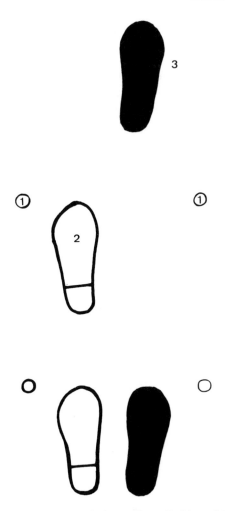

Fig. 7-3. Delayed three-point gait, left foot. (From Smidt and Mommens,[17] with permission.)

not even the limb load monitor. It is impossible to estimate visually if a patient places too much weight on the leg.[12–14,18]

Some investigators have tried to define partial weightbearing. The term touchdown ambulation, indicating a maximal floor reaction force (MVF) of up to 10 percent body weight, was described by Kathrins and O'Sullivan.[5] Marked step indicating a maximal vertical force of 17 percent body weight was based on Rydell's finding that vertical force corresponding to the weight of the affected lower extremity was mechanically less stressful to the hip joint than non-weightbearing.[19] Non-weightbearing and one-leg swing-through indicate that the involved leg is kept off the ground and the whole body weight is shared evenly between each walking aid. Throughout the gait cycle, the hip and knee joint of the affected leg are kept in flexed position. The muscle force required to keep the leg off the floor has a compressing effect on the hip joint, as shown by Rydell. It was less stressful for the hip when the leg rested toward the floor, indicating a maximal vertical force of 17 percent body weight, with 42 percent body weight taken by each crutch. This walking pattern, known as *marked step,* should be recommended to patients who are not to bear weight on the hip. Motion pattern will be more normal than in non-weightbearing, as knee extension and dorsiflexion at heel strike will be allowed.

Kathrins and O'Sullivan showed that oxygen consumption and systolic blood pressure are similar for non-weightbearing and touchdown ambulation with axillary crutches. Heart rate and myocardial oxygen consumptions were significantly higher during non-weightbearing ambulation due to greater upper- and lower-extremity isometric exercise.[5]

The peak vertical ground reaction force on the weightbearing leg during one-leg swing-through with axillary crutches increased by 21.6 percent body weight compared with normal walking in spite of the slower walking speed. This finding indicated that caution should be taken in the prescription of non-weightbearing ambulation in subjects with diseased bone and joints of the unaffected leg.[20,21]

Considering the arm strength, good technique, and physical condition needed to use touchdown ambulation, marked step, and non-weightbearing, as well as the lack of methods to control this, it seems reasonable to assume that patients often place more weight on the affected lower extremity than they should. It should be kept in mind that the more unloading required, the slower the patient must walk. Training to maintain the prescribed amount of unloading is necessary and, with increased skill, walking speed will increase. Walking speed in 24 healthy and well-motivated young people using marked step and forearm crutches for the first time was 0.36 m/s, which is one-fifth of normal free walking speed.[15]

SWING-THROUGH GAIT

Swing-through gait means that both crutches are lifted and placed on the ground in front of the body. The body swings through past the crutches so the feet land ahead of them (Fig. 7-4). This method of walking requires good balance, good arm strength, and full range of hip extension, or the gait pattern is described as swing-to gait. Swing-through gait is most frequently used as the primary means of mobilization by patients without voluntary control in the lower extremities (i.e., spinal cord injury patients). Waters and Lunsford[22] reported that oxygen consumption in 150 patients using swing-through crutch-assisted gait was 38 percent greater than required for normal walking. Shoup et al.[23] recommended three possible design improvement criteria: (1) to minimize the vertical motion of the body, (2) to minimize the shock associated with the planting of the crutch tips, and (3) to minimize the need for lateral motion of the crutch tips. Wells[24] suggested that a more "flowing" gait without the stop-start motion would be preferable from the point of view of reducing variations in body energy.

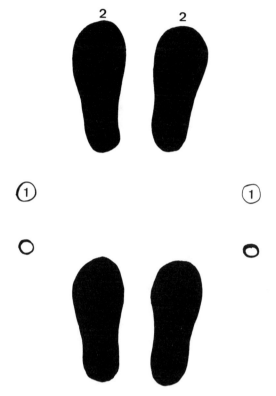

Fig. 7-4. Swing-through gait. (From Smidt and Mommens,[17] with permission.)

FOUR-POINT GAIT

Four-point gait indicates that the two walking aids are used one for each leg. The right waking aid is put forward, followed by the left leg, the left walking aid, and the right leg (Fig. 7-5). This is a safe gait indicating that there are always three points of support. The gait pattern when the reciprocal foot and aid are moved together is called two-point contralateral gait, or two-point alternate gait.

It should be kept in mind that four-point gait does not unload any leg. Patients with osteoarthritis of both hips using four-point gait did not unload in spite of weightbearing pain. The maximal vertical ground reaction force was between 95 and 100 percent body weight for both legs, because when each aid was moved forward, its contralateral leg was bearing almost all weight.[15]

Four-point gait should only be prescribed for balance, because unloading with four-point gait requires very strong upper extremities, great concentration and effort, and a very slow walking speed. In planning a surgical treatment that requires postoperative partial weightbearing, the surgeon should take into consideration that a patient who preoperatively uses four-point gait because of bilateral involvement probably will be unable to unload the operated leg.

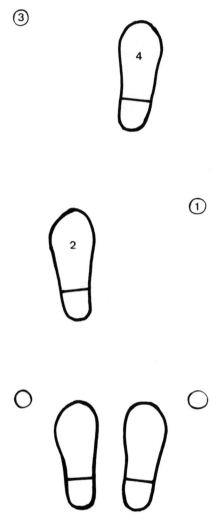

Fig. 7-5. Four-point gait. (From Smidt and Mommens,[17] with permission.)

UPPER-EXTREMITY LOADING

In non-weightbearing and in swing-through gait, the whole body weight must be shared between the arms. This creates moment values on the shoulder of similar magnitude to those at the hip in unaided gait.[8] Even partial weight-bearing gives cause for unfunctionally high loads on the upper extremities. Long-term use of assistive devices for the purpose of unloading implies a risk of degenerative or overuse symptoms from joints of the upper extremities. For this reason, it is important that patients be equipped with individually adjusted and proper assistive devices. Reisman et al.[10] investigated swing-through axillary crutch gait and found that the elbow should not be in more than 30° of flexion (otherwise the moment around the elbow would be too great) and that a small raise in handle position gave a great increase in elbow moment.[10]

The importance of a lightweight and biomechanically well-functioning walking aid is important in patients with rheumatoid arthritis. Lofkvist et al.[9] showed that 34 of 42 severely handicapped patients who were unable to use conventional walking aids were able to use individually molded handles and individually adapted lightweight walking aids[9] (Fig. 7-6A,B).

NEED FOR FURTHER STUDY

To improve assistive devices and their use, design improvements, more individually adjusted walking aids, and more relevant and thorough instructions on how to use them are needed. These adjustments should be based on further biomechanic studies with patients with different types of leg problems, rather than with able-bodied subjects with simulated leg impairments.

In spite of the many variations of the different assistive devices, the problems connected with the hand and hand piece seem to affect all of them. This applies not only to rheumatoid patients with hand involvement, but to almost everyone who has to place some of the body weight on arms and hands during walking.

For the large number of gait abnormalities for which assistive devices are indicated, criteria for prescriptive use are lacking. The effectiveness of assisted gait and various assistive devices in satisfying clinical objectives for gait has not been reported.

Because of the strain and effort connected with partial weightbearing as well as the influence of walking speed on the amount of weightbearing, there is reason to believe that patients often place more than the prescribed weight on their affected leg. This calls for a method to control the amount of weightbearing under clinical and dynamic conditions.

SUMMARY

Various types of assistive devices and their use are described. A system for clinical reporting for assisted gait is described and illustrated. Walking aids or assistive devices are commonly recommended for clinical problems of pain, fatigue, equilibrium, joint stability, muscular weakness, excessive structural loading, and cosmesis. Assistive devices used during gait have been shown to reduce walking velocity, energy expenditure, and floor reaction forces. However, because few studies have been reported on patients, the clinical value of assistive devices has not been well documented.

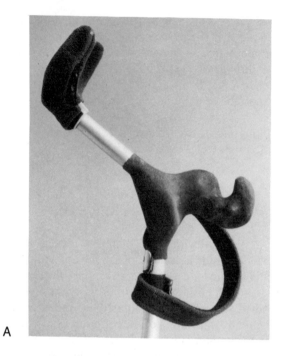

A

B

Fig. 7-6. **(A)** Assistive device for arthritic patients. **(B)** Assistive device in use by arthritic patient. (From Lofkvist et al.[9] with permission.)

REFERENCES

1. Bount WP: Don't throw away the cane. J Bone Joint Surg 38A:695, 1956
2. Brand RA, Crowninshield RD: The effect of cane use on hip contact force. Clin Orthop 147:181, 1980
3. Edwards BG: Contralateral and ipsilateral cane usage by patients with total knee or hip replacement. Arch Phys Med Rehabil 67:734, 1986
4. Ely DD, Smidt GL: Effect of cane on variables of gait for patients with hip disorders. Phys Ther 57:507, 1977
5. Kathrins BP, O'Sullivan SD: Cardiovascular response during nonweightbearing and touchdown ambulation. Phys Ther 64:14, 1984
6. Klenerman L, Hutton WC: A quantitative investigation of the forces applied to walking sticks and crutches. Rheumatol Rehabil 12:152, 1973
7. Murray MP, Seireg AH, Scholz RC: A survey of the time, magnitude and orientation of forces applied to walking sticks by disabled men. Am J Phys Med 48:1, 1969
8. Opila KA, Nicol AC, Paul JP: Forces and impulses during aided gait. Arch Phys Med Rehabil 68:715, 1987
9. Lofkvist UB, Brattstrom M, Geborek P, et al: Individually adapted light weight walking aids with moulded handles for patients with severely deforming chronic arthritis. Scand J Rheumatol 17:167, 1988
10. Reisman M, Burdett RG, Simon SR, et al: Elbow moments and forces at the hands during swing through axillary crutch gait. Phys Ther 65:601, 1985
11. Opila KA, Nicol AC, Paul JP: Upper limb loadings of gait with crutches. J Biomech Eng 109:285, 1987
12. Engel J, Amir A, Messer E, et al: Walking cane designed to assist partial weight bearing. Arch Phys Med Rehabil 64:386, 1983
13. Hirsch C, Lewenhaupt-Olsson E: Simple control devices in early ambulation following surgery of lower limbs. Acta Orthop Scand 40:119, 1969
14. Warren CG, Lehmann JF: Training procedures and biofeedback methods to achieve controlled partial weight bearing: An assessment. Arch Phys Med Rehabil 56:449, 1975
15. Olsson E: Partial weight bearing ambulation. The unloading effect of assistive devices and gait patterns. Unpublished data.
16. Schmitz TJ: Physical Rehabilitation. 2nd Ed. FA Davies, Philadelphia, 1988
17. Smidt GL, Mommens MA: System of reporting and comparing influence of ambulatory aids on gait. Phys Ther 60:551, 1980
18. Wannstedt G, Craik R: Clinical evaluation of a sensory feed back device: The limb road monitor. Bull Prosthet 8:49, 1978
19. Rydell NW: Forces acting on the femoral head prosthesis. Acta Orthop Scand Suppl 88, 37:107, 1966
20. Goh JC, Toh SL, Bose K: Biomechanical study on axillary crutches during single leg swing through gait. Prosthet Orthot Int 10:89, 1986
21. Stallard J, Dounis E, Major RE, et al: One leg swing through gait using two crutches. An analysis of the ground reaction forces and gait phases. Acta Orthop Scand 51:71, 1980
22. Waters RL, Lunsford BR: Energy cost of paraplegic locomotion. J Bone Joint Surg 67A:1245, 1986
23. Shoup TE, Fletcher LS, Merril BR: Biomechanics of crutch locomotion. J Biomech 7:11, 1974
24. Wells RP: The kinematics and energy variations of swing through crutch gait. J Biomech 12:579, 1979

8 | Gait in Children

Marilynn Patten Wyatt

Gait in children is a fascinating area of study because of the developmental changes that take place in the child. The toddler starts out with an awkward gait and develops the skill and strength to become a mature and efficient bipedal ambulator within a matter of months. Therapists, doctors, and others in the medical field are asked to evaluate the gait of children who exhibit motor disabilities. Techniques have been developed to measure the dynamic movements of children.[1,2] This chapter describes these movements in the gait of the developing child aged 1 to 7 years, in quantitative terms, as well as developmentally related changes. Clinical case studies are presented that contrast normal and abnormal gait.

NORMATIVE DATA

This chapter summarizes a study of gait in normal children that was completed at the Motion Analysis Laboratory at Children's Hospital and Health Center in San Diego. The details of the study can be found in the monograph, *The Development of Mature Walking*.[2]

Methods and Subjects

The subjects for this study were healthy, full-term children residing in the San Diego area. They were initially screened by means of a health history form that asked for birth history, medical history, orthopedic problems, and age at which they started walking. The criteria for inclusion in the study included whether the child (1) was the product of a full-term pregnancy, (2) walked independently by 14 months of age, (3) had no orthopedic problems or treat-

157

ments (including casts or special shoes), (4) displayed normal growth and development, and (5) experienced no major medical problems or hospitalizations.

The study group consisted of 309 normal children aged 1 to 7 years. Some children were studied more than once at different ages, for a total data set of 449 physical therapy examinations, 415 motion measurement studies, 430 time-distance parameter studies, 288 force-plate studies, and 369 electromyography (EMG) studies. There were 10 age groups of subjects: 1, $1\frac{1}{2}$, 2, $2\frac{1}{2}$, 3, $3\frac{1}{2}$, 4, 5, 6, and 7 years. The subjects were studied within 30 days either side of their birthday or "half-birthday." The number of boys and girls in each group was nearly equal. Analysis of the data revealed no differences between the sexes.

The movement measurement data were collected with three synchronized 16-mm motion picture cameras, running at 50 frames per second. The camera views were from each side and the front. The subjects were all barefoot and filmed at their free speed cadence. A piezoelectric force platform was at the center of the walkway, and force and motion data were collected on the same passages down the walkway. The film was projected on a Vanguard motion analyzer, and bony landmarks were digitized using a sonic digitizer. Twelve angular rotations were calculated for both the left and right side of the body. Complete descriptions of the measurement systems are presented in other publications.[2,3]

Age of Walking

The subjects' parents were asked to refer to baby books or to recall as accurately as possible the age at which their child began independent walking. The mean age of walking for our study population was 11.2 months. Descriptive data for independent walking by age group are presented in Table 8-1. Other investigators report children walking at 11.3 months, Denver Developmental Screening Test[4]; at 11.7 months, Bayley Scales of Infant development[5]; at 12

Table 8-1. Estimated Age of Independent Walking in Each Age Group

Age Group (years)	N	Age Started Walking (months)	
		Mean	SD
1	51	10.6	2.0
$1\frac{1}{2}$	40	11.8	1.5
2	45	12.1	1.5
$2\frac{1}{2}$	36	11.4	1.1
3	47	11.4	1.7
$3\frac{1}{2}$	40	11.1	2.0
4	39	11.3	1.6
5	42	10.6	1.8
6	44	10.7	1.6
7	46	10.9	2.4

(From Sutherland et al.,[2] with permission.)

months, Revised Denver Developmental Screening Test[6]; and at 15 months, Nelson Textbook of Pediatrics.[7] Our mean age of walking might be slightly younger than that reported in these references because we required subjects to have walked by 14 months of age for inclusion in the study.

Time/Distance Parameters by Age

In this chapter, gait cycle is defined as beginning and ending with foot-strike of the same foot. Foot strike (FS), and toe-off (TO) for each limb comprise the events that subdivide the cycle into initial double-limb support, single-limb stance (SS), second double-limb support, and swing phase. The right gait cycle begins with right foot strike, followed by left toe-off, which begins the period of SS. Single stance is ended by left foot strike, which begins the period of second double support. Right toe-off begins the swing phase for the right limb.[8]

The timing of these events is presented in Tables 8-2 to 8-4 for the 10 age groups. All the data were collected during free speed walking. The measurements are step length, stride length, opposite toe-off (OTO), opposite foot strike (OFS), toe-off (TO), duration of single-limb stance, cycle time, cadence, and walking velocity. Cycle time was measured in real time. The other time measurements were normalized by conversion to percentage of the gait cycle to facilitate subject-to-subject comparisons.

Table 8-2 presents the means and standard deviations for cycle time, cadence, and walking velocity for all 10 age groups. Note that the principal reduction in cadence occurs between ages 1 and 2 years, followed by gradual decrease. Walking velocity increases with age in a linear manner from ages 1 to 3 years, at a rate of about 11 cm/sec·year. From 4 to 7 years of age, the relationship remains linear, but the rate change diminishes to 4.5 cm/sec·year. The cycle time data show variability, but the median for the 1-year and the 1½-year age groups is 0.70 seconds; then, from age 2 years, it remains at approximately 0.80 seconds.

Table 8-2. Means and Standard Deviations for Cycle Time, Cadence, and Walking Velocity in Each Age Group

Age (years)	N	Cycle Time (sec) Mean	Cycle Time (sec) SD	Cadence (steps/min) Mean	Cadence (steps/min) SD	Velocity (cm/sec) Mean	Velocity (cm/sec) SD
1	51	0.68	0.09	176	24	64	16
1½	40	0.70	0.08	171	21	71	14
2	45	0.78	0.11	156	25	72	16
2½	36	0.77	0.08	156	17	81	15
3	47	0.77	0.07	154	16	86	14
3½	40	0.74	0.05	160	13	99	15
4	39	0.78	0.07	152	15	100	17
5	42	0.77	0.06	154	14	108	18
6	44	0.82	0.09	146	18	109	19
7	46	0.83	0.07	143	14	114	17

(From Sutherland et al.,[2] with permission.)

Table 8-3. Means and Standard Deviations for Height, Right and Left Leg Lengths, Right and Left Step Lengths, and Stride Length in Each Age Group[a]

Age (years)	N	Height Mean	Height SD	Right Leg Mean	Right Leg SD	Left Leg Mean	Left Leg SD	Right Step Mean	Right Step SD	Left Step Mean	Left Step SD	Stride Mean	Stride SD
1	51	74.5	3.0	31.6	1.4	31.6	1.4	21.6	3.9	21.4	3.5	43.0	6.7
1½	40	80.2	4.1	35.5	2.2	35.5	2.2	25.1	3.6	24.4	3.4	49.5	6.6
2	45	86.2	3.6	38.9	2.0	38.9	2.0	27.5	3.2	27.4	3.6	54.9	6.3
2½	36	89.9	3.9	41.4	2.5	41.5	2.6	30.7	3.9	31.1	3.6	61.8	7.4
3	47	94.8	3.3	44.3	2.1	44.4	2.1	32.9	3.6	33.9	3.7	66.8	7.0
3½	40	98.3	3.9	46.5	2.6	46.5	2.6	36.5	3.9	37.5	4.4	74.0	8.1
4	39	102.6	3.5	49.3	2.1	49.2	2.1	38.5	4.2	39.1	4.0	77.9	8.5
5	42	108.8	4.1	53.4	2.9	53.4	2.9	42.3	4.2	42.9	4.1	84.3	10.2
6	44	115.6	4.6	57.0	3.3	57.0	3.4	44.1	4.4	45.2	4.3	89.3	8.5
7	46	122.2	4.9	61.5	3.8	61.5	3.8	47.9	4.3	48.7	4.1	96.5	8.2

[a] All measurements are in centimeters (cm). (From Sutherland et al.,[2] with permission.)

Table 8-3 presents the data for means and standard deviation of the heights, right and left leg lengths, and stride lengths for the 10 individual age groups. Between ages 1 and 7 years, leg length and age are closely related. The correlation coefficient is 0.95. The correlation coefficient for step length versus height is 0.91. There is an obvious linear relationship between the means of step

Table 8-4. Means and Standard Deviations for Times of Gait Events, Expressed as Percentage of Gait Cycle[a]

Age (years)	N	Right OTO Mean	Right OTO SD	Left OTO Mean	Left OTO SD	Right OFS Mean	Right OFS SD	Left OFS Mean	Left OFS SD
1	51	17.1	4.2	17.9	3.6	49.2	2.1	50.4	2.1
1½	40	17.5	3.6	17.6	3.5	49.5	2.3	50.1	2.2
2	45	16.9	2.7	16.5	2.6	50.4	2.0	49.7	1.9
2½	36	15.5	2.5	15.6	2.3	50.3	1.2	50.2	1.3
3	47	15.6	2.2	15.4	2.3	50.4	1.4	50.2	0.9
3½	40	14.3	1.8	14.5	1.7	50.2	1.1	50.3	1.1
4	39	14.3	1.8	14.0	1.9	50.3	1.0	50.0	1.2
5	42	13.3	2.0	13.6	1.9	49.7	1.7	50.4	1.0
6	44	13.3	1.7	13.5	1.7	49.8	1.0	50.4	0.9
7	46	12.4	1.7	12.3	1.9	50.0	1.1	50.0	1.0

Age (years)	N	Right TO Mean	Right TO SD	Left TO Mean	Left TO SD	Right SS Mean	Right SS SD	Left SS Mean	Left SS SD
1	51	67.1	4.0	67.6	4.0	32.1	3.9	32.5	2.7
1½	40	67.6	3.9	67.6	3.4	32.1	3.6	32.4	3.5
2	45	67.1	2.7	66.6	2.6	33.5	3.0	33.3	2.7
2½	36	65.5	2.4	65.9	2.4	34.7	2.5	34.6	2.5
3	47	65.5	2.2	65.4	2.0	34.8	2.1	34.8	2.3
3½	40	64.6	1.7	64.3	2.0	35.9	2.0	35.8	2.2
4	39	64.2	1.8	63.2	4.8	35.9	1.9	36.0	2.0
5	42	63.4	2.1	63.5	2.1	36.6	2.1	36.8	1.8
6	44	63.5	2.0	63.7	1.7	36.5	1.7	36.6	2.1
7	46	62.4	1.7	62.4	1.9	37.6	1.7	37.8	1.6

[a] There are no significant differences in the mean values for left and right sides.
OTO, opposite toe-off; OFS, opposite foot strike; TO, toe-off; SS, single stance.
(From Sutherland et al.,[2] with permission.)

length and leg length between 1 and 7 years of age. This correlation coefficient is also 0.91.

The timing of the gait events for children aged 1 through 7 years is presented in Table 8-4. Duration of right and left single-limb stance, expressed as percentage of the gait cycle, is also presented. There were no significant differences in the mean values for right and left sides. One of the least variable gait events is the time of opposite foot strike, occurring regularly at around 50 percent of the cycle. Stance time is prolonged in children under $2\frac{1}{2}$ years of age, as indicated by the toe-off times of greater than 65 percent. The toe-off time declines gradually to a normal adult level, which is 62 percent, between 3 and 7 years of age. Note that the variability and duration of single-limb stance diminishes with age. The adult mean value for single-stance time is 38 percent; this value is approached when the child is $3\frac{1}{2}$ years old.

Important information can be obtained by assessing time-distance parameters. With increasing maturity, single-limb stance, step length, and walking velocity increase as cadence initial double support and second double support diminish. By 4 years of age, the interrelationship between the time-distance parameters is fixed through stride length, and walking velocity continues to increase with increasing leg length. Height and leg length are directly related to step length. Another important observation is that temporal and distance factors reflecting symmetry are essentially equal in normal children. Walking velocity increases with age in spite of decreasing cadence. This increase is due to increasing stride length. Cycle time bears an inverse relationship to cadence. Cadence decreases and cycle time increased rapidly between 1 and 2 years of age. A normal single stance time is an indication of stable weightbearing and ensures adequate time for opposite swing.

INDICATORS OF GAIT MATURATION

The presence or absence of heel strike and reciprocal arm swing, the ratio of the pelvic span over the ankle spread (P/A ratio), and the presence of the knee-flexion wave have been identified as possible indicators of gait maturation.[3] These indicators of gait maturation are defined and discussed individually below.

Foot Strike

Heel strike, or foot strike, is defined as the point in time at which the limb first touches the ground. The term foot strike is used more commonly because it can be used to describe all gait, normal and pathologic. Less than one-half of the 1-year-olds demonstrated heel strike, but by age $1\frac{1}{2}$ years, it was present in nearly all subjects. An important finding was that none of the subjects in this study, even the beginning walkers, demonstrated toe strike at the point of foot strike. All subjects contacted the floor with either the foot flat or a heel strike.

Reciprocal Arm Swing

In gait, reciprocal arm swing is defined as the moving forward in synchrony of the leg and the contralateral arm. None of the 1-year-olds had a reciprocal arm swing. Instead, they held their arms up in a high guard position. Reciprocal arm swing was demonstrated by 65 percent of the subjects at age 1½ years; between ages 2 and 3½ years, the proportion rose from around 92 percent to 98 percent. From age 4 years on, 100 percent of these normal subjects demonstrated reciprocal arm swing.

Knee-Flexion Wave

The knee-flexion/extension angular rotation curve is biomodal. The initial flexion wave in stance phase is defined as the knee-flexion wave. The knee-flexion wave was present in slightly less than one half the 1-year-olds, but by 1½ years, the proportion had risen to approximately 75 percent. A knee-flexion wave was established in most subjects by 2 years of age.

Pelvic Span over Ankle Spread Ratio

The pelvic span over ankle spread (P/A) ratio was calculated by first projecting the cinefilm at the point of double limb support and measuring the body width at the level of the anterior superior iliac spines in the coronal plane, then measuring the ankle spread as the distance between the left and right ankle centers. The ankle width value was then divided into the pelvic span value to obtain a ratio. At least five measurements were made for each subject, and a mean value was calculated to obtain a ratio for each individual subject. This P/A ratio turned out to be an important barometer of mature gait. It is an indication of a wide- or narrow-based gait. When a child begins to walk, the base is very wide for stability; as strength and coordination are developed, the base narrows. Young children walk with a wide base, producing a low P/A ratio (close to 1.5); when the gait matures, the base narrows and the P/A ratio increases roughly linearly from age 1 to 3 years, remaining constant thereafter at about 2.5.

ELECTROMYOGRAPHY

Surface electrodes were used to study seven muscles or groups in a total of 369 subjects. The muscles we studied were tibialis anterior, vastus medialis, gluteus medius, medial hamstrings, lateral hamstrings, gluteus maximus, and gastrocnemius-soleus. Since stance is more prolonged in the younger age groups than in the more mature walkers, the duration of muscle phasic activity was presented as a percentage of the stance phase or swing phase rather than of the gait cycle as a whole. This method of data displays simplified comparisons of the changes in phasic activity across the different age groups.

The activity of the tibialis anterior was strikingly different in the 1 and
1½-year-old subjects compared with the 2- to 7-year-olds (Fig. 8-1). The 1-year-
olds lacked initial heel strike, landing foot flat, so the stance phase activity of the
tibialis anterior was prolonged. There also was a delay in the onset of swing-
phase activity demonstrating this immature pattern. Activity in the 1½-year-olds
was very similar, but with somewhat less stance phase prolongation. Then, from
2 to 7 years of age, the EMG phasic activity was nearly constant, demonstrating
a mature pattern with onset just before toe-off and full swing-phase activity
continuing to approximately the 40 percent point of stance phase.

The other muscle group that showed striking differences in the pediatric
population was the gastrocnemius-soleus. Swing phase activity, not usually
present in the adult, was commonly seen in our subjects, particularly in the
younger age groups. We found two patterns that require separate descriptions.
The first we termed the immature pattern, because it showed the greatest
variation from that of the normal audit controls. This immature pattern occurred
in a very high percentage of 1- and 1½-year-olds and in approximately one fourth
of the subjects in the remaining age groups. This immature pattern is a wrapa-
round pattern beginning near the middle of swing phase and ending with opposite foot strike. Sixty-seven percent of the 1-year-olds and 63 percent of the
1½-year-olds demonstrated this immature pattern (Fig. 8-2). There was a drop in
the proportion of subjects with this pattern at 2 years; however, at 2 years and
older, approximately one fourth of our subjects still demonstrated this immature

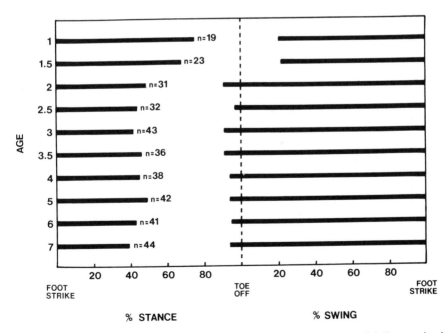

Fig. 8-1. Mean times of onset and cessation of EMG activity in the tibialis anterior in
each of the 10 age groups.

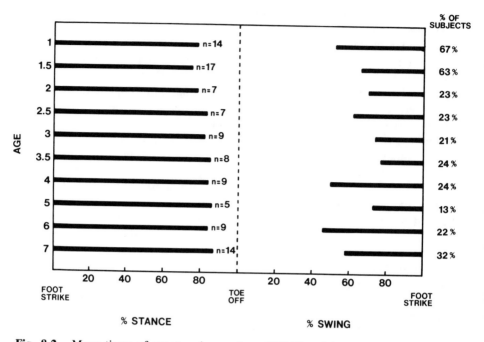

Fig. 8-2. Mean times of onset and cessation of EMG activity in the gastrocnemius-soleus (immature pattern).

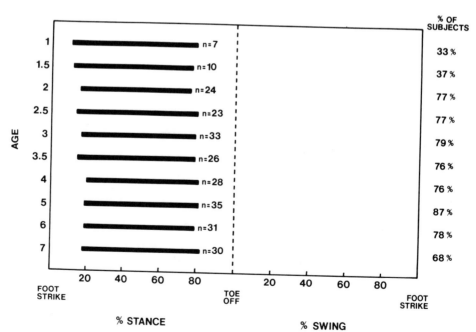

Fig. 8-3. Mean times of onset and cessation of EMG activity in the gastrocnemius-soleus (mature pattern).

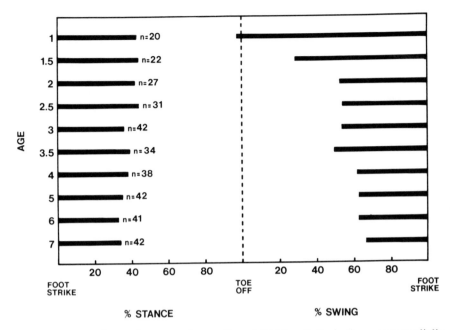

Fig. 8-4. Mean times of onset and cessation of EMG activity in the vastus medialis.

pattern. In the mature pattern, activity of the gastrocnemius-soleus is confined in the single stance portion of the stance phase, resembling the adult pattern. The mature pattern was present in approximately one-third of the 1- and 1½-year-olds and in about three fourths of the older children (Fig. 8-3).

The vastus medialis showed prolonged activity in swing phase in the younger age groups. A slight prolongation of activity during stance phase also was evident in the 1- to 2½-year-old subjects in comparison with the older children. Again, these differences are probably related to delayed maturation of the control system, resulting in some lack of precision in movement. By the age of 4 years, a mature pattern had emerged with the onset of muscle activity in late swing at around 60 percent of the gait cycle, continuing into stance phase to approximately 35 percent (Fig. 8-4).

The gluteus medius showed little change in stance phase dynamic EMG across the 10 age groups (Fig. 8-5). There was a trend toward reduction of activity in swing phase after the age of 4 years. The mature pattern consists of onset at approximately 60 percent of swing continuing to approximately 60 percent of stance.

The medial hamstrings showed stance-phase activity prolongation in the 1-year-olds. By age 2 years, a mature pattern was present, with activity commencing at about 50 percent of swing and continuing to approximately 55 percent of stance (Fig. 8-6).

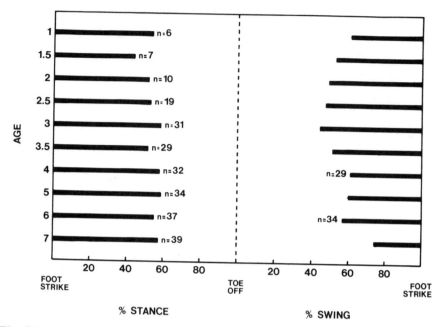

Fig. 8-5. Mean times of onset and cessation of EMG activity in the gluteus medius. (As indicated, no swing-phase activity was recorded in three 4-year-olds and in three 6-year-olds.)

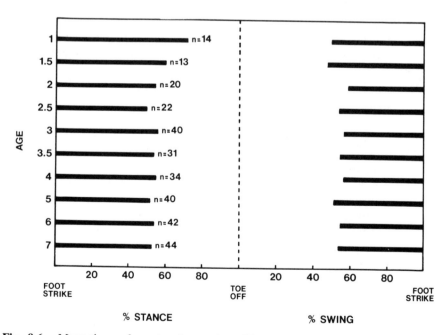

Fig. 8-6. Mean times of onset and cessation of EMG activity in the medial hamstrings.

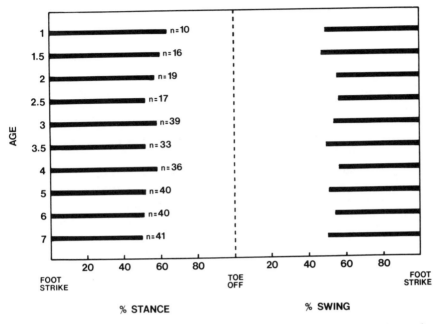

Fig. 8-7. Mean times of onset and cessation of EMG activity in the lateral hamstrings.

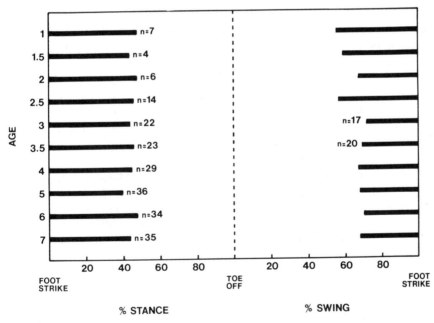

Fig. 8-8. Mean times of onset and cessation of EMG activity in the gluteus maximus. (As indicated, no swing-phase activity was recorded in five 3-year-olds and in three 3½-year-olds.)

The dynamic phasic activity of the lateral hamstrings is very similar to that of the medial hamstrings (Fig. 8-7). The two youngest age groups showed slightly more prolonged activity in stance phase, again demonstrating an immature pattern. The mature pattern, first seen at 2 years, consists of onset at about 55 percent of swing continuing to around 60 percent of stance.

All age groups showed similar stance-phase activity of the gluteus maximus. In the 1-, 1½, and 2½-year-olds, swing-phase activity was slightly more prolonged than in the 2- and 3-year-olds. A fully mature pattern was evident by 3 years of age, with onset of activity by 65 percent of swing, continuing to about 50 percent of stance (Fig. 8-8).

The prolongation of EMG activity in the youngest children is not a surprise. They walk with a wide-base gait, their coordination is yet to be refined, and their foot-strike pattern might be foot-flat rather than heel-strike. Along with maturation of the nervous system and perfection of an adultlike gait pattern, the EMG patterns turn to what we know as adult patterns.

JOINT ANGLES

Twelve joint angles were calculated for left and right sides of the subjects from points digitized off the cine film. A total of 415 movement measurement studies were completed. Close to equal numbers of boys and girls were studied. The data were analyzed for possible sex differences; as none was found, the data were combined and analyzed by age group. There were about 40 studies per age group with 49 studies in the 1-year-old age group. The joint angle data for the 1-, 1½-, 2-, and 7-year-old age groups are presented in this chapter (Figs. 8-9 to 8-12). Mean joint angles of rotation, film tracings, and time/distance parameters are presented for these groups. In other publications on these data, a statistical technique is presented that calculates 95 percent prediction regions around the mean curves.[2,9] This provides a gait laboratory with a method to compare a subject's data not only with a mean curve, but with a region around the mean curve that encompasses normal limits.

Several changes are to be noted in the joint angles from age 1 to 2½ years and then very slight changes up to age 4, when gait demonstrates a mature pattern. The 1-year-olds have a wide base of support, outstretched or high guard arms, lack of reciprocal arm swing, and flat foot strike. These toddlers demonstrate a large pelvic tilt angle. There is only a hint of the knee-flexion wave, and the legs and feet are externally rotated (Fig. 8-9).

At age 1½, there is heel strike, the base of support has narrowed, and reciprocal arm swing has made an appearance in 65 percent of subjects. There is still an increased pelvic tilt, and the knee-flexion wave following foot strike is increased by 4 or 5 degrees; thus, there is a knee-flexion wave, although it is still immature. The external rotation of the lower extremity and foot has decreased over age 1 but is still −10 degrees of neutral (Fig. 8-10).

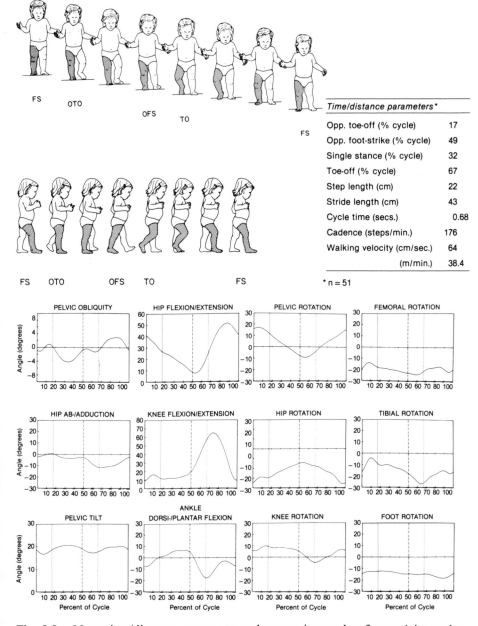

Time/distance parameters*	
Opp. toe-off (% cycle)	17
Opp. foot-strike (% cycle)	49
Single stance (% cycle)	32
Toe-off (% cycle)	67
Step length (cm)	22
Stride length (cm)	43
Cycle time (secs.)	0.68
Cadence (steps/min.)	176
Walking velocity (cm/sec.)	64
(m/min.)	38.4

*n = 51

Fig. 8-9. Mean time/distance parameters and composite graphs of mean joint angles (right side) for 1-year-old normal subjects, plus cine-film tracing (front and right-side views) of the gait cycle of a representative 1-year-old. Note wide base of support, outstretched arms, lack of reciprocal arm swing, and flat foot strike. FS, foot strike; OTO, opposite toe-off; OFS, opposite foot strike; TO, toe-off.

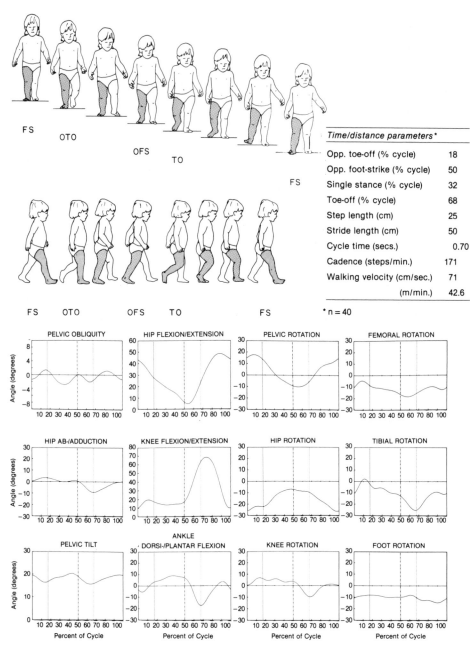

Time/distance parameters*	
Opp. toe-off (% cycle)	18
Opp. foot-strike (% cycle)	50
Single stance (% cycle)	32
Toe-off (% cycle)	68
Step length (cm)	25
Stride length (cm)	50
Cycle time (secs.)	0.70
Cadence (steps/min.)	171
Walking velocity (cm/sec.)	71
(m/min.)	42.6
* n = 40	

Fig. 8-10. Mean time/distance parameters and composite graphs of mean joint angles for 1½-year-old normal subjects, plus film tracings of representative 1½-year-old. Note that there is much less plantar flexion at foot strike than at age 1 year. The arms are much lower and reciprocal arm swing is making an appearance.

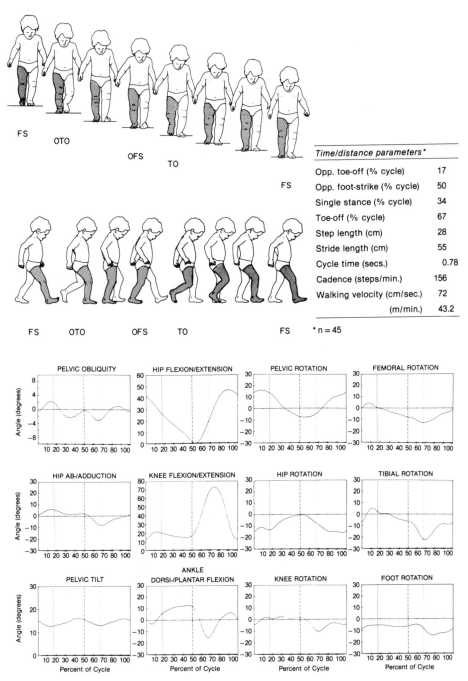

Time/distance parameters*	
Opp. toe-off (% cycle)	17
Opp. foot-strike (% cycle)	50
Single stance (% cycle)	34
Toe-off (% cycle)	67
Step length (cm)	28
Stride length (cm)	55
Cycle time (secs.)	0.78
Cadence (steps/min.)	156
Walking velocity (cm/sec.)	72
(m/min.)	43.2

*n = 45

Fig. 8-11. Mean time/distance parameters and composite graphs of mean joint angles for 2-year-old normal subjects, plus film tracings of representative 2-year-old. Changes by comparison with the 1½-year-olds include more clearly defined knee-flexion wave and heel strike (plantar flexion following foot strike), increased hip adduction in stance, and decreased external rotation of the hip.

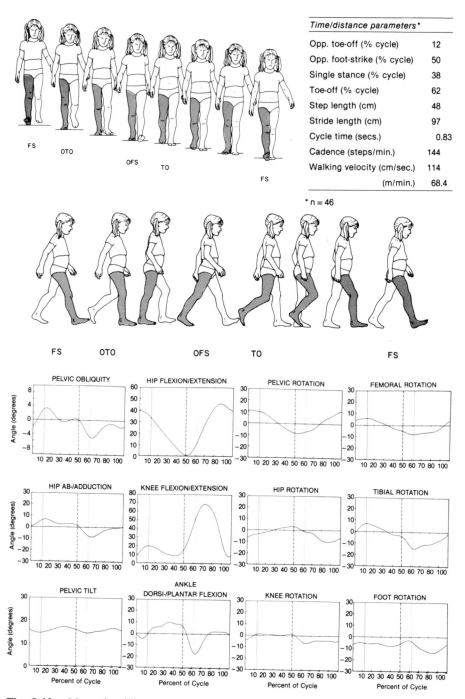

Time/distance parameters*	
Opp. toe-off (% cycle)	12
Opp. foot-strike (% cycle)	50
Single stance (% cycle)	38
Toe-off (% cycle)	62
Step length (cm)	48
Stride length (cm)	97
Cycle time (secs.)	0.83
Cadence (steps/min.)	144
Walking velocity (cm/sec.)	114
(m/min.)	68.4

* n = 46

Fig. 8-12. Mean time/distance parameters and composite graphs of mean joint angles for 7-year-old normal subjects, plus film tracings of representative 7-year-old.

By age 2 years, there is a more clearly defined knee-flexion wave and heel strike, increased hip adduction in stance, and a decreased external rotation of the hip (Fig. 8-11). We saw irregularity of foot rotation in swing up to age $2\frac{1}{2}$ years. By age 4, the knee-flexion wave demonstrates a totally mature pattern in stance phase. Ankle dorsiflexion also demonstrates a mature pattern.

The data for 7-year-olds are presented to demonstrate a set of mature graphs for the angular rotations (Fig. 8-12). We found very few differences between these data and our adult laboratory normal data.

GROUND REACTION FORCES

Ground reaction force data were obtained for as many subjects as possible. A clear piezoelectric force platform was built into the floor at the center of the walkway. The children were asked to walk across the window in the floor so that we could take a picture of the bottom of the foot. In this way, we avoided targeting the plate.

We collected measurements of the vertical force, the vertical ground reaction force, fore/aft shear, the ground reaction force acting horizontally in the line of progression of the child's walk, and medial/lateral shear, the ground reaction force acting horizontally, perpendicular to the line of progression of the child's walk. We refer to the shear forces from the subject's point of view, hence the fore(forward) shear when the foot is pushing ahead. All these force measurements were normalized by conversion to percentage of body weight. Because the children were small and our force plate was large, we often had double foot strikes on the force plate and could not always obtain a clean signal. The statistical analysis was done from foot strike or 0 percent of the gait cycle to 50 percent of the gait cycle (approximately opposite foot strike). A cubic spline technique was used to analyze the force data.[2] Force data from the 1- and $1\frac{1}{2}$-year-olds were obtained for only a small portion of the studies and could not be properly analyzed with this technique.

VERTICAL FORCE

The vertical force data are presented in Figure 8-13 for the 2-, $2\frac{1}{2}$-, 3-, $3\frac{1}{2}$, 4-, 5-, 6-, and 7-year-olds. As indicated, the data end at 50 percent of the gait cycle; although incomplete, they show the loading portion, the midstance trough, and most but not all of the second peak. The decline in the force that occurs during second double support is missing due to this analysis technique. The mid-stance trough occurred regularly at 30 percent of the gait cycle. The trough appears to be less well developed in the younger age groups than in the more mature children. The trough demonstrates increasing definition as the children get older, measuring 17 to 24 percent of body weight in 2- to 3-year-olds, 30 percent in $3\frac{1}{2}$- to 5-year-olds, and about 40 percent in the 6- to 7-year-olds. This was attributed to the increasing single limb stance, stride length, and walking veloc-

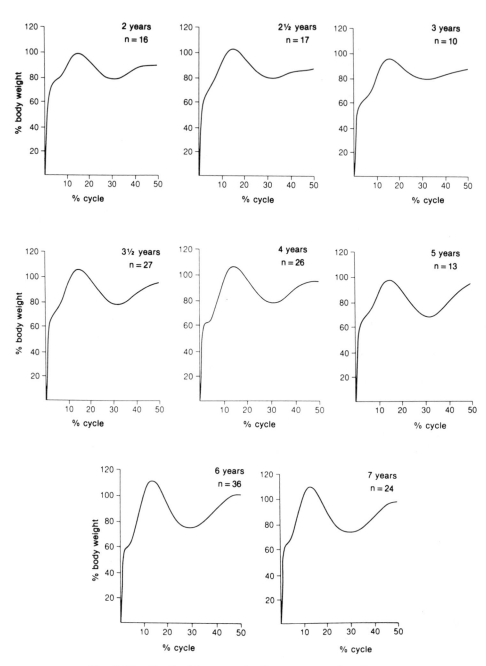

Fig. 8-13. Vertical force graphs for age groups 2 to 7 years.

ity. Mean vertical force at 50 percent of the gait cycle was consistently less than peak force in the loading phase in all age groups. The mean loading peaks were around 110 percent of body weight (Fig. 8-13). These are lower than the 120 percent measured in normal adults.

FORE/AFT SHEAR

The differences in fore/aft shear from ages 2 to 7 years are minimal. The times of direction change are remarkably constant across all age groups. The peak of forward shear occurs at 10 percent of the gait cycle. The time of reversal of fore/aft shear occurs after 30 percent of the cycle in all age groups. The pattern of pediatric fore/aft shear is very similar to that of adults.

MEDIAL/LATERAL SHEAR

The differences in medial/lateral shear from ages 2 to 7 years are very few. The lateral shear force peaks at around 20 percent of the gait cycle. This is the same for adult data. The presence of well-defined lateral shear by age 2 indicates that stable weightbearing is achieved early. We were unable to define any maturational changes in medial/lateral shear in this study.

CASE PRESENTATIONS

How are these normative data used? Most laboratories have a practice of comparing a subject's data with a set of normative data. By superimposing the two plots on a single graph, a visual comparison can be made. At the Children's Hospital Motion Analysis Laboratory, we plot pediatric patients' data against the age-matched control data; we then plot various conditions against one another. For example, we will plot normal data, patient data barefooted, and then patient data braced, or preoperative data and postoperative data will be plotted against normal data. Data from patients over the age of 7 years are compared with adult data. We are in the process of updating our format so that the calculated prediction regions generated from these data will also be plotted on the graphs around the mean curve. When this process is finalized, we will have a better visual presentation of the range of normal for various ages and will be able to identify easily the data points that fall out of that range. Two cases are presented below to give the reader an example of data presentation and analysis from this laboratory.

The first case is of a young child, D.F., who presented with severe bowlegs at age 22 months. He started walking at 10 months of age, and his parents noted an exaggerated bowleg tendency at 15 months. His supine intercondylar distance measured 6 cm. By radiologic evaluation and results of an initial gait study, it was determined that the child had physiologic genu varum rather than

Blount's disease. The orthopedist's recommendation was to observe the child with subsequent gait analysis; studies at 6-month intervals showed gradual improvement of his genu varum.

The initial and final data were selected for presentation to demonstrate the spontaneous resolution of his physiologic genu varum. Figure 8-14 is a film tracing from the front camera that shows the genu varum alignment of this patient at age 2 years. His gait demonstrates that of an immature pattern for his age exemplified by (1) poorly developed reciprocal arm swing, (2) increased knee and ankle flexion during stance, (3) absence of the knee-flexion wave, (4) decreased step length, (5) increased internal foot rotation, and (6) increased external hip rotation, (Fig. 8-15). At age 4 years, a well-developed reciprocal arm swing is apparent, along with less hip external rotation and foot external rotation replacing the earlier pattern of internal rotation (Figs. 8-14 and 8-15). The child's alignment and movement measurements were considered normal by age 4 years.

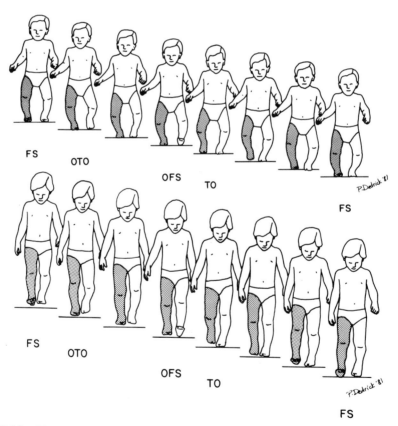

Fig. 8-14. Frontal view film tracings of patient D.F. at 22 months and 4 years. Full spontaneous resolution of physiologic genu varum. FS, foot strike; OTO, opposite toe-off; OFS, opposite foot strike; TO, toe-off.

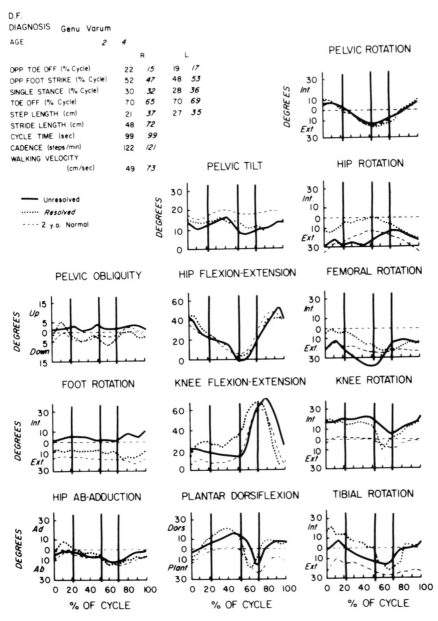

Fig. 8-15. Joint-angle rotations of patient D.F. at 22 months and at 4 years shown together with mean rotations of 2-year-old normal data.

The gait findings that differentiate Blount's from physiologic genu varum are (1) excessive external rotation of the femur and hip joint, (2) excessive internal rotation of the knee joint, and (3) a peculiar lateral thrusting movement of the knee during single-limb support.[10] This latter finding can be seen in exaggerated vertical and medial/lateral force curves. This child had only a moderate increase in hip external rotation and knee internal rotation but lacked the exaggerated force measurements and knee thrust. This alignment improved without therapeutic intervention and was measured by objective criteria.

The second case study is of a patient, J.W., who was noted to have right hemiparesis in the first year of life. His developmental milestones were mildly delayed, and his treatment had consisted of both physical and occupational therapy. At age 4 years, he underwent a right heel cord lengthening. His equinus contracture recurred, and he was referred for gait analysis at the age of 9 years. Characteristic features of hemiplegia are seen in tracings of film from the right side and front views (Fig. 8-16). The major movement measurement abnormalities were (1) the right ankle in equinus at the time of foot strike and the marked equinus persisting throughout stance and swing phases, (2) increased anterior pelvic tilt, and (3) internal rotation of the foot (Fig. 8-17). The EMG findings demonstrated premature onset of firing of the tibialis posterior and the soleus.

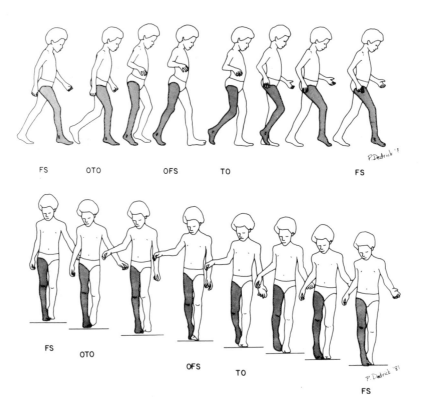

Fig. 8-16. Patient J.W. Preoperative film tracing from side and front cameras.

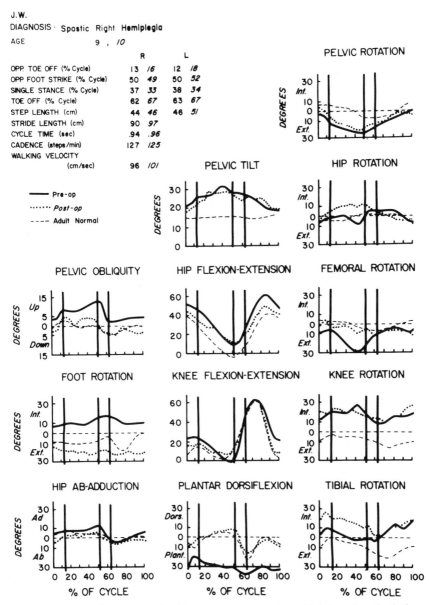

J.W.
DIAGNOSIS : Spastic Right Hemiplegia
AGE   9 , 10

	R		L	
OPP. TOE OFF (% Cycle)	13	16	12	18
OPP. FOOT STRIKE (% Cycle)	50	49	50	52
SINGLE STANCE (% Cycle)	37	33	38	34
TOE OFF (% Cycle)	62	67	63	67
STEP LENGTH (cm)	44	46	46	51
STRIDE LENGTH (cm)	90	97		
CYCLE TIME (sec)	.94	.96		
CADENCE (steps/min)	127	125		
WALKING VELOCITY (cm/sec)	96	101		

——— Pre-op
········· Post-op
– – – Adult Normal

PELVIC ROTATION

PELVIC TILT

HIP ROTATION

PELVIC OBLIQUITY

HIP FLEXION-EXTENSION

FEMORAL ROTATION

FOOT ROTATION

KNEE FLEXION-EXTENSION

KNEE ROTATION

HIP AB-ADDUCTION

PLANTAR DORSIFLEXION

TIBIAL ROTATION

% OF CYCLE   % OF CYCLE   % OF CYCLE

Fig. 8-17. Pre- and postoperative linear measurements and joint-angle calculations for right lower extremity of patient J.W. compared with adult normal values.

The tibialis anterior showed relatively normal phasic activity. Additionally, stance phase activity of the lateral hamstrings, vastus medialis, and vastus lateralis was prolonged (Fig. 8-18). The force-plate recordings showed rapid and excessive loading, early shear, and concentration of the center of pressure in the forefoot on the sound left limb (Fig. 8-19). The right lower extremity force data showed rapid loading, increased forward shear, absent lateral shear and concentration of the center of pressure in the forefoot (Fig. 8-19).

The recommendations from the study findings were to lengthen the Achilles tendon and the tibialis posterior. The referring physician chose to transfer the tibialis posterior to the dorsum of the foot and lengthen the Achilles tendon.

The 1-year postoperative results are plotted against the normal and preoperative graphs (Fig. 8-17). The movement measurements show the ankle curve to be normal, foot rotation external rather than internal, and the pelvic tilt unchanged. The film tracings show heel strike, correction of equinus, and improvement in arm position (Fig. 8-20). The EMG activity in the tibialis posterior is unchanged, but the soleus and quadriceps EMG activity has changed to a more normal pattern (Fig. 8-18). The postoperative ground reaction measurements showed considerable improvement and were all close to normal (Fig. 8-19).

By objective criteria, this treatment was successful and the patient is improved. The study recommendation was to continue following the patient because of the concern that the tibialis posterior transfer will cause an increase in valgus alignment of the foot and an alteration of the mediolateral balance due to the loss of the medical stabilizing effect.

SUMMARY

The development of gait in children aged 1 to 7 years is summarized and two case studies of children with pathologic gait are presented. The average age of walking in this population was 11.2 months. There were equal numbers of boys and girls, and no statistical differences accountable to sex or differences in left and right side were found.

Several age-related differences were found in time-distance parameters partially because these parameters are so closely related to leg length. Walking velocity increases linearly with age, and cadence decreases significantly between ages 1 and 2 years, after which it gradually continues to decrease after age 2. Single-limb stance and step length increase with maturity. These normal children showed symmetry from side to side. Stance time was prolonged in children under $2\frac{1}{2}$ years of age, indicating that swing phase was diminished. The more stable the child's gait becomes, the faster he or she can walk and the less time needs to be spent in stance phase. By age 4, the interrelationship between time-distance parameters is fixed, although stride length and walking velocity continue to increase with increasing leg length.

Time-distance parameters are a sensitive measure of gait abnormalities and often show asymmetry, prolonged stance phase, decreased velocity, and in-

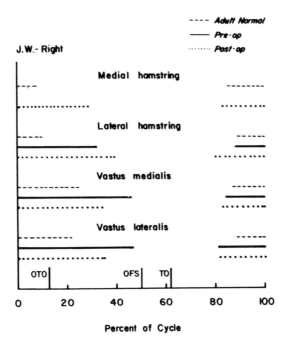

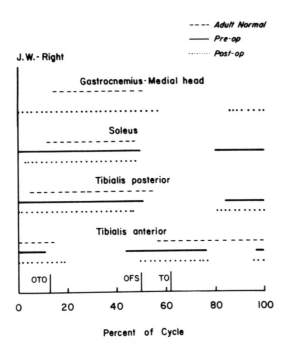

Fig. 8-18. EMG tracings for patient J.W. pre- and postoperative phase EMGs compared with adult normal values.

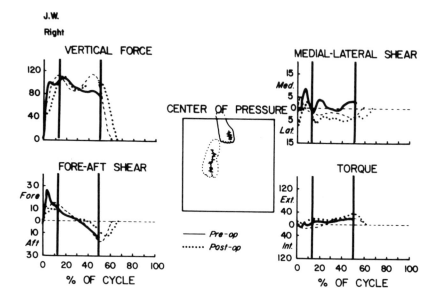

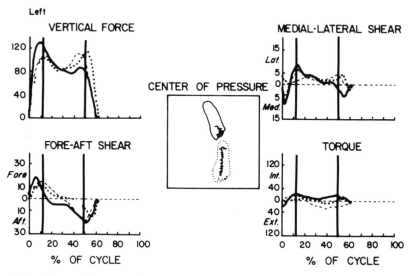

Fig. 8-19. Force-plate recordings for patient J.W. pre- and postoperatively with adult normal values for comparison.

creased cadence in children with pathology. Normal pediatric values should be used when interpreting pathologic gait studies of children.

Other indicators of gait maturation are the presence of reciprocal arm swing (100 percent of children by age four), knee-flexion wave (present by age 2), pelvic span over ankle spread ratio (adultlike by age three), and heel strike

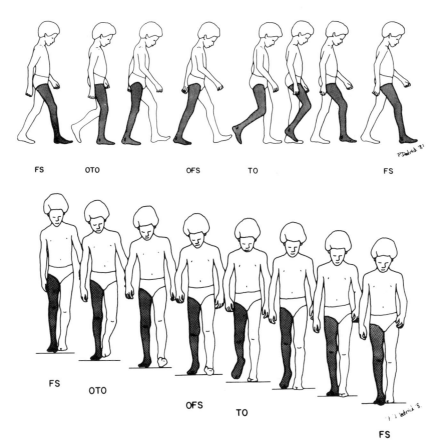

FS   OTO   OFS   TO   FS

FS   OTO

OFS   TO

FS

Fig. 8-20. Film tracings from side and front cameras of patient J.W. taken from postoperative gait study.

(present by age 1½). These are also good parameters to evaluate while assessing a pathologic gait pattern.

Electromyographic timing patterns are presented for seven muscle groups studied by surface electrodes. General prolongation of activity was seen in younger children. This needs to be taken into account when evaluating children with pathologic gait. The prolongation of muscle activity might be due to immaturity rather than strictly to pathology.

The joint angles comparison across ages shows maturational changes from age 1 to 2½ and then minor refinement until age 4, when mature patterns are present. Age-related changes in the ground reaction forces were found in vertical force but were minimal in fore/aft and medial/lateral shear.

Normative data are very helpful when interpreting pathologic gait. Normal values and their ranges are available[2] for children aged 1 to 7 years and can be used for more accurate comparisons and interpretations of pathologic gait in patients within this age group.

ACKNOWLEDGMENTS

This work was supported by grants 5R01 HD 08520 and 5 R01 HD15801 from the National Institutes of Health. I would also like to extend my appreciation to Sherill Marciano for assistance in preparation of this manuscript.

Figures 8-1 through 8-13 are reproduced from Sutherland et al.[2] with permission (Figures 8-9 through 8-13 have been modified). Figures 8-14 through 8-20 are reproduced from Sutherland[10] with permission.

REFERENCES

1. Sutherland DH, Hagy JL: Measurements of gait movements from motion picture film. J Bone Joint Surg 54A:787, 1972
2. Sutherland DH, Olshen RA, Biden EN, Wyatt MP: The Development of Mature Walking. MacKeith Press, Oxford, 1989
3. Sutherland DH, Olshen RA, Cooper L, Woo S-L: The development of mature gait. J Bone Joint Surg 62A:336, 1980
4. Frankenberg WK, Dodds JB: The Denver developmental screening test. J Pediatr 71:181, 1967
5. Bayley N: Manual for the Bayley Scales of Infant Development. Psychological Corporation, New York, 1969
6. Frankenberg WK, Fandel AW, Sciarillo W, Burgess D: The newly abbreviated and revised Denver development screening test. J Pediatr 99:995, 1981
7. Vaughan VC, Litt IF: Developmental pediatrics. p. 6. In Behrman RE, Vaughan VC (eds): Nelson Textbook of Pediatrics. 13th ed. WB Saunders, Philadelphia, 1987
8. Sutherland DH: The events of gait. Bull Prosth 10:35,312, 1981
9. Olshen RA, Biden EN, Wyatt MP, Sutherland DH: Gait analysis and the bootstrap. Ann Stat 17:1419, 1989
10. Sutherland DH: Gait Disorders in Childhood and Adolescence. Williams & Wilkins, Baltimore, 1984

9 | Aging and Gait

Gary L. Smidt

THE AGING PROCESS

In the aging process among old people, the probability of death has been shown to increase in proportion to decreasing degree of mobility to include walking.[1] Environmental conditions likely affect the aging process as well. Other influences, such as disease, trauma, and biologic deterioration, seem to reduce length of life. Successful combative efforts on these influences have led to a rising life expectancy. It is hoped that this rise will continue for several centuries into the future. Whatever the case, walking ability is a critical quality-of-life factor for the aged irrespective of life expectancy. To this end, retention and rehabilitation of walking ability in the aged are universally important.

Today, Isaacs[2] recommends that the elderly be subdivided into three age groups: 65 to 74, 75 to 84, and 85 years and over. However, to understand the aging process in a pure sense, biologic deterioration should be studied in people living in healthy environmental conditions in the absence of disease and trauma. This pure approach may not be attainable. However, for the biologic and functional areas, differentiation between changes associated with age-related and disease/trauma-related influences on the aging process appears to be a worthwhile pursuit.

Physiologic Changes

Payton and Poland[3] have, for several organ systems of the body, nicely summarized the physiologic changes that take place with aging. Some of these changes are thought to predispose to disease entities. With age, muscles appear to atrophy, weakness occurs, and there is decreased speed of contraction. Decreased speed of nerve transmission at the myoneural junction, loss of num-

185

ber and size of muscle fibers in mitochondrial enzymes, and replacement of muscle by fibrous tissue have been implicated. Also, ligaments, tendons, joint surfaces, and other connective tissues tend to lose some of their shock-absorbing capability with age. The cause of these muscular and connective tissue changes may in large measure be due to decreased physical activity.

Continuing with the scientific-based summary, Payton and Poland[3] review the cardiopulmonary changes accompanying the aging process. There is a tendency for an increased blood pressure and decreased stroke volume. Cardiac reserve and sympathetic nervous system responsiveness decrease as well. The lungs demonstrate significant reduction in maximal voluntary ventilation and vital capacity, with consequent reduced tolerance to physical stress. Furthermore, pulmonary gas exchange, cardiac output, and maximum pulmonary ventilation are reduced.

Payton and Poland[3] indicate that the influence of age on the nervous system is demonstrated by decreased brain weight, probably because of neuronal atrophy and reduction in the total number of brain cells.[3] Nerve conduction velocities, rate and magnitude of reflex responses, as well as sensory function all decrease. Peripheral vision and simple reaction time are negatively affected. Visual acuity also declines as age increases.[4] Lack of ability of the aged to maintain bodily homeostasis is thought to be affected by changes in the endocrine system.

GAIT AND AGE-RELATED CHANGES

The elderly commonly complain about difficulty with walking.[5] It has been estimated that in the absence of specific disease or "normal" aging, disturbances of gait produce disability in approximately 13 to 15 percent of older adults.[6,7] The characteristic smooth, cyclic, and reproducible normal gait patterns appear to be retained until at least the seventh decade.[8] It should be pointed out that during the early decades of life, minor traumatic insults, such as sprains, strains, bumps, and bruises, as well as illnesses, such as influenza, measles, head colds, and fevers, may very well hasten the aging process. An attempt to study the aging process in humans in the absence of these natural expected onslaughts on the body is probably unrealistic. Gait among the elderly who have not experienced significant function depreciating disease or trauma is described and discussed below.

Temporal and Distance Factors

Several investigators have studied the gait of men and women along an age range of 20 to 87 years.[7-19] The investigative environments permitted acquisition of data in some cases for a few strides on a laboratory walkway to a large number of strides on a long walking course or treadmill. Some trends are apparent from these studies. Whether walking at a self-selected or preferred velocity, the subjects in groups over age 60 tend to walk more slowly than their younger counterparts, although some studies show no difference (Table 9-1). The same is true when subjects were instructed to walk fast. One study showed that the self-selected walking velocity for the old and young is statistically equal (119 and 121 cm/sec, respectively).[7] Another study showed that similar results and differences resulted only when subjects were asked to walk as fast as they possibly could.[12] Although the differences in most studies were statistically significant between the walking velocities, the differences in a practical sense are not particularly impressive. Old subjects in the main chose to walk at a moderate self-selected rate and, when asked to walk at a fast rate, were able to do so (see the categories presented in Table 1-2).

It is important to consider the large variability among subjects in the old and young groups. For example, calculations from the Murray data[19] reveal that more than 20 percent of subjects in the old group walked faster than the average self-selected and fast velocities for the young group (<60 years). However, the walking velocity of the old group should not be construed as abnormal. Any ambulatory velocity differences between the old and young may not be justifiably attributable to physiologic causes. For example, Imms and Edholm[20] showed that chosen walking velocities are influenced more by customary activity than by age.

Perhaps a more enlightening finding is the manner in which the old increase their walking velocity. When normalized or equated for walking velocity, the older group (>60 years) in comparison with the younger group (<60 years) seem to walk faster by relying more on increasing cadence or step frequency and less on increasing stride length. It may very well be that changes in the nervous system or foreshortening of muscular collagenous structures (e.g., anterior hip joint structures) are responsible for limiting increases in stride length, so that increasing the cadence is the only available alternative.

Rhythmicity or the ability to reproduce successive foot placement has been shown to be the same for young (21 to 47 years) and old (66 to 84 years).[15] The factors used in the comparison were step length, stride time, step width, and double stand time. Another study[19] also reported that rhythmicity was the same for the old and young until beyond 80 years, when step length and foot angles were dissimilar among successive steps in walking. In general, variability among all subjects is low for successive step length and stride time measures, while step width and double support times are highly variable.[15] Therefore, inclusion of step width and double-support time measures in clinical studies should be viewed with caution.

Women tend to walk slower and with shorter step lengths.[11] However, when normalized to appropriate segment lengths or body height, temporal and distance measures have been shown to be similar between the sexes.[17]

One practical consideration involving temporal and distance factors is the nature of the indoor walking surface. For 58 hospital patients (mean age 76 years), Willmott[21] compared walking characteristics on carpeted and vinyl floor. The patients walked faster and with longer steps on the carpet. Some of the patients expressed a fear of walking on the vinyl surface but were confident walking on carpet. This finding has obvious implications, particularly in the homes and health care institutions for the elderly.

Table 9-1. Summary of Temporal and Distance Measures for Normal Young and Old Subjects

Investigators	No. of Subjects	Age (yr)	Sex	Walking Velocity[c] (cm/s)	Cadence (steps/min)	Stride Length (cm)	SL/LEL SL/Ht	Stride Width (cm)	Foot Angle (degrees)	Cycle Time (sec)	Stance Phase (% Cycle)	Swing Phase (% Cycle)	Double Stance (% Cycle)
Chao et al. (1983)[11]	21	19–32	M	Free 120 (21)	100 (13)	138 (9)	1.46[a]	—	—	1.20	60	40	20
	32	32–85	M	Free 127 (21)	104 (8)	146 (8)	1.56[a]	—	—	1.15	59	41	18
	20	19–32	F	Free 102 (18)	102 (8)	120 (7)	1.38[a]	—	—	1.18	59	41	19
	37	32–85	F	Free 112 (18)	112 (8)	122 (8)	1.40[a]	—	—	1.07	60	40	20
Cunningham et al. (1982)[12]	43	19–49	M	Slow 108 (12)	95	132 (8)	0.76[b]	—	—	1.27	—	—	—
	41	55–66	M	Slow 104 (12)	95	132 (6)	0.76[b]	—	—	1.27	—	—	—
	43	19–49	M	Free 139 (10)	108	154 (6)	0.87[b]	—	—	1.11	—	—	—
	41	55–66	M	Free 133 (9)	109	146 (5)	0.84[b]	—	—	1.10	—	—	—
	43	19–49	M	Mod/Fast 171 (12)	119	172 (7)	0.99[b]	—	—	1.01	—	—	—
	41	55–66	M	Mod/Fast 160 (10)	120	160 (5)	0.92[b]	—	—	1.00	—	—	—
	43	19–49	M	Fast 225 (21)	144	188 (7)	1.06[b]	—	—	0.83	—	—	—
	41	55–66	M	Fast 193 (14)	135	172 (6)	0.99[b]	—	—	0.89	—	—	—
Finley et al. (1969)[14]	12	18–38	F	Free 82 (10)	105 (9)	94 (11)	—	—	—	1.14	63	37	—
	23	64–84	F	Free 70 (14)	109 (13)	76 (12)	—	—	—	1.10	67	33	—
Gabell et al. (1984)[15]	32	21–47	?	Free 137	108	152	—	8	—	1.10	—	—	24
	32	66–84	?	Free 119	112	128	—	10	—	1.08	—	—	24

188

Study	N	Age	Sex	Velocity									
Gifford and Hughes (1983)[16]	69	20–59	?	Free 130 (20)	109 (11)	140 (0.9)	0.83 (0.09)[b]	—	—	—	1.11	55	45	—
	21	60–79	?	Free 118 (14)	110 (9)	122 (0.6)	0.76 (0.06)[b]	—	—	—	1.10	57	43	—
Hageman et al. (1986)[00]	13	20–35	F	Free 160 (16)	119	163 (11)	1.87[a]	8 (3)	—	—	1.01	—	—	—
	13	60–80	F	Free 132 (24)	120	135 (15)	1.55[a]	10 (4)	—	—	1.00	—	—	—
Himann et al. (1988)[8]														
Jansen et al. (1982)[17]	20	20–29	M, F	Fixed 110	131	101 (8)	0.59[b]	—	—	—	—	69 (4)	31 (4)	36 (4)
	20	60–69	M, F	Fixed 110	135	98 (10)	0.59[b]	—	—	—	—	69 (4)	31 (4)	36 (4)
Larish et al. (1988)[7]	11	26	M, F	Free 119	—	—	—	—	—	—	—	—	—	—
	17	71	M	Free 121	—	—	—	—	—	—	—	—	—	—
Murray et al. (1964)[18]	48	20–55	M	Free 152	117	157	0.90[b]	8 (3)	6 (5)	1.03 (0.1)	61	39	—
	12	60–65	M	Free 147	115	153	0.87[b]	7 (4)	10 (7)	1.04 (0.1)	61	39	—
Murray et al. (1969)[19]	32	20–55	M	Free 152 (23)	111	154 (16)	0.90[b]	9 (4)	6 (7)	1.04 (0.1)	61	39	—
	32	60–87	M	Free 126 (23)	111	139 (26)	0.82[b]	9 (4)	9 (7)	1.13 (0.1)	60	40	—
	32	20–55	M	Fast 215 (40)	132	185 (26)	1.08[b]	10 (4)	4 (7)	0.88 (0.1)	57	43	—
	32	60–87	M	Fast 175 (40)	132	160 (26)	0.94[b]	10 (4)	10 (7)	0.94 (0.1)	59	41	—

[a] SL/LEL, stride length divided by lower-extremity length.
[b] SL/Ht, stride length divided by standing height.
[c] Free connotes self-selected walking velocity.

189

Another practical consideration has to do with the ambulation requirements within a community setting. In studies of small, medium, and large communities, the range of walking velocities required to cross a street safely at a stop light was 45 to 132 cm/sec.[22-24] Walking distance requirements in a variety of environmental conditions ranged from 39 for the post office to 417 for a shopping mall. There is a need to evaluate gait with home and community constraints in view.

Kinematics

As with temporal and distance factors, the body segment movement patterns during gait are remarkably similar among all subjects.[8] This similarity has been shown for lower-extremity joint motion for the young and old.[14] A study of multiple kinematic variables reported some differences between the old and the young.[19] The groups over 65 years of age tended to have reduced sagittal motion at the hip, knees, and ankles; less vertical displacement of the head; and reduced transverse rotation of the pelvis. The lateral excursion of the head was greater for the old; for the 81 to 87-year age group, there was decreased heel rise during swing phase. Since no numerical data were shown and the old subject groups walked slower, these results should be viewed with caution. The same can be said for another study,[25] which reported less motion for the old (60 to 84 years) than for the young (20 to 35 years). The average difference was 4.7° for a pelvic obliquity measure and 6.0° for sagittal plane ankle motion.

More convincing are the reports of upper-extremity motion and "out of phase" upper/lower-extremity movements. In an old subject group (81 to 87 years), there was a much less elbow flexion/extension excursion. Shoulder extension was greater and shoulder flexion less. Typically, the reversal of contralateral upper- and lower-extremity sagittal motion occurred near heel strike. For the groups over 65 years of age, this reversal varied from 0.3 seconds before and 0.4 seconds after heel strike. This latter finding may have ramifications for neuromuscular control.

Using a group of subjects ranging from 19 to 85 years, Chao et al.[11] concluded that for adult gait, gender-related variation was more significant than age-related variation. Among other factors, angular motion in three planes was studied. The salient differences between the gait of the very old and young are depicted in Figure 9-1.

Kinetics

Components of floor reaction forces have been compared between old and young adults.[7,11] In one study evaluating performance and time of onset of peak vertical, fore-aft, and mediolateral forces, no difference between groups was

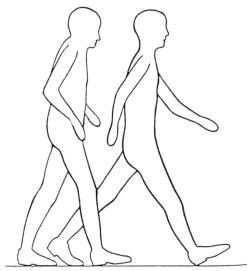

Fig. 9-1. Illustration of foot placement and kinematic gait differences between the young and very old (≥75 to 80 years). Differences in the sagittal and plane positions of the body of older (above left) and young (above right) men at the instant of right heel contact. The older men show shorter step lengths; decreased hip flexion-extension motion; decreased plantar flexion and elevation of the heel of the trailing limb; decreased elevation of the forefoot of the forward limb, decreased shoulder flexion on the forward arc of the swing, and decreased elbow extension on the backward arc. (From Murray et al.,[19] with permission.)

noted.[11] For frame of reference, descriptive data from 107 subjects are provided: initial peak vertical floor reaction force, just after heel strike, 108 ± 8 (percent BW), at midstance 75 ± 8 (percent BW), and just before toe-off 112 ± 8 (percent BW). The initial peak aft force just after heel strike was 2 ± 2 (percent BW), followed by a retarding force of 16 ± 5 (percent BW), and a propulsion force of 18 ± 5 (percent BW) just before toe-off. Just after heel strike, the average medial force was 4 ± 2 (percent BW), followed by a lateral force of 5 ± 2 (percent BW) and another peak lateral force of 4 ± 2 (percent BW) just before toe off.[11] The subjects walked on average at 113 ± 18 cm/s.

At controlled walking velocities of 81 and 134 cm/s, some differences in peak vertical and fore-aft floor reaction forces were found between the young males (average 26 years) and old physically active males (average 71 years).[7] In this study, statistically significant differences were found to be greater in the younger group for the aft-retarding force. The initial peak vertical floor reaction force was higher for the young group walking at the faster rate. These differences between the groups were quite small with the average vertical force difference range of 1.0 to 3.0 percent body weight and a difference of 0.1 to 0.4 percent body weight for the fore-aft floor reaction measures. From a practical vantage point, these small differences make any age-related inference tenuous.

Crowninshield et al.[25] compared a small group of 11 young subjects (mean age 24 years) and 15 old subjects (mean age 71 years). No significant difference was found in the hip joint resultant force (net force occurring between the thigh and pelvis). A range of five walking velocities from 30 to 150 cm/s and a regression analysis were used. However, Crowninshield et al. show that the peak resultant joint moment and hip joint contact force were proportionately smaller for the older group. For the latter findings, the shorter stride length and lesser hip muscle action are implicated in the older group.

Energy Expenditure

There is some evidence to show that a person tends to have, if not one specific walking velocity, certainly a small range whereby he or she is able to walk most economically from an energy expenditure point of view (see Ch. 1). With energy expenditure normalized to body weight and distance walked, no difference was found between the most economical walking velocities for old men (mean age 71 years) and young men (mean age 26).[7] The most economical imposed walking velocities were 107 and 134 cm/s.

Cunningham et al.[12] measured maximum oxygen uptake in three age groups: 19 to 29, 39 to 49, and 55 to 66 years. The subjects were asked to walk at four different rates according to the following instructions: (1) rather slowly (slow), (2) at normal pace (normal), (3) rather fast but without overexerting yourself (fast), and (4) as fast as you can (very fast), during which time heart rates were obtained via telemetry. After controlling for age, height, weight, and fitness in a multiple regression model VO_2 max was significantly related to the three fastest walking velocities. Cunningham et al. concluded that self-selected walking velocity was associated with maximal aerobic power independent of age.

Simply being a middle distance runner in earlier years does not appear exclusively useful for aerobic efficiency in later years.[26] The aerobic efficiency during walking was compared between former competitive runners and non-athletes aged 47 to 68 years. No differences between the groups were found.

In a study of 60 to 80-year-old healthy women, a non-weightbearing gait using a walker was evaluated.[27] The average heart rates rose 49 beats/min for an average of 83 percent of their age-predicted heart rate. The subjects' average walking velocity was 20 cm/s. The extra cardiovascular demands imposed by various assisted-type gates are important considerations in the care and ambulatory training of the elderly.

Neural Related Factors

Apart from the basic neurophysiologic changes with aging, a paucity of work is done involving neural factors, aging, and gait as a functional activity. Integrated electromyographic (EMG) signals from muscles of the trunk and lower extremity have been reported to be higher among the elderly.[14] The same study found that the location of the center of gravity relative to a person's body height was significantly higher in the elderly. This latter finding would tend to increase the demand for balance retention and control in the elderly.

FALLS IN THE ELDERLY

Gait and Falls

Because of the high incidence of falls among the elderly, some discussion is warranted here.[3,28–32] Overstall[33] defines a fall simply as an uncorrected displacement. He elaborates that walking is hazardous because it imposes a complicated range of displacements. An age-matched group of one-time fallers and nonfallers over age 65 were compared using selected gait characteristics. Compared with nonfallers, the fallers as a group demonstrated the following characteristics: slower walking velocity (34 versus 21 cm/s), shorter step length (38 versus 22 cm), wide range of cadence, and large variability in step length.[34]

It appears either that impaired gait may precipitate falling or that falling may cause an impaired gait, even in the absence of physical injury or pathology, or both. Prevention of falling is a crucial focus, since it is a recurring problem among the elderly. Twenty-five percent of all falls have been reported to occur on stairs.[35] Therefore, it is appropriate to provide some information on walking stairs that can be used by clinicians in an educational sense to help prevent falls in the elderly.

Walking Stairs

Walking on a level surface, ascending stairs, or descending stairs is carried out under normal conditions with similar repetitive and cyclic body movements.[36] Even the contraction of various lower-extremity muscles is repetitive and cyclic, irrespective of whether the person is an athlete or not.[37] Level walking, ascending stairs, and descending stairs are in a real sense a repeated, controlled fall whereby the body's center of gravity is located just in front of the base of support at the foot-walking surface interface.[38] Some key normal conditions that permit these desirable repeatable, cyclic body movements are (1) level walking surface for level walking, (2) steps that are equal in dimensions for a particular flight of stairs, and (3) sufficient friction between the foot and support surface to provide a stable base of support.

Walking stairs is considerably more demanding on the body as compared with level walking: More physiologic energy,[39] lower-extremity joint motion[1,40] and larger forces at joints.[41,42] Muscle action of the upper extremities has not been shown to be different,[43] while lower-extremity muscle action is greater.[44] Forces and moments at the hip and knee are greatest for descending stairs. To provide an objective sense of the kinetic and kinematic demands of stair walking, some examples of increases over the requirements for walking include: approximately 25 degrees of knee motion, 50 percent in lower-extremity moments of force, 12 to 25 percent tibial femoral contact force, and 7 times greater force at the kneecap.

Increased step heights require commensurate increases in knee and thigh movement.[45] Thus, high steps can be expected to be more demanding than are low inclined steps. Although stair movements are cyclic and repetitive, the variability is higher for descending stairs as compared with ascending. As such, it might be inferred that step heights in a staircase should be precisely equal in order to minimize the variability in movement.

People normally use visual guidance when initiating the descent of a flight of stairs. However, during subsequent steps in the descent, the nervous system tends to control movement at the subcortical or unconscious level, presumably because movement requirements are predictably repetitive and cyclic. If a person expects a differing step height, the muscles of the calf tend to contract, thereby absorbing the shock imposed on the body. Nevertheless, the smooth body movement is disrupted by the perturbation imposed by the step of differing height and additional nonrepetitive neuromuscular and biomechanical events occur.[46]

With unanticipated changes in step height (e.g., 5 cm), it has been shown that ankle and knee joint angles were increased and that an abnormally large upward thrust on the body tended to accelerate the body mass upward. There was also an associated increase in muscle activity.[47]

When a person begins to fall forward out of control, several neuromuscular events occur in rapid-fire order. The immediate mechanical reflex eliciting compensatory muscle action has been shown to occur at 91 milliseconds (ms), the lead foot brakes the forward fall in 184 to 237 ms, and the trail foot begins to come forward in 236 to 328 ms. Following the initial reflex action, the response to falling is believed to be influenced by a combination of cortical (voluntary) and (subcortical) involuntary factors. Furthermore, the subjects demonstrated considerable elbow flexion.[48,49] In most cases, a flat surface 36 inches long in the direction of the path of the impending fall was required for successful negotiation of a balance recovery step.[50]

SUMMARY AND CLINICAL IMPLICATIONS

At various stages beyond age 65, as compared with their younger counterparts, the healthy elderly groups studied show the following tendencies:

1. Walk at somewhat slower self-selected walking velocity
2. Are less capable of walking extremely fast
3. Increase walking velocity by increasing step frequency to a greater extent than increasing stride length
4. Demonstrate gender differences in step length and some biomechanical variables
5. Walk with less angular movement at the joints
6. Consume more energy while walking

When present, differences between the young and old were small, and large variability revealed overlap between the two groups. Among the variables studied, there were often far more similarities than differences between the young and old groups.

By and large, some preliminary age-related gait aberrations begin to appear around age 60, but more profound alterations in gait are delayed until at least 75 to 80 years of age. Clinical implications can be important. First, in dealing with the healthy old from a preventive vantage point, the targeted expectations for gait training as an exercise should be little, if any, less than for a young adult. To this end, it is important to have medical confirmation of good health, proper warmup exercise, and extended gradual increases in exercise intensity, frequency, and duration.[51] A second implication applies to the finding that the healthy old emphasize cadence rather than step length in walking fast. Therefore, it is advisable to evaluate for shortened hip flexor/anterior hip structures and hamstring muscles, triceps surae, and pelvic rotators, any of which could diminish step length.

A third clinical implication is that because the differences in gait between the young and healthy old are small, the clinician should not feel constrained by the age of the patient. That is, the clinician should feel free to dedicate his or her attention to the many other factors that may have a negative effect on gait. Musculoskeletal, neuromuscular, and cardiopulmonary afflictions frequently affect gait (these areas are addressed in subsequent chapters of this book). In addition, gait is likely affected by other factors, such as current physical activity level, physical activity history, body weight, attitude, motivation, mental state, footware, hearing status, vision, mobility environment, nutrition, and the nature of the instructions provided to the patient.

A fourth implication is that the ability of the elderly person to walk in a test should be judged against the domiciliary and community requirements. The healthy elderly groups discussed earlier demonstrated the ability to walk fast enough and far enough to satisfy these requirements.

Finally, a fall has been defined as an uncorrected displacement. Falls are a frequent cause of injury among the elderly and may point to unsuspected pathology. A high percentage of falls occur while walking stairs. Foot placement, joint motion, forces encountered, and movement control are markedly greater for walking stairs as compared with walking on a level surface. To help prevent falls, the capability of the elderly to walk stairs should be maintained. Furthermore, as with level walking, it would appear advisable that the elderly retain familiarity with ascending and descending stairs.

REFERENCES

1. Brauer E, Mackeprang B, Bentzon MW: Prognosis of survival in a geriatric population. Scand J Soc Med 6:17, 1978
2. Isaacs B: Has geriatric medicine advanced? p. 1. In Isaacs B (ed): Recent Advances in Geriatric Medicine. Churchill Livingstone, Edinburgh, 1978
3. Payton OD, Poland JL: Aging process: implications for clinical practice. Phys Ther 63:41, 1983
4. Milne JS: Longitudinal studies of vision in older people. Age Aging 8:160, 1979
5. Barron RE: Disorders of gait related to the aging nervous system. Geriatrics 22:113, 1967
6. Koller WC, Glatt SL, Fox JH: Senile gait. Clin Geriatr Med 1:661, 1985
7. Larish DD, Martin PE, Mungiole M: Characteristic patters of gait in the healthy old. In Joseph JA (ed): Central Determinants of Age Related Declines in Motor Function. The New York Academy Sciences, New York. Ann NY Acad Sci 515:18, 1988
8. Himann JE, Cunningham DA, Rechnitzer PA, Patterson DH: Age related changes in speed of walking. Med Sci Sports Exerc 20:161, 1988
9. Bassey EJ, Bendall MJ, Pearson M: Muscle strength in the triceps surae and objectively measured customary walking activity in men and women over 65 years of age. Clin Sci 74:85, 1988
10. Bassey EJ, Fentem PH, MacDonald IC, Scriven PM: Self-paced walking as a method for exercise testing in elderly and young men. Clin Sci Mol Med 51:609, 1976
11. Chao EY, Laughman RK, Schneider E, Stauffer RN: Normative data of knee joint motion and ground reaction forces in adult level walking. J Biomech 16:219, 1983
12. Cunningham DA, Rechnitzer PA, Pearce ME, Donner AP: Determinants of self-selected walking pace across ages 19 to 66. J Gerontol 37:560, 1982
13. Drillis RJ: The influence of aging on the kinematics of gait: Geriatric review. Report on a Conference Sponsored by the Committee. National Research Council. Committee on Prosthetics Research and Development, NAS-NRC 919, 1961
14. Finley FR, Cody KA, Finizie RV: Locomotion patterns in elderly woman. Arch Phys Med Rehabil 50:140, 1969
15. Gabell A, Nayak USL: The effect of age on variability in gait. J Gerontol 39:662, 1984
16. Gifford G, Hughes J: A gait analysis system in clinical practice. J Biomed Eng 5:297, 1983
17. Jansen EC, Vittas D, Hellberg S, Hansen J: Normal gait of young and old men and women: Ground reaction force measurement on a treadmill. Acta Orthop Scand 53:193, 1982
18. Murray MP, Drought AB, Kory RC: Walking patterns of normal men. J Bone Joint Surg 46A:335, 1964
19. Murray MP, Kory RC, Clarkson BH: Walking patterns in healthy old men. J Gerontol 24:169, 1969
20. Imms FJ, Edholm OG: Studies of gait and mobility in the elderly. Age Aging 10:147, 1981
21. Wilmott M: The effect of a vinyl floor surface and a carpeted floor surface upon walking in elderly hospital in-patients. Age Aging 15:119, 1986

22. Lerner-Frankiel MB, Vargas S, Brown MB, et al: Functional community ambulation: What are your criteria? Clin Mgmt 6(2):12, 1986
23. O'Dwyer KO: Gait and the elderly. Graduate Program in Physical Therapy, University of Iowa, 1988
24. Robinett CS, Vondran M: Functional ambulation velocity and distance requirements in rural and urban communities: A clinical report. Phys Ther 68:1371, 1988
25. Crowninshield RD, Brand RA, Johnston RC: The effects of walking velocity and age on hip kinematics and kinetics. Clin Orthop 132:140, 1978
26. Robinson S, Dill DB, Robinson RD, et al: Physiological aging of champion runners. J Appl Physiol 41:46, 1976
27. Baruch IM, Mossberg KA: Heart-rate response of elderly women to nonweight-bearing ambulation with a walker. Phys Ther 63:1782, 1983
28. Isaacs B: Clinical and laboratory studies of falls in old people: Prospects for prevention. Clin Geriatr Med 1:513, 1985
29. Wild D, Nayak USL, Isaacs B: Characteristics of old people who fell at home. J Clin Exp Gerontol 2:271, 1980
30. Wild D, Nayak USL, Isaacs B: Description, classification and prevention of falls in old people at home. Rheumatol Rehabil 20:153, 1981
31. Wild D, Nayak USL, Isaacs B: How dangerous are falls in old people at home? Br Med J 282:266, 1981
32. Wild D, Nayak USL, Isaacs B: Prognosis of falls in old pepole at home. J Epidemil Community Health 35:200, 1981
33. Overstall PW: Falls in the elderly—Epidemiology, aetiology and management. p. 61. In Isaacs B (ed): Recent Advances in Geriatric Medicine. Churchill Livingstone, Edinburgh, 1978
34. Guimaraes RM, Isaacs B: Characteristics of the gait in old people who fall. Int Rehabil Med 2:177, 1980
35. Nickens H: Intrinsic factors in falling among the elderly. Arch Intern Med 145:1089, 1985
36. Townsend MA, Tsai TC: Biomechanics and modeling of bipedal climbing and descending. J Biomech 9:227, 1976
37. Townsend MA, Shiavi R, Lainhart SP, Caylor J: Variability in synergy patterns of leg muscles during climbing, descending and level walking of highly-trained athletes and normal males. EMG Clin Neurophysiol 18:69, 1978
38. Pedotti A: A study of motor coordination and neuromuscular activities in human location. Biol Cybern 26:53, 1977
39. Dean GA: An analysis of energy expenditure in level and grade walking. Ergonomics 8:31, 1965
40. Laubenthal KN, Smidt GL, Kettelkamp DB: A quantitative analysis of knee motion during activities of daily living. Phys Ther 52:34, 1972
41. Andriacchi TP, Andersson GBT, Fermier RS, et al: A study of lower limb mechanics during stair climbing. J Bone Joint Surg 62A:749, 1980
42. Reilly DT, Martens M: Experimental analysis of the quadriceps muscle force and patello-femoral joint reaction force for various activities. Acta Orthop Scand 43:126, 1972
43. Hogue RE: Upper-extremity muscular activity at different cadences and inclines during gait. Phys Ther 49:963, 1969
44. Lyons K, Perry J, Gronley JK, et al: Timing and relative intensity of hip extensor and abductor muscle action during level and stair ambulation. Phys Ther 63:1597, 1983

45. Grieve DW, Leggett D, Wetherstone B: The analysis of normal stepping movements as a possible basis for locomotor assessment of lower limbs. J Anat 127:515, 1978

46. Freedman W, Wannsted G, Herman R: EMG patterns and forces developed during step down. Am J Phys Med 55:275, 1976

47. Nashner LM: Balance adjustments of humans perturbed while walking. J Neurophysiol 44:650, 1980

48. Dietz V, Noth J: Preinnervation and stretch responses of triceps brachii in man falling with and without visual control. Brain Res 142:576, 1978

49. Do MC, Brieniere Y, Brengui ER: A biomechanical study of balance recovery during the fall forward. J Biomech 15:933, 1982

50. Cavagna GA, Margaria R: Mechanics of walking. J Appl Physiol 21:271, 1966

51. deVries HA: Tips on prescribing exercise regimens for your older patient. Geriatrics 34(4):75, 1979

10 | Gait in Musculoskeletal Abnormalities

Gary L. Smidt

When elements of the musculoskeletal system are adversely affected, gait abnormalities frequently result. Gait is a needed and commonly used function that, if less than optimal, is justifiably a concern of patients and clinicians alike. A plethora of publications directly address or allude to abnormal gait resulting from musculoskeletal disease or trauma. In a variety of ways, these gait abnormalities have been described, the effect of treatment intervention has been reported, and the use of gait analysis as a diagnostic tool has been purported. Confounding influences such as wide variability in degree of involvement, health history, type of therapeutic intervention, and levels of clinical skill make it difficult to paint a neat rhetorical picture of gait abnormalities in the form of pathologic categories. This variability should be accepted as a clinical reality. Lack of standardization in assessing gait also adds to the difficulty, but this problem can be resolved.

Cognizance of confounding influences has been borne in mind in carrying out the mission of this chapter: to review gait abnormalities according to selected musculoskeletal pathologic groups, and identify and comment on clinical implications and issues. Some of the musculoskeletal aspects are clarified elsewhere in this volume. As a consequence, pediatrics and energy expenditure are not included in this discussion.

CHRONIC ARTHRITIS

Two common arthridites are rheumatoid (RA) and osteoarthritis (OA). Osteoarthritis is a disease of the articular cartilage, while in the rheumatoid case the focus of the pathology is the synovial lining, a nonarticular structure. Investigations involving therapeutic intervention and gait have been dominated by surgical approaches. Very little has been reported on the impact of postsurgical rehabilitation and noninvasive conservative techniques as primary forms of treatment.

Hip

Classic Gait Abnormalities

During the early 1960s, Calve et al.[1] describe the "limp of coxalgia." The limp is characterized by excessive lateral displacement of the head and upper trunk toward the involved weightbearing side. On the basis of observation, the stance time on the affected side is quick and the step lengths are unequal. What is the hip condition that causes this gait abnormality? Is it a foreshortened lower extremity, or ankylosis, or a deformity? Calve believed that the articular surface and joint capsule of the hip joint were compromised and the abnormal upper body movement was a reflex defense to bring the center of gravity over the hip, thus reducing the force at the joint. This abnormal gait pattern has been commonly referred to as an antalgic gait which in effect is not necessarily a painful gait but rather a pattern resulting from cyclical attempts to avoid pain (Fig. 10-1).

In contrast to the antalgic gait, a Trendelenburg gait is characterized by an excessive downward rotation of the pelvis on the side opposite the involved stance limb (Fig. 10-1). The key word is excessive since, in the normal case, the pelvis rotates a few degrees downward in the coronal plane. The cause of the Trendelenburg gait is classically believed to be the inability of a weakened gluteus medius to prevent the excessive pelvic rotation.

Bechtol[2] advocated teaching a dynamic balance gait for patients with either a Trendelenburg or antalgic gait. The dynamic balance gait is employed to balance the trunk and reduce hip pain by substituting the inertia of the body to shift the upper body's center of mass laterally over the affected hip. The method is dynamic because it must be employed during the act of walking, not standing. The key purported elements of instruction to the patient are to (1) walk with a slightly wider base, (2) increase the lateral shift of entire body toward the affected side during stance, and (3) shift the pelvis toward the affected side during ipsilateral stance. This advocated technique appears to be a complementary maneuver to the body's involuntary gait adjustments to joint pathology. Tesio et al.[3] demonstrated that the limping arthritic patient has a greater transfer between kinetic and potential energy of the center of gravity on the involved stance limb. The clinical relevance of this finding is that the work performed by the affected limb is small. In a compensatory way, most of the

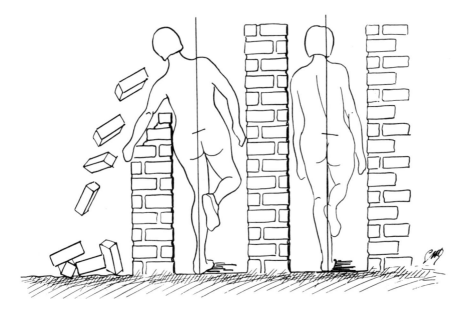

Fig. 10-1. Illustration of antalgic gait on left and Trendelenburg gait on right. (From Calve et al.,[1] with permission.)

work is done by the muscles of the sound limb and, in the case of the advocated dynamic balance maneuver, the trunk as well.

Pain and function continue to be the primary concerns in the evaluation and treatment of osteo and rheumatoid arthritis. Advances in technology have permitted description of gait abnormalities in quantitative terms. This objective information should enhance the understanding of abnormal gait and aid in the assessment of various surgical and nonsurgical treatment approaches.

Rating Scales

Rating scales have been used to assess patients with hip disease. D'Aubigne and Postel[4] included pain, joint range of motion, and gait in their rating scale. Gait was given 33 percent of the total possible points. Larson[5] included pain, function, joint range, motion, deformity, and gait as separate categories. Gait was given 10 percent of the total. Another frequently used rating scale by Harris[6] included pain, function, joint range of motion, and absence of deformity. Gait was awarded 33 percent of the total.

As an alternative to surgical implant treatment for hip disease, the girdlestone approach has been used for patients with arthritis. As compared with preoperative status, long-term follow-up of 54 patients revealed improved gait in 72 percent of cases, but all patients continued to walk with a limp.[7] Postoperative weightbearing was started at 3 months. Before the advent of total joint implants, the cup arthroplasty was a commonly performed surgical technique. In a study of 251 cup arthroplasty patients with OA and RA, Johnston and Larson[8] used the Iowa Hip Rating scale. At the 3- to 16-year follow-up examination, approximately 96 percent walked with a limp and 10 percent used crutches. Compared with preoperative status, gait was improved in 56 percent and the same in 27 percent, and 17 percent were worse.

In a clinical follow-up study of predominantly osteoarthritic patients who had total hip replacements, Johnston[9] reported on 256 patients (326 hip replacements). The patients were assessed at 6, 12, and 24 months postoperatively. Both Larson and Harris hip-rating scales yielded similar results. Some interesting results relative to gait were reported. Preoperatively, pain during every walking step was experienced by 80 percent of the patients. Parenthetically, others[10] have rated pain as it was experienced during the act of walking. Postoperatively, the patient's limp and reliance on assistive devices were impressively decreased. The patient's ability seemed to level off at 1 year postoperatively and remained the same during the second postoperative year (Table 10-1). Immediately after surgery, patients were placed in balanced suspension and were taught crutch walking within the first 4 to 7 days. Patients walked with crutches for 6 months after discharge from hospital and then usually switched to a cane for 1 to 6 months until they could walk well without support. The side of hip involvement for this large group of patients was distributed equally between right and left, a finding that refutes speculation by Neumann and Cook[11] that the side of occurrence of osteoarthritic hip disease is related to the use of the dominant upper extremity.

A wide variety of total joint implants have been used. Because of the large number of confounding variables in any gait study, it is difficult to make definitive statements about the efficacy of various implants for restoring walking. In a 47-month follow-up of 78 OA patients with McKee Farrar implants, Baldurson[12] reported that, compared with the preoperative picture, gait was improved in 50 percent and remained the same in 42 percent, and 8 percent were worse.

The need for the patient's use of walking aids is included in the rating scales.[13] With Charnley total joint implants in 66 OA and RA patients, 89 percent required assistive devices, whereas 96 percent did not walk with assistive devices postoperatively.[14] In another study, 14 patients with OA received a Charnley prosthesis; postoperatively, 57 percent walked without aid, and the

Table 10-1. Pain with Activity[a]

Degree of Pain	Preop (%)	Postop (%)
None	3	76
Mild	1	18
Moderate	16	6
Severe (every step)	80	0

[a] Gait results for total hip replacements ($N = 256$).

(From Johnston,[9] with permission.)

Table 10-2. Assistive Devices Used[a]

| Assistive Device | Number of Patients[a] | | Code |
	Preop	Postop	
Walker	4	0	1
Two crutches	13	2	2
Two canes	2	1	3
One crutch	1	1	4
One cane	4	7	5
None	1	14	6
	25	25	

[a] Mean preop: 3.5; mean postop: 5.3.
(From Stauffer et al.,[17] with permission.)

remaining 43 percent used one assistive device.[15] Fifty months after receiving a Monk total joint, 34 percent of 36 OA patients used walking aids.[16] Gradations of assistance from walking aids have been reported for 25 OA and RA patients who received a Charnley implant. On the whole, the patients used two assistive devices or a walker preoperatively and at 6 months postoperatively they walked with one or no assistive devices[17] (Table 10-2). In the situation in which surgical revision occurred, the positive results are compromised (e.g., 79 percent used walking aids).[18] In 8 patients with severe RA, 75 percent were nonambulatory, and at 16 to 40 months postoperatively 50 percent could walk without aid and 50 percent used walking aids.[19] In this study, patients received both hip and knee implants.

Retention of the benefit of walking improvement from total hip arthroplasty surgery has been shown.[20] The walking ability of patients at 36 months and 72 months postoperatively was essentially the same.

Improvement in gait function from total joint implant surgery probably results primarily from a pre- versus postoperative change in pain. For example, in the Stauffer, Smidt, Wadsworth study, all 25 patients had severe pain (14 also reported rest pain) preoperatively, 6 months later, 18 were pain free and only one had pain that limited function.[17]

Deviations from Normal

Patients with OA and RA at the hip tend to walk slower than normal. From several gait studies of OA and RA, the average walking velocity ranged from 36 to 67 cm/s[17,21–27] (see Ch. 1, Table 1-2, for guidelines on categories of walking velocity and Ch. 14, Table 14-2, for grades of walking ability using Smidt's Number). The average fast walking velocities in patients with arthritic hips have ranged from 69 to 94 cm/s.[21,24,28] Hip disease patients tend to spend a disproportionate amount of time in single limb stance (average 71 percent of cycle).[27] In a study of unilaterally involved patients, the majority (85 percent vs. 13 percent) spent less time on the involved side (in comparison with less involved) during stance phase.[29]

Angular hip motion is reduced particularly in the sagittal plane (Fig. 10-2).[17,21,27,30-33] Floor reaction forces in all directions on the side of the involved hip are also reduced, [17,22,24,26,34] and acceleration patterns are altered (Figs. 10-3 to 10-5).[35] In a study of men with unilateral hip pain, Murray et al.[32] characterized the gait abnormalities as follows:

> Irregularity and asymmetry in the following gait components during successive phases of weight-bearing on the painful and sound limb: duration of the weight bearing periods; step length; vertical and forward motion of the head; lateral displacement of the head, trunk, upper limb or

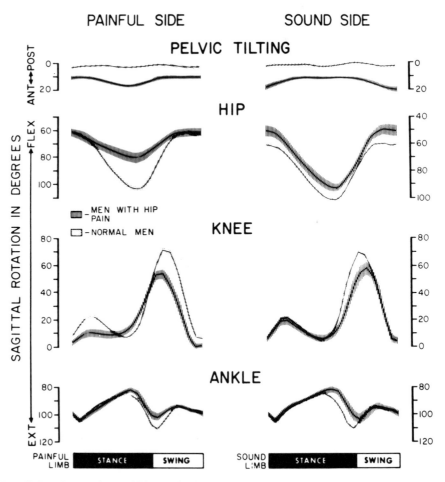

Fig. 10-2. Comparison of kinematics between painful and sound side in patients with unilateral hip pain. (From Murray et al.,[32] with permission.)

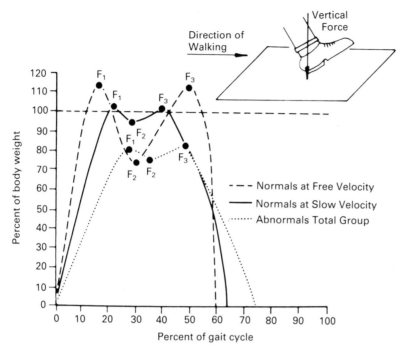

Fig. 10-3. Vertical floor reaction force for normals and arthritic patients. N=26 Patients and 64 normal men. Shaded areas represent 2 SEs above and below the mean. (From Smidt and Wadsworth,[26] with permission.)

some combination of the three; and sagittal rotation of the shoulders and elbows. The following components were significantly less than normal: walking speed; step length; cadence; maximum extension of both hips and both ankles during the late stance phase; maximum flexion of both knees during swing; shoulder flexion during the forward arc of arm swing; and elbow extension during the backward arc. The following components were significantly greater than normal: lateral motion of the head; anterior pelvic tilting; and transverse rotation of the pelvis.

Locomotor function reflects severity of pain.[36] However, once pain is alleviated, joint deformity, muscle weakness, abnormal joint motion, neural control deficits, and multiple joint involvement can, in a residual sense, contribute significantly to walking abnormalities in patients with hip disease (Fig. 10-2).

Effects of Therapeutic Intervention

The lion's share of investigations of treatment effects has involved surgery. During the mid-1960s, patients with severe hip joint destruction and pain were treated surgically with a cup arthroplasty while during the past two decades or so, both acetabular and femoral components have been implanted.

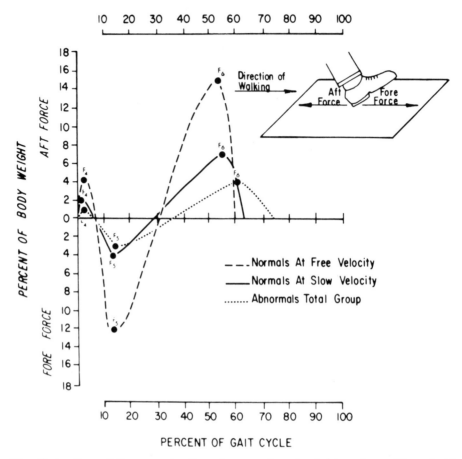

Fig. 10-4.   Fore-aft floor reaction force for normals and arthritic patients. (From Smidt and Wadsworth,[26] with permission.)

It appears that compared with preoperative status, the walking ability of total joint implant patients improves considerably. At 6 months postoperatively, the average increase from preoperative self-selected walking velocity has been shown to range from 4 percent to 49 percent.[17,21,24,27,31] From 6 months to 12 to 24 months, the gains are smaller but not plateaued, with a range of 5 percent to 18 percent.[21,24,31] Preoperative/postoperative changes are reported for other temporal and distance factors, but one must hedge on interpretation because walking velocity was often dissimilar over time.

For an ankylosed hip, Hauge[37] stated that the most ''normal'' gait can be obtained with the hip in 15° flexion, 3 to 5° adduction, and 5 to 10° external rotation. One study[38] reported on the ability to walk long distances in 28 patients who were surgically treated with hip fusion. In a 5- to 10-year follow-up of 47 predominantly osteoarthritic patients with unilateral hip disease, Perrin et

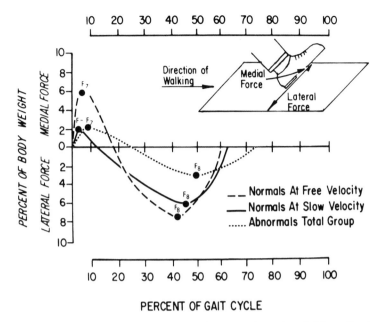

Fig. 10-5. Mediolateral floor reaction force for normals and arthritic patients. (From Smidt and Wadsworth,[26] with permission.)

al.[39] indicated that over the 2- to 4-month postoperative period, patients' self-selected walking velocity was 80 percent of normal. These patients, who received total hip arthroplasties, were reported to have progressively improved stance time symmetry over the 5-year postoperative period, but no data were provided. Thirty-seven months after having the original total joint surgically revised, Carlsson et al.[40] reported that of the 57 OA and RA patients, 32 percent could walk more than 12.0 km, 49 percent 0.5 to 2.0 km, 16 percent 0.1 to 0.5 km, and 4 percent less than 0.1 km. Seventy-one percent reported that they could walk more than 1 mile and 21 percent between $\frac{1}{2}$ to 1 mile, and 8 percent were limited to less than $\frac{1}{2}$ mile. Rather than direct measurement, reports from patients were typically relied upon for this important factor of walking distance capability.

By and large, positive preoperative/postoperative functional changes have been reported for a number of important mechanical variables: increased angular hip motion predominantly in the sagittal planes[17,21,23,24] and increased floor reaction forces.[17,24] Displacement of the head[23] and center of gravity[22] during walking has been shown to decrease (Table 10-3). Mechanical energy used is also decreased.[22]

Of 294 total hip patients interviewed, 95 percent indicated preoperatively that they could not walk a 0.5-km distance.[42] Following surgery, only 12 percent reported a 0.5-km constraint.

Table 10-3. Results of Various Gait Parameters in Patients with Unilateral Total Hip Replacements[a]

	Unit	Preoperation	Post-THR (18–24 months)	Control (Normal Female)
N		9	9	25
Clinical score[c]		50.6 ± 10.3	93.3 ± 5.7	
Age (range)	yr	60.1 (53–67)	62.3 (54–69)	39.2 (21–62)
Body weight	kg	49.6 ± 5.7	51.5 ± 5.3	50.9 ± 6.3
Stride	cm	91.9 ± 11.3[b]	105.9 ± 10.5	114.1 ± 7.6
Cadence	steps min^{-1}	94.7 ± 13.2[b]	113.9 ± 10.7	123.4 ± 8.0
Velocity	m min^{-1}	43.4 ± 8.5[b]	57.6 ± 8.0[b]	70.4 ± 6.9
Displacement width of COG				
Lateral	$\lvert Dx\rvert$ cm	4.4 ± 1.6[b]	3.3 ± 0.8	3.2 ± 0.7
Fore-aft	$\lvert Dy\rvert$ cm	2.8 ± 1.1[b]	2.0 ± 0.7	1.7 ± 0.4
Vertical	$\lvert Dz\rvert$ cm	4.3 ± 1.6[b]	2.7 ± 0.8	2.7 ± 0.6
Total	D_{total}(cm)	11.5 ± 3.8[b]	8.0 ± 1.8	7.6 ± 1.0
Displacement volume DV	(cm^3)	68.4 ± 27.7[b]	19.0 ± 13.7	14.9 ± 7.0
Energy variation/ 1 cycle				
PE	$\lvert PE\rvert$ J	21.1 ± 7.9[b]	13.1 ± 3.8	13.4 ± 2.9
KE	$\lvert KE\rvert$ J	8.3 ± 2.8[b]	11.1 ± 3.1	12.8 ± 2.7
TE	$\lvert TE\rvert$ J	16.3 ± 8.3[b]	11.3 ± 3.1	10.0 ± 2.5
Total internal work Wt kg^{-1} m^{-1}	J kg^{-1}m^{-1}	0.78 ± 0.30[b]	0.56 ± 0.12	0.54 ± 0.10

[a] Results are mean ± SD.
[b] $p < 0.01$ when compared with control (analysis of variance using Scheffe's method).
[c] Score of Japanese Orthopaedic Association.
(From Iida and Yamamuro,[22] with permission.)

From total joint surgery, the end result for walking seems to be highly satisfactory but considerably short of normal. Such an outcome can logically be expected, since the patients are typically severely debilitated before surgery.

One study was located in which the effect of nonsteroidal anti-inflammatory drugs (NSAIDs) (aspirin) was assessed in patients with active RA disaese.[43] Sixteen subjects completed a double-blind study in which aspirin treatment was administered over a 2-month period. The patients reported decreased day and night pain, joint stiffness, and swelling. Their average self-selected velocity increased from 85 to 93 cm/s, and the relative increase in heart rate was desirably decreased while walking.

There is a glaring absence of nonsurgical or so-called conservative treatment reports for gait in musculoskeletal disorders. Even in studies involving surgical intervention, the postoperative rehabilitation program is often reported in benign brevity, if at all. Some are of the opinion that ambulation is the only necessary exercise for these patients and that the weakest of the muscle groups are the hip abductors.[44] These claims have not been tested in the crucible of research. There is a need to assess preventative measures short of surgery as well as the effects of short-term and long-term rehabilitation programs for arthritic patients receiving surgery. The difficulty of such studies should not be minimized. The general medical and physiologic status of the patient, health history, integrity of the musculoskeletal system (e.g., muscle strength, bone mineral density), specificity of diagnosis, quality of the evaluation methods, skill of the surgeon, and skill of the rehabilitation specialist are, to name a few, important issues that could profitably be addressed in future clinical investigations.

For example, static stretching exercise of foreshortened hamstring and hip flexor muscle groups has been demonstrated to improve significantly the physiologic economy for walking in asymptomatic males.[45] What impact can such indirect forms of intervention have on prevention and restoration of hip abnormalities?

Relationship of Clinical and Gait Measures

In an effort to determine the relevance of gait assessment in patient care, investigators inquired about the association of clinical signs and symptoms and measures of gait. In a study of 92 RA patients, Spiegel et al.[46] demonstrated that maximum walking velocity was significantly related to joint deformity, but change in maximum walking velocity was unrelated to change in clinical signs and symptoms. For this group of patients, walking velocity was a good indicator of disease activity but not of clinical change. For example, the average maximum walking velocity for patients with minimal lower-extremity joint deformity was 117 cm/s, 72 cm/s for moderate deformity, and 60 cm/s for severe deformity.

Smidt[25] demonstrated that, in normal subjects, hip motion during gait increases in concert with increased walking velocity. This relationship seems to hold for the sagittal plane in patients who have adequate available pelvifemoral motion. In the Gore study,[21] the patients increased in both walking velocity and sagittal plane motion. However, for patients with hip disease, there seems to be a poor correlation between clinical measures of range of motion and the amount of motion used during gait.[17] As such, it would appear to be incumbent on the clinician to consider gait-training methods so that patients might optimally use the hip motion available to them.

Self-selected walking velocity has been shown to be unimpressively associated with the composite score on the Iowa Hip Rating Scale.[47] For patients assessed preoperatively and five times postoperatively, the r values were 0.35, 0.33, 0.19, 0.32, 0.07, and −0.98 for patients with unilateral total hip replacements; for bilateral hip replacements, the r values were 0.68, 0.19, 0.64, −0.43, 0.11, and 0.14. Two problems come to mind in this type of study: (1) the rating scales used have typically not been validated, so their use as a gold standard for reflecting a patient's functional status can be questioned; and (2) gait occupies only a portion of the composite score from a rating scale, so it may not be appropriate to hypothesize a strong relationship with objective measures of gait.

Olsson[24] reported several clinically relevant associations for gait: (1) increased weightbearing pain and decreased vertical floor reaction force, (2) a severe limp and a long weight acceptance time preoperatively, (3) improved walking distance with most gait variables, and (4) the faster the time to ascend stairs the better the values of gait performance. A summary of the correlation between clinical and gait variables are shown in Table 10-4.

In addition, Wadsworth et al.[27] showed that the degree of aid to gait with assistive devices was unrelated to hip motion for hip disease patients, while a statistically significant relationship ($P < 0.05$) was found for selected temporal and distance factors: cadence ($r = 0.83$), walking velocity (0.70), swing/stance ratio ($r = 0.46$), and stride-length/lower-extremity-length ratio ($r = 0.40$).

Knee

Relationship of Clinical and Gait Measures

As with the hip, rating scales have been employed to assess outcomes of intervention, primarily surgical, for arthritis at the knee joint. These rating scales vary in the weighting of items evaluated and in the items included. Some include a mixture of classic clinical assessment items (e.g., pain, range of motion, deformity) and gait.[47] By contrast, Wilson[49] believes that rating scales should reflect the status of only the knee(s) being assessed and should not include such functions as gait, which require the use of multiple joints. Common to all scales, however, is the highest weighting or most points given for pain, an inclusion that is consistent with Laskin's[50] conviction. Laskin stated that the primary indication for total knee replacement surgery is pain and that such factors as restoration of stability and increasing knee motion, although desirable, will rarely represent justification for surgery.

Rating scales have also been used to help determine associations between clinical and gait measures. Using rating scale[4] data (preoperatively, and 6 and 36 months postoperatively) for knee arthroplasty patients, pain and walking ability are depicted[51] (Fig. 10-6). In the same study, increased knee motion in the sagittal plane during gait was associated with decrease in pain. The composite score from the Larson scale yielded statistically significant correlations (r values) for walking velocity (0.43), cadence (0.37), stride length (0.37), and cycle time (−0.35) in 17 total knee arthroplasty patients.[52]

Objective data for gait have enabled investigators to make clinically relevant observations. Andersson[53] stated that walking ability of arthritic knee patients was related to pain, limp, and ability to walk distances. Range of motion (ROM), muscle strength, and pain, as well as multiple upper- and lower-extremity locations in 72 OA patients were related to walking velocity and cadence.[54] Statistically significant but weak correlations were found between these two gait parameters and pain ($r < -0.30$), ROM ($r < 0.30$), and strength ($r < 0.30$).

In 45 OA patients, rating scale composite scores were related to a number of gait variables.[55] Pre- and postoperatively significant ($P < 0.05$) correlations

Table 10-4. Correlation Between Gait Variables and Clinical Examination for Total Hip Patients (n = 119)[a]

Variables	Subjective Opinion		Pain in General		Pain on Weightbearing		Limp		Walking Distance		Harris's Score	
Velocity	***		*		*		***		***		***	
	-.34	-.41[c]	.19	.31	-.21	-.33	.49	.58	.44	.58	.56	.63
			**		**		***		***		***	
Step rate	**				*		***		***		***	
	-.34	-.47	.24	.37	-.25	-.34	.44	.57	.46	.59	.51	.62
					*				**			
Step length (mean)	***		*		**		***		**		***	
	-.27	-.29			-.19	-.24	.40	.43	.30	.46	.43	.45
							***		***		***	
Gait cycle	***		*		**		***		**		***	
	.29	.37	-.21	-.31	.24	.25	-.38	-.52	-.41	-.55	-.45	-.58
							***				***	
Single stance percent gait cycle[b]	-.36	-.41	.19	.27	-.28	-.36	.31	.35	.27	.47	.34	.48
Stance phase percent gait cycle[b]	***						***		***		***	
							-.38	-.43	-.29	-.49	-.33	-.50
							**		***		***	
Weight acceptance percent gait cycle[b]	.33	.38	-.28	-.42	***		*		***		***	
	***		**									
Maximum vertical force percent body weight[b]	-.51	-.52	.23	.60	-.36	-.41	-.41	.62	.41	.49	.49	.69

[a] Weight acceptance was studied in 78 patients.
[b] Of involved leg.
[c] In the numbered pairs, the first correlation value is for the preoperative case, and the second, for the postoperative case.
* The single correlations comprised $p < 0.05$, $p < 0.01$ and $p < 0.001$, ** $p < 0.01$ and $p < 0.001$, *** all single correlations $p < 0.001$.
(From Olsson and Barck,[63] with permission.)

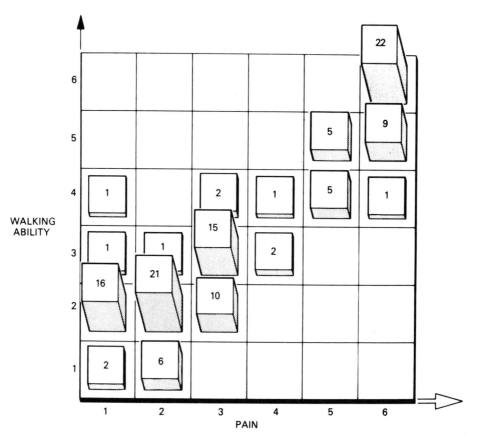

Fig. 10-6. Relationship between pain and walking ability for total knee patients. Figures in the graph indicate the number of observations. Merle d'Aubigne classification (modified) for grading pain and walking ability. (From Kolstad et al.,[51] with permission.)

were reported for walking velocity, lateral head motion, and pain. Smoothness of fore-aft body movement and sagittal motion during gait were significant only for the postoperative stage. For OA and RA patients who had received a total knee, an extremely high relationship was found between measured sagittal plane knee ROM and the motion used during gait.[56] Preoperatively, the correlation was found to be 0.97 and at 12 months postoperatively 0.87. This finding shows that patients with more available knee motion use more motion during gait. By contrast, Minns et al.[57] reported a poor relationship between passive ROM and sagittal motion used during gait. Whether patients optimally use the available motion during gait may be open to question. For example, RA patients have been shown to use only 25 percent of available knee motion during gait compared with 46 percent in normals.[58] Gait-training methods may succeed in improving the use of available knee motion.

From a kinetic viewpoint, varus deformities produce an expected elevation in adductor moment of force during gait in both OA and RA patients.[59] It should be borne in mind that varus deformities are far more common for OA. Excessive force concentrations at the medial compartment also occur in varus knees during gait.[57] For gait, the relative magnitude of the force load at the medial compartment of the knee has been shown for 87 OA and RA patients to be highest in varus knees.[60] Clayton et al.[61] advocate the use of soft tissue release and patellar realignment to aid in the operative achievement of desireable varus-valgus alignment.

Table 10-5 summarizes the results of three studies[58,62,63] showing statistically significant relationships ($P < 0.05$). Among a variety of objective gait measures (temporal and distance factors, kinematics, and kinetics) and clinical findings, several clinically relevant observations can be drawn from this summary. First, the movement behavior of OA and RA appears to differ considerably and, as such, these two entities probably should not be combined into one group when studied. Furthermore, could it be that distinctly different restoration and rehabilitation programs need to be developed for each diagnostic group? In effect, there are probably functional and diagnostic subsets to consider. Second, the commonly assessed clinical measures (e.g., pain, ROM, muscle strength, and deformity) appear frequently in Table 10-5, but with no clear-cut pattern. Since both involve the same function (gait), we should expect the clinical measures and objective measures of gait to be correlated. In addition, the vast majority of correlations reported were far too low to permit prediction of gait ability from clinical findings or vice versa. Therefore, it seems that neither objective gait measures nor clinical measures best reflect a patients' status independently; rather, the two need to be judiciously combined and applied to patient care such that clinical outcomes can be rendered for clearly identified clinical problems.

Deviations from Normal

In studies of patients afflicted primarily with OA and RA, temporal and distance factors, knee motion, and selected floor reaction force measures appear to be discriminating of abnormality. One study cites decreased joint motion alone.[58] Andriacchi et al.[65] found that the key indicators were shorter step length, higher cadence, decreased swing, and stance time. The medially directed floor reaction force in patients was higher. The patterns for moment of force in the sagittal plane were found to be abnormal. Chao et al.[66] cited single-limb support, decreased joint motion in three planes during stance, and three components of the vertical floor reaction force curve (peak and location of the second peak and the location of the trough).

In general, patients walk slower, with more asymmetry, with less joint motion in the involved joint, and with less forward and lateral smoothness during progression, and the rate and release of limb loading are decreased. Numerical data are provided to illustrate some of the deviations from normal[67] (Tables 10-6 and 10-7).

Table 10-5 Summary of Significant Relationships Between Objective Gait Measures and Clinical Findings for the Knee Joint[a]

Gait variable	Gyory et al.[62]	Kettelkamp et al.[58]	Olsson and Barack[63]
	65 OA 43 bilateral age 67 ± 16 22 unilateral, age 65 ± 6 30 RA 24 bilateral, age 54 ± 14 6 unilateral, age 60 ± 22	41 RA 14 bilateral 13 unilateral Age range 34–73	21 OA Postop TKR Age 72 (62–86)
Self-selected walking velocity	OA out of chair Limp (–) Passive ROM Walking distance Muscle strength RA Out of chair	RA	OA postop ROM Rating scale function (–) Walking distance Max. walking velocity Stairclimbing
Cadence	OA Out of chair Walking distance Limp(–) Walking pain (–)		ROM Pain (–) Pain after walking (–) Pain at rest (–) Flex contracture Rating scale–function Joint instability Walking distance
Cycle time			Pain Pain after walking Flex. contracture (–) Rating scale function (–) Walking distance (–) Max. walking velocity (–)
Stride length/lower-extremity length	Sag. motion in stance Limp (–) Muscle strength Medial stability Lateral stability	Pain (–) Standing flex. (–) Joint abn; x-ray	ROM Max. walking velocity
Stance phase (% cycle)	Standing knee flexion Joint abn: x-ray Out of chair		Pain after walking ROM (–) Rating scale–function Walking distance (–) Up stairs (–)

Gait parameter				
Sagittal motion during stance	Passive ROM	Quad strength; Walking pain	Pain (−); Flex. contracture (−); Standing flex. (−); ROM; Varus-valgus angle (−); Joint abn; x-ray (−)	Up stairs
Sagittal motion during swing			Pain (−); Flex. contracture (−); Standing flex (−); ROM; Varus-valgus angle (−); Joint abn; x-ray (−)	
Sagittal motion during cycle		Quad strength		ROM; Sit down; Down stairs
Abduction during cycle			Joint abn; x-ray (−); Varus-valgus angle (−)	
Adduction during cycle	Out of chair		Flex. contracture (−); Varus-valgus angle	
Internal rotation during cycle				
External rotation during cycle				
Weight acceptance time to peak vert. floor reaction force (% cycle)				Pain after walking; Strength (−); Rating scale function; Walking distance (−); Up stairs
Peak vert floor reaction force (% body weight)	Out of chair	Walking pain (−); Ant. instability (−)	Pain (−); Varus-valgus angle (−); joint abn; x-ray	Pain after walking; Rating scale function; Walking distance; Max. walking velocity

[a] $P < 0.05$.

OA, osteoarthritis; RA, rheumatoid arthritis; postop, postoperative; ROM, range of motion; Sag., sagittal; (−), negative relationship with gait variable.

Table 10-6. Comparison of Temporal and Distance Factors (Mean ± 1SD) Between Normal Men and Men with Knee Pain

Gait Component	Normal Men	Men with Knee Pain
Velocity (m/min)		
Free	91 ± 12	57 ± 13[a]
Fast	131 ± 15	81 ± 19[a]
Cadence (steps/min)		
Free	113 ± 10	94 ± 8[a]
Fast	138 ± 10	113 ± 11[a]
Stride length		
In centimeters		
Free	156 ± 13	117 ± 19[a]
Fast	186 ± 16	136 ± 23[a]
In percentage of stature		
Free	89 ± 6	68 ± 11[a]
Fast	107 ± 9	79 ± 13[a]
Absolute difference in successive steps (cm)		
Free	3 (0–3)	5 (0–18)[b]
Fast	4 (0–14)	8 (0–25)[b]
Stride width (cm)		
Free	7.7 ± 3.5	13.2 ± 4.0[a]
Fast	9.1 ± 4.1	13.2 ± 4.1[a]

[a] Patients significantly different from normal ($P < 0.01$).

[b] Patients significantly different from normal ($P < .05$). Values in parentheses indicate range.

(From Murray et al.,[67] with permission.)

Table 10-7. Comparison of Temporal and Distance Factors (Mean ± 1 SD) in Sound Side, Painful Side, and Normal Controls

Gait Component	Normal Men	Men with Knee Pain	
		Sound Side	Painful Side
Foot angle (degrees)			
Free	6.3 ± 5.7	4.6 ± 6.9	10.2 ± 8.7[c]
Fast	5.3 ± 5.5	5.2 ± 7.4	9.3 ± 8.0[c]
Stance phase (sec)			
Free	0.65 ± 0.07	0.86 ± 0.13[b]	0.78 ± 0.09[b]
Fast	0.49 ± 0.05	0.68 ± 0.11[b]	0.62 ± 0.08[b]
Swing phase (sec)			
Free	0.41 ± 0.04	0.42 ± 0.05	0.49 ± 0.05[b]
Fast	0.38 ± 0.03	0.39 ± 0.04	0.44 ± 0.05[b]
Double-limb support (sec)[a]			
Free	0.12 ± 0.03	0.15 ± 0.04[b]	0.21 ± 0.08[b]
Fast	0.06 ± 0.03	0.10 ± 0.04[b]	0.13 ± 0.05[b]

[a] Values for painful side represent the double-limb-support period when the painful limb is forward; for the sound side when the sound limb is forward.

[b] patients significantly different from normal ($P < 0.01$).

[c] Patients significantly different from normal ($P < 0.05$).

(From Murray et al.,[67] with permission.)

One study[68] found that the average elderly person on holiday takes 6,000 steps per day. Eleven total knee patients averaged 7,950 steps per day over a 1-week period, demonstrating a reasonable postoperative activity level.[69]

Effects of Therapeutic Intervention

Reminiscent of the hip, most publications on the knee involve surgical intervention. With rapid and dominating insurgence of knee-replacement surgery, no attempt will be made to report on the plethora of implant hardware types. Sufficient is the following summary statement; studies[65,70–73] have endeavored to identify effects of various implants on gait and that the newer generation of implants seem to provide better functional results.[70]

Compared with preoperative status for total knee replacement patients, postoperative gait assessment 6 months and beyond has yielded the following results.[53,56,64,74] They walked faster, walked farther, with longer and more rapid steps, improved temporal symmetry, smoother head and body motion, and increased knee motion. In these studies, the improvement was short of normal. Even patients who were asymptomatic postoperatively have been shown to exhibit abnormal gait.[65] In two other studies, the primary gain was in knee motion.[66,70] Most improvement was acquired within the first 6 postoperative months. Some additional gains and losses have been reported for the 6-month to 2-year postoperative period.[75]

The magnitude and pattern of sagittal plane motion are among the most improved parameters of gait following total knee replacement (Fig. 10-7). In an interesting study by Brinkman and Perry,[76] the angular velocity of the knee motion was also evaluated in OA and RA patients. Extrapolating from the curves provided, it appears that the angular velocity rates, when adjusted for walking velocity, were normal both pre- and postoperatively for both groups. Descriptive data shown in Table 10-8 also illustrate a common finding, a deficit in terminal knee extension during gait. These patients have a deficit in knee range of motion, with the passive motion often significantly exceeding the active motion, a situation which is commonly referred to as extensor lag. Clearly, although not adequately addressed in the literature, preventative and restorative intervention for OA and RA patients should emphasize retention and/or acquisition of terminal knee extension both actively and passively. This terminal knee extension should then be transferred for use at the late stance/early swing period of the gait cycle. With limited success, posterior capsulotomies can be performed on patients with severe flexion contractures. However, the functional outcome in 37 patients ranged from ability to walk with two crutches to bed rest for most patients. The number able to walk without assistive devices increased from 5 to 12.[77]

Rheumatoid arthritic patients receiving total knee replacements tend to be more severely involved and improve proportionately (pre- vs. postoperatively) a greater amount. However, they do not tend to reach the level of gait perfor-

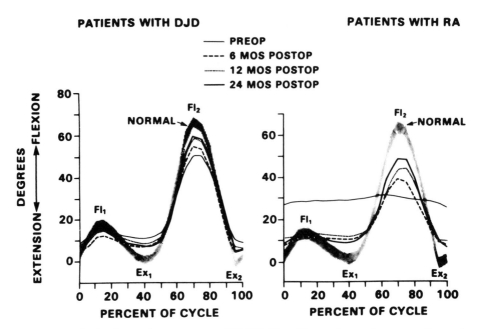

Fig. 10-7. Sagittal plane knee motion in DJD (OA) and RA patients who received a total knee replacement. (From Murray et al.,[75] with permission.)

mance as the OA patients.[75] Severity of involvement and disease of patients needs to be seriously considered when expectations and clinical objectives are identified. For example, Simon et al.[78] compared the gait characteristics of 12 unilateral patients with OA and an age-matched control group. The patients were a select group in the sense that they had only one knee joint involved; as such, their level was representative of only 2.5 percent of a large OA arthritic data base. At 2 years postoperatively, no differences were found between the control and patient group for any of the gait parameters considered: walking velocity, stride length, angular knee motion at knees and ankles, muscle action potential, and amount of mechanical work at the lower extremities. By contrast, Collopy et al.[56] studied patients who in the main had multiple joint pathology bilaterally, and the resulting postoperative status of patients was far removed from normal. Variability among the patients was also great. For example, the preoperative walking velocity ranged from 5 to 67 cm/s and 15 to 150 cm/s postoperatively.[56]

Berman et al.[79] subdivided OA patients into three groups: (1) unilateral total knee replacement with no symptoms in contralateral knee, (2) unilateral total knee replacement with asymptomatic contralateral knee, and (3) arthritis bilaterally treated with total knee replacement. The gait of each group improved, but groups 1 and 3 improved more than did group 2. It was concluded that asymptomatic arthritis can impair gait. Skinner et al.[52] indicated that the OA and RA disease processes are responsible for a loss in proprioceptive joint position

Table 10-8. Knee Kinematics in Normal and Arthritic Patients

Subject	Gait Velocity (m/min)	Maximum Extension (Flexion)[a]	Maximum Flexion (°)	Range (°)	Flexion Rate (°/sec)	Extension Rate (°/sec)
Healthy free speed	80 (±10)	2 (±5)	62 (±6)	60 (±7)	344 (±64)	344 (±58)
Rheumatoid arthritic						
preop	27 (±15)	21 (±13) (0)[a]	36 (±13) ⟨50⟩	15 (±14) ⟨50⟩	82 (±79) ⟨198⟩	83 (±88) ⟨213⟩
postop	43 (±16)	6 (±8) ⟨0⟩	42 (±13) ⟨52⟩	36 (±13) ⟨52⟩	201 (±79) ⟨226⟩	211 (±87) ⟨238⟩
Osteoarthritic						
preop	38 (±12)	6 (±9) ⟨0⟩	39 (±8) ⟨52⟩	33 (±14) ⟨52⟩	154 (±66) ⟨226⟩	196 (±99) ⟨238⟩
postop	52 (±14)	8 (±8) ⟨0⟩	47 (±14) ⟨55⟩	40 (±13) ⟨55⟩	237 (±84) ⟨263⟩	227 (±93) ⟨276⟩

[a] Number in brackets, ⟨ ⟩, indicates value of healthy subjects ambulating at gait velocity similar to arthritic group. (From Brinkman and Perry,[76] with permission.)

sense. A clinical implication from these works is to consider incorporating biofeedback in the prevention and restoration programs. Training to achieve designated knee motion and strength targets may aid in the augmentation of limited existing or auxiliary neurosensory mechanism toward improved function.

Again, reminiscent of the lack of attention devoted to the rehabilitation aspects of the treatment of total knee patients, only Simon et al.[78] described the postoperative program in an investigative study. Active assisted exercise and weightbearing was initiated on day 2 and gait training started during days 8 to 10 postoperatively. Following discharge, the patients rode a stationary bicycle without resistance for a minimum of 20 min/day. Landon and Richtsmeier[80] reported on an impressive postoperative physical therapy program to include consideration of assistive devices, but the program has apparently not been reported in a prospective study involving patients.

The total knee operation carries with it a risk of complication. By way of consolation, Heywood and Learmonth[81] reported that a tibiofemoral arthrodesis as a salvage procedure improved the walking ability of all patients made worse by complications of the arthroplasty. The optimal knee angle for arthrodesis is reported to be 30° flexion, and the advantages of the procedure are the ability of the patients to perform rigorous activity with full stability and freedom from pain.[82] Gait has been characterized in nine patients with knee resection arthrodesis.[83] The average self-selected velocity was 93 ± 16 cm/s. There was a higher step time with the fused limb (0.61 vs. 0.51 second) to allow the fused limb to swing. The stance time on the sound side was higher (42 vs. 32 percent). Increased dorsiflexion and delayed hip extension in late stance were used to compensate for the lack of knee flexion. Increased pelvic obliquity, hip abduction, and ankle plantar flexion permitted the clearance of the fused limb. The vertical component of the floor reaction force was decreased for the fused limb during gait.

Force of the medial tibial plateau is significantly influenced by the presence of varus or valgus deformity (Fig 10-8). High tibial osteotomy is an operative procedure for correction of varus deformities at the knee. Using dynamic mechanical analyses of force plate and light emitting diode data, Prodromos et al.[84] demonstrated that the osteotomy significantly reduced the adductor (varus) moment of force during gait (Fig. 10-9).

The nonoperative treatment options which can effect gait in patients are diverse, but the number of studies in the literature is scant. As a general guideline, rest is advised for the RA patient when the disease is active and the joints inflamed and during the nonacute stage walking is a desirable form of exercise. Nonetheless, the specific role of rest and exercise in RA is unclear.[85] Walking is a critical function to be retained. Barraclough et al.[86] used hydrotherapy, gradual progression of walking with walking aids, optional footware and correction of ankle deformities in a rehabilitation effort for 32 severely involved rheumatoid arthritics who were unable to walk. Following the rehabilitiation effort, most of the patients were able to attain a useful degree of independence.

Wedged insoles is a conservative treatment for patients with medial knee

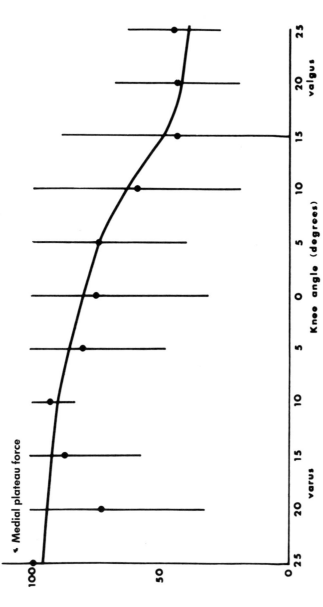

Fig. 10-8. Percentage medial plateau load during stance phase plotted against varus-valgus knee angle. Vertical lines represent 1 SD from the mean. (From Johnson and Waugh,[60] with permission.)

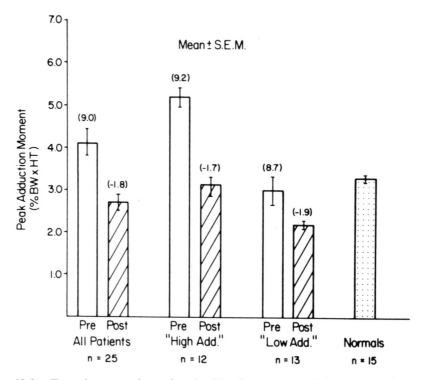

Fig. 10-9. For gait, comparison of peak adduction moments of force at knee between patients grouped together, and for patients with high and low adduction moments. Numbers in parentheses are the average alignments of the knee preoperatively and postoperatively. A positive number indicates varus alignment and a negative number valgus alignment. (From Prodromos et al.,[84] with permission.)

joint pain and OA.[87] Lateral wedges and indomethacin was the treatment in 67 patients and indomethacin alone was given to 40 patients in the control group. The treatment group's decrease in pain and increase in walking distance ability was statistically superior to the control group. For example, the average change in pain was from mild—moderate to none—mild. Walking distance capability increased from 0.5—1.0 km to 1.0—unlimited km. No change in radiographic findings was found (e.g., widening of the medial joint space). The wedged insole was most successful for patients with mild OA involvement (radiographic staging categories I, II, and III).

Thirty-four nonacute RA patients were divided into two groups who each performed 15 to 20 minutes of ordinary physical training five times per week for 6 weeks.[88] The treatment group performed 20 to 40 minutes of additional exercise consisting of resistive exercise for the quadriceps and interval training on a bicycle ergometer. As part of the evaluation process, patients were asked to walk an 850-m course as fast as possible before and after the exercise training program. The treatment group increased their maximum walking velocity from 151 to 177 cm/s, 12 percent superior to the control group. This study demonstrates that selected forms of exercise can have a positive indirect effect on gait.

In a study of cadaveric knees, Seedholm et al.[68] discovered that articular cartilaginous lesions at the patellofemoral joint were localized in the range of 40 to 80° of knee flexion. These workers hypothesized that high joint force at the knee during such activities as negotiating stairs and ramps may be responsible for the lesions, particularly in people in poor physical condition, a state that seems to characterize most of our current society. By way of clinical consideration, the key question is this: is it possible to optimally condition articular cartilage to withstand the microtrauma and occasional modest forceful insults encountered in daily life? Rehabilitation tends to focus on muscle strength, neural control, bone strength and cardiopulmonary efficiency. In the case of arthritis, why not include the health of the articular cartilage?

In an early study, Moll et al.[89] reported that a favorable total knee replacement result was demonstrated by the increase in the number of patients who were able to walk without assistive devices (17 to 37 percent). Eighty-eight percent of patients judged the treatment intervention successful, while 12 percent considered the outcome unsuccessful. Judgment of treatment success or lack of same was made by each patient, a rendering that may too often be overlooked. Perhaps more credence should be overtly given to the patient's self-assessment of treatment outcome. Family members, therapists, nurses, and physicians also tend to make independent evaluations of treatment outcome, thus confounding the efficacy of treatment picture. As we have seen in this section on the knee, gait can be a form of treatment or a function evaluated to assess treatment outcome. At this point, there is no available gold standard against which rating scales and/or objective gait assessment methods can be judged. It is my conviction that such a standard or standards will not be forthcoming without a considerable amount of creative work. Whatever the approach, the assessment of gait must be easily interpreted[90] and contributory to a diagnosis and/or solution to a clinical problem.

Ankle

One treatment for severe involvement of the arthritic ankle has been surgical arthrodesis. Boobbyer[91] reported on postoperative status (1 to 17 years) for ankle arthrodesis patients whose most common indication for surgery was post-traumatic OA. Thirty-three percent had no limp, 33 percent a slight limp, and 34 percent a distinct limp. On the fused side, RA patients in one study tended to minimize heel-toe and heel-off to toe-off periods of stance phase.[92] Taking into consideration bilateral knee and ankle motion for 19 patients with ankle arthrodesis, the ideal position for fusion of the ankle was found to be neutral flexion, that is, 0 to 5° valgus angulation of the hindfoot, and 5 to 10° of external rotation.[93] This position was claimed to permit the greatest compensatory motion at the foot and exerted the least strain on the knee. Following triple arthrodesis, 80 percent of 58 patients walked without a limp when wearing shoes.[94] In another study, 12 post-traumatic arthritic patients were evaluated 8 years after arthrodesis.[95] The walking velocity for the group was 113 ± 18 cm/s.

Small foot placement asymmetries were found; single-limb stance 37 percent on sound side, 33 percent on fused, and step lengths of 63 cm with the sound lead leg and 63 cm for the fused side. Interestingly, when walking with shoes on, the sagittal motion magnitude and patterns for the pelvis, hip, knee, and ankle were essentially the same on both sides. Unshod, the patients were slightly slower (103 ± 15 cm/s), and other parameters of gait were also altered in a negative sense. In effect, the shoe and the articular motion in the small joints of the foot were the key compensators for the loss of ankle motion (Fig. 10-10). As a consequence, motion testing of these small foot joints, and, if necessary, passive mobilization, should be considered in the evaluation and treatment of arthritic patients so that the quality of gait is maximized.

The results of the total ankle replacement operative procedure were found to be disappointing when compared with prosthetic replacements at other joints.[96] Abnormal gait patterns were said to be associated with muscle weakness, particularly the plantarflexors. The issue of postoperative rehabilitation was raised.

Rheumatoid arthritis involvement at the ankle and subtalar joints can lead to decreased walking velocity and single limb support time. Application of rigid orthoses for these cases has been shown to reduce pain, and allow greater walking velocity and a more normal single limb support time.[97]

Foot

By virtue of the large number of bones and joints in the foot, it is several orders of magnitude more complex than the other lower-extremity articulations. Scranton et al.[98] reported 23 different diagnoses in 96 patients who presented

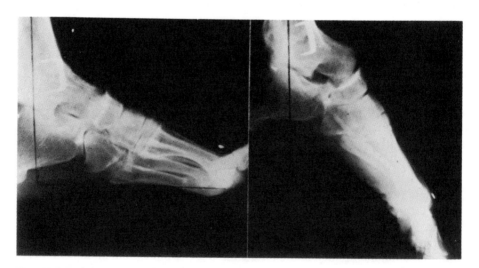

Fig. 10-10. Lateral roentgenogram of a fused ankle with dorsiflexion (left) and plantar flexion (right) stress applied. Note the displacement of the nonfused joints of the foot. (From Mazur et al.,[190] with permission.)

with painful foot problems. The subtalar joint is responsible for transferring the axial rotation of the tibia to the foot. While there is little or no motion at the intertarsal and tarsal metatarsal joints,[99] extension of the toes causes the plantar fascia to become taut.[99] In late stance during walking, the toes extend to ~60 to 65 degrees in the normal case,[100] and the resulting tautness of the plantar fascia provides dynamic stability for the foot.

Far beyond the scope of this book is a presentation of foot abnormalities. The reader is directed to a number of reviews which appear in the literature.[101–104]

Deviations from Normal

As we might expect, a problem at the hindfoot manifests itself in a decreased floor reaction force at the initial peak, whereas the peak during late stance is decreased for patients with forefoot anomalies.[105] The same results seem to hold for the RA patient.[106]

Studies of RA patients and gait have demonstrated that, compared with normals, in stance phase the center of pressure tends to shift laterally on the plantar surface of the foot.[106–108] At late stance, the focus of force moves from under the toes and first metatarsal to the outer three metatarsal heads (Fig. 10-11, Table 10-9). The forces at the metatarsal heads during gait are two to three times more than normal.[107]

Minns et al.[107] also found a strong relationship between the static (standing) and dynamic (walking) pressure distributions at the plantar surface of the foot. Whether such a relationship holds for the flatfoot or cavus problems is unclear. Simple footprints and use of the arch index[109] (Fig. 10-12) could provide a means of investigating this issue in the clinical realm. Stewart[110] has suggested that wearing shoes in childhood may be the cause of problem feet. In a fascinating multiethnic study, he has found that unshod children tend not to have symptomatic foot problems, whether they have flatfeet or not.[111]

Therapeutic Intervention

In a group of subjects with flexible flat feet, low-dye taping, and a heel cup caused a decrease in force at the midfoot but shifted the center of pressure medially. While the medial arch support shifted the center of pressure lat-

Table 10-9. Gait Comparison of Location of Maximum Force at Plantar Surface of Foot in Normal and Rheumatoid Patients

	No. of Feet	
	Normal (%)	Rheumatoid (%)
First metatarsal	81 (60)	51 (37)
Second and third metatarsal	36 (27)	22 (16)
Fourth and fifth metatarsal	17 (13)	65 (47)

(From Minns and Braxford,[107] with permission.)

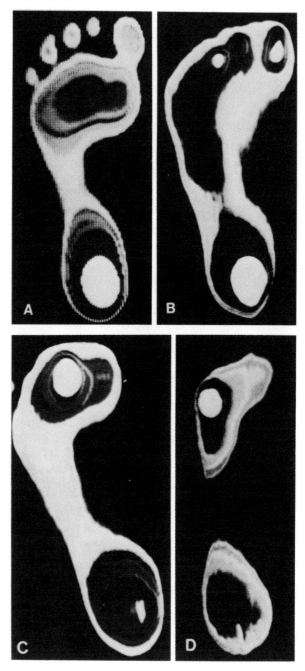

Fig. 10-11. Pedobarograph foot pressure distribution during midstance. A, the normal foot; B, maximum pressure at first metatarsal area; C, maximum pressure at second and third metatarsal areas; D, maximum pressure in the forth and fifth metatarsal areas. (From Minns and Braxford,[107] with permission.)

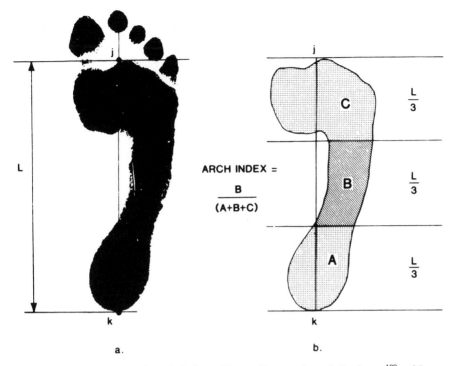

ARCH INDEX =

$$\frac{B}{(A+B+C)}$$

Fig. 10-12. Illustration of arch index. (From Cavanagh and Rodgers,[109] with permission.)

erally.[98] Walking casts have been effective in reducing pressure at the first and third metatarsal heads in patients with Hansen's disease.[59] The heel cup has been shown to be effective in relieving symptoms in the case of the painful heel syndrome probably because the force distribution during stance is distributed over a larger area.[112] In contradistinction, the heel cup was not effective for plantar fasciitis.

Simple, forgiving, and supple footware has been advocated for RA patients to attain greater pressure distribution.[113] Clearly, various types of footware significantly influence the heel to toe center of pressure pattern during gait (Fig. 10-13).

Erosion of the joints produces a variety of joint deformities at the foot. These deformities contribute to abnormal gait, consisting of decreased velocity, cadence, stride length, poor heel-toe pattern, and abnormal weightbearing. Nonsurgical intervention may include joint stabilization methods, assisted gait devices, orthotics, and physical therapy procedures[114] (Table 10-10).

Excessive foot-pronation may cause the patella to track laterally, or perhaps sublux over the femoral groove and cause irritation and articular degeneration.[115] A medial heel wedge is deemed appropriate for correcting this gait abnormality.[115] Also soft or resilient heels have been shown to reduce by 50

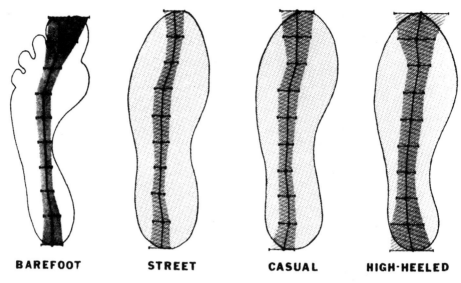

BAREFOOT   **STREET**   **CASUAL**   **HIGH-HEELED**

Fig. 10-13. Mean center of pressure patterns in normal subjects wearing different shoe types. The width of the pattern represents ±1 SD. Note that 10 discrete points are delineated for comparison. (From Katoh et al.,[191] with permission.)

percent the "shock" at heel strike, a reduction that may help avert joint degeneration.[116]

Walking velocity, cadence, step length, percentage support phase, and percentage stance phase were reported as less than normal for patients who received an osteotomy surgical procedure for hallux valgus.[117] When compared preoperatively and postoperatively, 21 female hallux valgus patients did not demonstrate a significant difference in objective temporal and distance gait measures. However, 19 of the 21 patients were satisfied with the results of the osteotomy so the authors speculated that the patients' satisfaction could be attributed to improved cosmesis and reduction of pain during walking.

Fractures and Gait

Very little objective and detailed information could be found on gait as it was associated with fracture outcome. This section briefly describes the rationale for fracture care and report on some studies involving fractures at selected lower-extremity sites.

Basic medical principles of fracture care are centered around acquisition and maintenance of bony alignment, immobilization and restoration of function.[118] Pain, swelling, and infection are other clinical concerns.

The biologic events following the initial insult of bone deformity, hemorrhage, edema, tissue necrosis, and inflammation are complex. Sequential events are proliferation of repair tissue, organization and removal of dead tissue, entry of bone-forming cells, bridging the fracture gap with fibrocartilaginous tissue to establish union, and finally healing by remodeling of the bridged fracture gap and reorganization of newly formed bone tissue.[119]

At some point in the sequence of bone healing, exercise and walking are typically initiated. A seemingly unanswered question is how (1) bony union and healing and (2) restoration of function can be achieved in the shortest optimal period of time and minimize tissue atrophy? Should walking be used to prevent the retardation process as well as restore function?

For 2 to 4 weeks following a fracture, loading of bone is probably of little benefit in facilitating bony union.[120] It is clear, however, that bone repair is desirably effected by compressive loading and not tension. Therefore, until the bone is healed, it would appear prudent to train patients to walk flatfooted with minimal lower-extremity joint movement during any level of partial weightbearing and in so doing minimize the bending moment of force at the bone (see Fig. 10-14). Cyclic bending of the fractured bone as might occur during partial or full "heel-toe" weightbearing gait in the early healing phase could result in a stress fracture "conversion of soft fiber bone to fibrous tissue."[113] Training toward quality of walking to include a heel-toe gait should be reserved for the time when the fracture is indisputably healed.

Pelvic Fractures

Motor vehicle and motorcycle accidents were the most frequent cause of pelvic fractures in 84 patients, 53 of whom were diagnosed as having Malgaigne fractures,[121] whereby there was a longitudinal fracture through the sacrum and through the ipsilateral superior and inferior pubic rami. At 2- to 12-year follow-up, 30 percent of the patients assessed had a gait abnormality.

Hip Fractures

This area is also addressed in Chapter 9 (Aging and Gait). Barnes[122] reported that 40 to 50 percent of the noninstitutionalized elderly patients with hip fractures reclaim their prefracture walking ability level. Positive outcome is expressed in another way using the D'Aubigne scale for 69 patients, in that the post-treatment quality of gait was poor (7 percent), fair (12 percent), good (51 percent), and excellent (26 percent).[92] Results for the institutionalized elderly are disheartening. In a study of 188 patients, 37 percent died within 6 weeks and only 20 percent ultimately achieved ambulatory status.[13] For hip fractures, the key predictors of poor outcome are age over 75 years, cerebral dysfunction, multiple secondary problems, and low prefracture functional status.[123] These outcome studies on function to include gait have implications for health care planning and budgeting. During rehabilitation, the quality of gait as reflected by temporal and distance factors has been shown to improve during crutch walking but not when the transition was made to walk with canes.[124] The optimal

Table 10-10. Gait Deviations, Physical Examination Findings, and Treatment Goals for Selected Foot Problems

Gait Deviations	Physical Examination Findings	Treatment Goals
Pronated foot	Tenderness over subtalar midtarsal area	Relieve subtalar and midtarsal joint stresses
Shuffled progression	Limited inversion range	Increase ankle inversion
Decreased step length	Weak and painful posterior tibialis muscle	Strengthen posterior tibialis muscle
Initial contact with medial border of foot	Pronated weightbearing posture of foot	Stabilize hypermobile joints with rigid orthosis
Decreased single-limb balance	Lax medial collateral ligament of knee	Maintain neutral alignment in stance by foot positioning
Prolonged double-support phase		
Late heel rise		
Plantarflexion of ipsilateral limb in swing		
Genu valgus with weightbearing		
Hallux valgus	Lateral deviation of great toe	Accommodate foot with wide toe box shoe
Lateral and posterior weight shift	Swelling of first MTP joint	Increase extension of great toe
Late heel rise	Shortening of flexor hallucis brevis muscle	Relieve weightbearing stresses
Decreased single-limb balance	Tenderness of great toe	
	Weakness of great toe abduction	
Metatarsophalangeal joint subluxation	Painful MTP heads with weightbearing	Redistribute pressure with metatarsal bar
Diminished rolloff	Callus formation over MTP heads	Relieve pressure with soft cutout shoe insert
Decreased single-limb stance		

Gait/Functional	Clinical Findings	Treatment
Apropulsive progression Decreased single-limb balance	Ulcerations over MTP heads Limited MTP flexion Prominent MTP heads	Increase flexion mobility of MTP joints Accommodate foot with extradepth shoe
Hammer or claw toes Diminished rolloff Decreased single-limb stance Apropulsive progression Decreased single-limb balance	Posture of MTP joint hyperextension with proximal and distal interphalangeal joint flexion Posture of MTP and distal interphalangeal joint hyperextension with proximal interphalangeal flexion Callus formation at plantar tips and dorsum of proximal interphalangeal joint Limited MTP flexion	Improve toe alignment with metatarsal bar Accommodate foot with extradepth shoe Diminish pressure with soft shoe Increase toe mobility
Painful heel Toe-heel pattern No heel contact in stance Decreased stride length Decreased velocity Plantarflexion of ankle in swing Increased hip flexion in swing Decreased step length of contralateral limb	Painful active plantar flexion Painful passive and active dorsiflexion Swelling and pain at Achilles insertion Tenderness over spur Decreased ankle dorsiflexion range	Decrease inflammation with steroid injection or modalities Relieve weightbearing stress Decrease pressure over spur with soft shoe insert Maintain ankle mobility

(From Dimonte and Light,[114] with permission.)

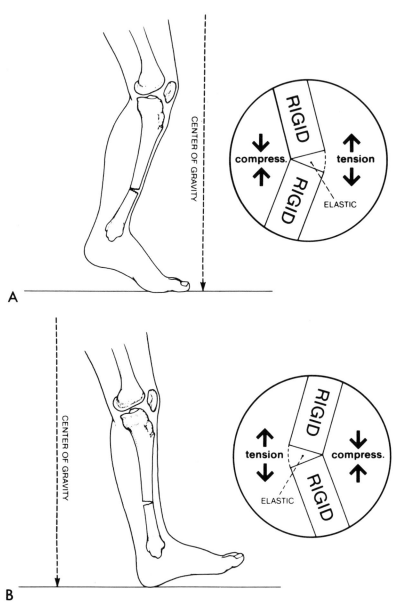

Fig. 10-14.   Illustration of the ill effects of heel-toe gait on ununited fractures. Note differences between bending moment effects at fracture site during late stance and early stance. (From Bassett,[120] with permission.)

progression and associated guidelines for assisted gait in rehabilitation hip fracture patients have apparently not been developed and used to assess changes in patient status and outcome. Gait training in the home environment following hospital discharge is needed. For example, 68 hip fracture patients whose mean age was 79 years were able to walk without an assistive device or walked with a cane and yet more than 50 percent of the group did not leave the home to go shopping.[125]

Femoral Fractures

A cast brace with plaster of paris cylinders around the thigh and shank with an intervening hinge at the knee has become a popular form of treatment for femoral shaft fractures.[125-129] This form of treatment permits early ambulation and ostensibly permits compression force at the fracture site to promote healing. The fractured femur is placed in traction until the third week.[30] In a study of 79 cases of femoral shaft fracture, the cast brace was applied and early walking was initiated over a wide range of postinjury times (72 percent up to 42 weeks and 28 percent after 28 weeks). Again, guidelines for gait training and associated walking ability outcomes have not been reported and evaluated. Farrell[130] described the cast-brace treatment from a nursing perspective.

Tibial Fractures

Drennan et al.[131] stated that for tibial fractures weightbearing should be avoided for 12 to 16 weeks postinjury to permit cancellous and fibrocartilaginous callus to form. On the other hand, early ambulation has also been advocated.[132,133] In a follow-up study of 26 tibial fracture patients for which Hoffman external fixation was used, 65 percent walked with no limp, 12 percent with a slight limp, 4 percent with a moderate limp, and 19 percent with a severe limp.[134] In a rarely found discourse on postinjury rehabilitation procedures, Brown and Urban[135] reported on 63 tibial fractures suffered by military personnel. The patients were casted to the level of the hip, partial weight bearing crutch walking as tolerated was started the second postinjury day, cast was removed in 6 to 8 weeks and the patient remained at bedrest for 2 to 10 days until the knee flexion of 60° and knee extension with a 10-pound weight was demonstrated. Progressive weightbearing gait with crutches was used. The criteria for cast removal were radiographic evidence of mature bridging callous and lack of tenderness at the fracture site. The patient was progressed to walk with a cane when he could extend the knee with a 15-pound weight. Unfortunately, the rationale for the association between knee extensor strength and gait training progression in the rehabilitation of the patient was not provided. The only outcome reported which related to gait was that 57 of the 63 patients ended up with no disability.

Ankle Fractures

Osteochondral fractures of the talus yield a disconcerting outcome. In one study 31 percent were unable to run and 74 percent reported a problem with pain.[136] Rowley et al.[137] compared open reduction with internal fixation and closed manipulation techniques in management of 42 ankle fractures. Foot angle and step length measures of gait did not meaningfully discriminate between the two techniques.

Rehabilitation Following Fractures

Gait training protocols with guidelines and rationale have apparently not been developed, established and evaluated in the context of postfracture care. The load limb monitor seems to offer promise as a gait training method to target prescribed levels of dynamic weightbearing force during the post fracture rehabilitation period.[138] This method has been shown to be valid and reliable basically as a footswitch device for obtaining temporal and distance factors.[139,140] Wolf and Binder-Macleod[140] simultaneously obtained floor reaction force measures from a force plate and a load limb monitor and concluded the load limb monitor as ineffective for measuring force. However, I believe that the load limb monitor may have enough accuracy and precision to permit weight bearing force surveillance for desired ranges of targeted force. The study by Wolf and Binder-Macleod[140] involved normal subjects and associated vertical floor reaction force patterns for normal subjects. The load limb monitor in postfracture care seems to have potential value during the early gait-training period, when the patient may be instructed to walk with a partial weightbearing gait and maintain a foot-flat position during stance. For this type of intended use, the load limb monitor may be a valid force sensing treatment modality in postfracture care.

Soft Tissue Injuries

"Garden variety" aches and pains probably resulting from chronic static and dynamic overuse of body tissue may very well affect gait in subtle ways. Carried a step further, pain, effusion, and overload resulting from overuse injuries may occur because of slightly repetitive subtle abnormal movement patterns which may produce undue force on body structures.[141] Whether gait-training methods can be identified and demonstrated helpful for the above situation is open to question. This section presents several common soft tissue injuries in association with gait.

Cruciate Ligaments Injuries

Compensatory alterations in gait seem to be imposed by abnormal knee mechanics in the cruciate deficient knee. Compared with normal controls, anterior cruciate ligament (ACL) deficient knee subjects during gait demonstrated

(1) increased A-P tibiofemoral translation,[142] (2) decreased medial lateral translation,[143] (3) increased adduction (varus) during midstance and external rotation during the transition from swing to stance,[143] (4) at early stance decreased muscle activity (EMG) at the quadriceps and increased activity of the biceps femoris, and (5) at mid- to late stance decreased hamstring activity.[144] Surgically transferred pes anserine muscles have been shown to be highly active during stance phase, thus appropriately aiding in control of anteromedial rotary instability of the knee.[145] From a rehabilitation standpoint, it should be remembered that increased compressive loading (which can be provided by co-contraction) has been shown to significantly increase the stability of the knee joint.[146] Comparing ACL results and normal, one study[147] did not find any muscle action differences, and another[148] no differences in angular motion in any of the three planes. Walking velocity seems to be unaffected[143,144]; however, temporal and distance indices of symmetry were not assessed. Use of the Lenox Hill brace for unstable knees increased energy cost by 5 percent.[72]

Chondromalacia Patellae

Kinematic analyses were performed for treadmill walking to compare knee movement patterns between symptomatic females with chondromalacia patellar and normal subjects.[149] Compared with normals, the chondromalacia subjects exhibited less flexion during stance phase and a sharp inward femoral rotation immediately preceding heel strike. Increased lateral femoral rotation was found during swing phase during level walking and down a 15° slope (Fig. 10-15). This demonstrated abnormal tibiofemoral motion no doubt influences the tracking of the patella in the intercondylar groove potentially creating undesirable joint stress on the femoral and/or patellar component of the articulation. Ramig et al.[115] observed that one cause of lateral patellar tracking is excessive foot pronation during stance. Walker[150] reported on patients with passive hyperextension (3 to 20°) of the knees who were diagnosed with chondromalacia. The excessive knee extension tended to carry over to late stance phase of gait. This abnormality was effectively corrected and symptoms reduced with the use of a heel lift in patients with hyperextension of 10° or less (Fig. 10-16). Using a force plate, it has been demonstrated that unilaterally high medial pronation forces occur in subjects with one extermity longer than the other. Correction of the leg length inequality with a heel lift reduced slightly this medial force.[151] A recently developed kinematic magnetic resonance imaging (MRI) technique capable of dynamically quantifying patellar movement with respect to the femur may prove helpful in better diagnosis and treatment of anterior knee pain problems.[152]

Shinsplints

DeLacerda[153,154] showed in isolated cases that shinsplints are associated with pronated feet. There is a tendency for displacement of the navicular bone

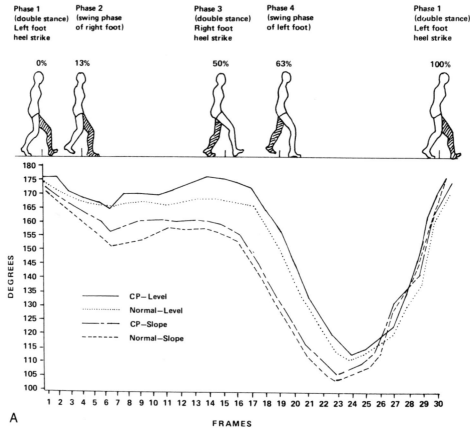

Fig. 10-15. **(A)** Gait comparison of knee flexion and extension between normals and patients with chondromalacia patellae (cp). (From Dillon et al.,[149] with permission.) *(Figure continues.)*

and longitudinal arch. The hypothesis here is that excessive stress occurs in the resulting distended tibialis anterior muscle during gait.

Achilles Tendon

Achilles tendinitis is an overuse type of injury. Tenderness seems to occur at the medial aspect of the insertion so that foot pronation has again been implicated as a cause.[155] Mixed results for walking ability were found following different combinations of ultrasound, exercise and heel pad treatment intervention. Unfortunately, the walking velocity was not reported for the three groups in this study of Achilles tendinitis. In the case of Achilles tendon rupture, controversy exists regarding the best form of post injury treatment (surgery or conservative approach to include casting).[156] EMG was used to illustrate indi-

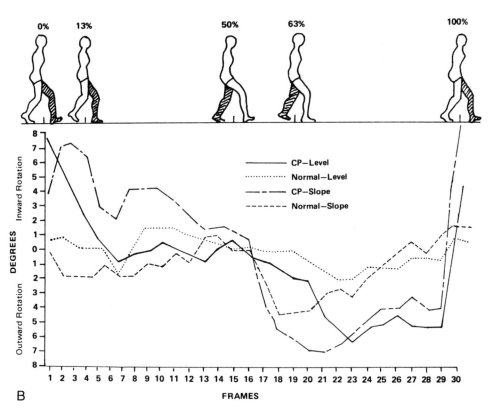

Fig. 10-15. (*Continued.*) **(B)** Gait comparison of femoral axial rotation between normals and patients with chondromalacia patellae (cp).

rectly that a person can walk in a cast without risking excessive tension along the Achilles tendon.[157]

Ankle Sprain

The lateral collateral ligament is an ankle structure frequently injured. Glick et al.[158] suggested an association between lateral collateral ankle injuries and the tilt of the talus. Adhesive taping is a common form of treatment for stabilization. Following rigorous exercise, taping has been shown to lose 40 percent of its support.[159] Taping may provide sensory stimulation of peroneus brevis to provide ankle support.[158] In a fine study by Laughman et al.[160] ankle motion was shown to be reduced by 27 percent during gait; following exercise, the motion reduction was acceptably retained at 19 percent. In this study walking velocity, cadence, step length, percentage stance, percentage single limb support, and percentage double limb support were not affected by taping the ankle. In another experimental study, Carmines et al.[161] applied a closed basketweave with

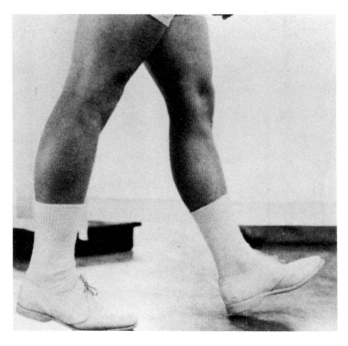

Fig. 10-16.   Illustration of knee hyperextension during late stance. (From Walker and Schreck,[150] with permission.)

a heel lock taping approach. As a result, the subjects walked with a 20 percent reduction in sagittal plane ankle motion. With taping, the foot flat to heel-up point in the gait cycle occurred 5 percent earlier in stance, and phalangeal extension was higher (7°). There was no difference in the floor reaction force patterns, but taping seemed to reduce the impulse at the heel and forefoot while increasing the impulse at the midfoot. An air stirrup in conjunction with ice massage and dorsiflexion exercise has been reported as a form of treatment for ankle sprains.[162] The air stirrup must be worn with high-top shoes in order to be effective. The stirrup purportedly permits sagittal plane motion but limits inversion and eversion. The recommended progression for gait was a three-point gait, two-point gait, and no assistive device when the patient was able to walk without a limp.

Contractures

Perry maintains that traditionally rest, as a form of treatment for musculoskeletal injuries and postoperative care, has been unduly emphasized with the associated risk of impaired physical function. Evidence is provided that physiologic positioning of inflamed or swollen joints to minimize tissue strain introduces motion restrictions at 15° plantar flexion and 30° flexion at the hip and knee. Hip joint hypomobility manifests observable gait abnormalities (Figs. 10-17 to 10-19). A simulated gait-training technique for patients with plantar flexor foreshortening is shown in Figure 10-20.[163]

Spinal Abnormalities

The literature has a sparse number of reports on gait and spinal abnormalities, despite the fact that the trunk is a weightbearing region of the body.

Acute and chronic low back pain and gait have received some attention in recent years. Thomas et al.[164] assessed physical therapy intervention consisting of twice-daily mat exercise, targeted walking distance, and targeted cycling for chronic low back pain patients (pain duration 6 months or more). Following this inpatient program, patients showed improvement in the following ways: walking velocity (increased 35 percent), cadence (increased 15 percent), and energy expenditure (decreased 18 percent). Apart from walking slow (average 74 cm/s),[165] 30 patients with lumbosacral problems showed no other gait abnormalities

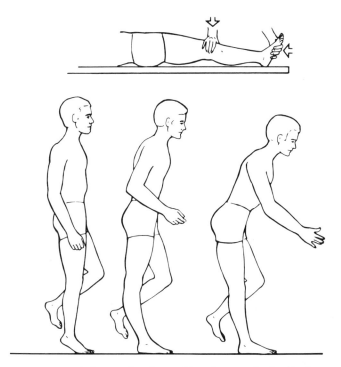

Fig. 10-17. Illustration of abnormal gait resulting from a plantar flexion contracture. Clinical finding is shown at top. Abnormal gait is characterized by premature heel-off during stance (left), genu recurvatum at midstance (center figure), and excessive forward trunk movement with hip flexion during mid to late stance (right). (From Perry,[192] with permission.)

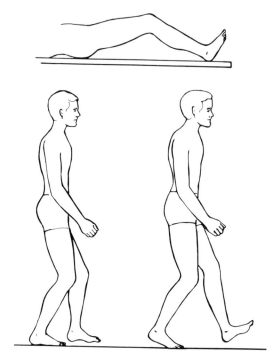

Fig. 10-18. Illustration of abnormal gait resulting from a knee flexion contracture. Clinical finding is shown at top. Abnormal gait is characterized by excessive dorsiflexion during late swing-early stance on the uninvolved side and early heel-off during midstance. (From Perry,[192] with permission.)

in terms of temporal and distance or floor reaction force asymmetry between sides. From a series of studies, it appears that back pain patients have less inherent ability to attenuate the forces imposed on the body at heel strike.[166-168] An accelerometry method was used in which a ratio was the quotient from peak acceleration at the femoral condyle over the acceleration at the forehead. Voloshin and Wosk make a case for using Viscoelastic inserts for back pain patients by virtue of their findings that the inserts spare the body of some imposed shock.[167] In a rating scale approach in evaluating 382 black pain patients, 79 percent reported good to excellent results by wearing the inserts compared with 44 percent good to excellent results for the controls.[168]

An exciting study of 18 chronic low back pain patients and 18 normals reported that pain behaviors (guarding, bracing, rubbing painful area, grimacing, sighing) during gait were significantly correlated with very few temporal and distance factors.[169] Only step-length difference (r = 0.67), R-L step length (r = −0.53), and L-R step length (r = −0.55) significantly ($P < 0.05$) related with back pain while walking velocity, stride length, swing times, stand times, and single limb support times were not significant. However, differences in favor of the normal group occurred for all the above mentioned variables except

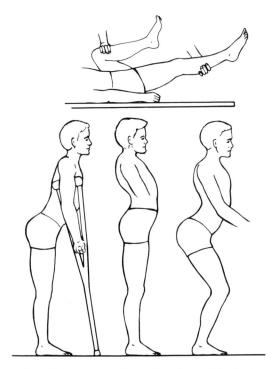

Fig. 10-19.   Illustration of abnormal gait resulting from a hip-flexion contracture. Clinical finding is shown at top. (Left) Crutch support for forward trunk. (Center) Lordosis to place trunk weight behind the hip joint axis. (Right) Combined knee flexion and lordosis. (From Perry,[192] with permission.)

right single limb support, left stance time, and step time difference. The study of overt pain behaviors during gait may prove useful toward improved assessment of back pain patients.

Carrying objects while walking may contribute to musculoskeletal problems. Wells et al.[170] showed that letter carriers had significantly more back problems than did their counterparts whose jobs required very little walking. Carrying objects on one side of the body could precipitate or aggravate low back dysfunction because of increased unilateral trunk and hip muscle action,[11] and thus increasing in an asymmetric fashion the demand for the lumbar erector spinae muscles to perform their main function, which is to restrict excessive trunk movements, particularly in the coronal plane in walking.[171] It follows that for asymmetric carrying, the maximum compressive loading of approximately 1.0 times body weight[20] found in normal gait would be asymmetrically elevated.

Mechanical disruption of lumbosacral movement can produce gait abnormalities. In a study of 10 spondylolisthesis patients, 9 of whom had a 50 percent forward displacement of the L5 vertebrae on S1, a peculiar gait was observed. These patients walked with a posterior tilt of the pelvis, hyperlordosis of the lumbar spine and flexed hip and knee joints. The authors attributed the lordosis to the forward displacement of the L5 vertebrae and the remainder of the gait abnormalities to tight hamstring muscles. Normal gait was restored within 6 months following surgical decompression and fusion.[172] The effectiveness of posture and therapeutic exercise in the prevention and control of unstable spinal segments needs to be addressed.

Controlled spinal movement during gait is a worthy goal. Without spinal movement, as in patients who received Harrington distraction instrumentation, which essentially immobilized their spine for treatment of lumbar fractures, compensatory body adjustments were made in walking.[173] When hip hyperextension motion was available, it was the favored adaptation for loss of lumbar lordosis. If not, the patients walked with a forward trunk lean with the hips in flexion.

Motivation of the patient to walk should be addressed. A patient with bilateral hip and knee fusions in a structurally asymmetric orientation serves to illustrate. He walked by actually rotating his body on his weightbearing side. Although his step times were unequal, stance time was 76 percent of the cycle and his body movements excessive, his forward walking velocity was within normal limits.[174] Matsunaga et al. attributed this patient's walking ability to his "rigorous and strong desire to overcome the hardship of immobilization."

Poliomyelitis

Before the Salk vaccine, poliomyelitis epidemics in the United States left thousands of debilitated persons in their wake. Immunization remains a need in developing countries.[175] The triple arthrodesis for muscle-deficient feet and ankles helps improve and retain gait function over the long term.[142] More than 30 years following initial poliomyelitis, patients are now experiencing new weakness, fatigue and muscle pain in what is being called *the postpolio syndrome*.[176] Electromyographic[176] and energy expenditure[177] studies indicate that the remaining nonparalyzed muscles work harder to carry out the walking act. By inductive reasoning, it makes sense to associate the relative high muscle activity over decades of gait function with overuse and then predicate this association as the cause for postpolio symptoms. Until such time as the concept of "overuse of the neuromuscular machinery" is more clearly understood, the cause for postpolio symptoms affecting gait should be considered tenuous.

Osteoporosis

Bone mass is approximately 30 percent higher in men than in women.[178] Peak bone mass is achieved at about 35 to 40 years of age for cortical and earlier for trabecular bone.[179,180] A few years after peak adult bone mass occurs, sooner in women than men, age-related bone loss begins and continues throughout life. In women the average loss is approximately 1 percent of peak adult bone mass per year for both cortical and trabecular bone,[180,181] accelerated for 3 to 7 years after menopause[178] and decelerated somewhat thereafter.[180,182]

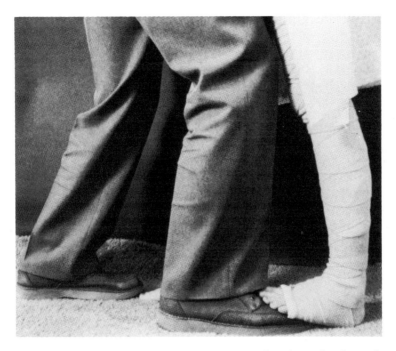

Fig. 10-20. Gait-training technique for plantar flexor foreshortening for early stance. Left ankle is in dorsiflexion with complete knee extension. (From Duncan,[163] with permission.)

Numerous risk factors have been suggested for postmenopausal osteoporosis; ethnicity, premature menopause—either surgical or natural, sedentary lifestyle, low calcium intake, slender body build, family history, alcohol consumption and cigarette smoking.[160,183,184] Exercise, estrogen therapy, and nutrition regimen have been a widely used three-dimensional approach for prevention and management of postmenopausal osteoporosis.[185–187] Walking as a therapeutic adjunct seems to be beneficial in effecting bone mineral content.[188,189] However, walking is typically included as part of a broad intervention program so its independent effect on the bone mineral content of the lower extremities and axial skeleton are not yet clear. However, walking as an exercise is advised for women at risk of osteoporosis. Whether other forms of exercise are superior is open to question.

SUMMARY

A review of gait studies plus clinically relevant illustrations and comments are provided for a variety of musculoskeletal abnormalities. When sufficient data were available, the summaries were divided into three areas: (1) deviation from normal, (2) relationships between clinical and gait measurements, and (3) effects of therapeutic intervention.

Data for a variety of temporal and distance, kinematic, and kinetic variables are reported. No generic set of measures seem to best discriminate between normal and abnormal or determine treatment efficacy. Part of the problem seems to be that there is wide diversity among patients' walking ability, even for those in the same medical diagnostic categories. Kinetic and kinematic measures offer promise, but simple measures such as normal walking velocity, maximum walking distance, indices of symmetry, and levels of assisted gait used are the measures that most frequently discriminated among walking abnormalities.

Surgical outcomes were by far the most reported in the gait literature. In most cases, the patients showed significant short-term improvement. Few long-term studies of several years were found. Investigations of conservative treatment to include exercise and gait training for musculoskeletal abnormalities are few and far between. The benefits of gait as a therapeutic entity are well documented from a cardiovascular standpoint, in contrast to the musculoskeletal area, in which little has been reported.

REFERENCES

1. Calve J, Galland M, De Cagny R: Pathogenesis of the limp due to coxalgia: The antalgic gait. J Bone Joint Surg 21(A):12, 1939
2. Bechtol CO: Correction of gluteus medius gait: Dynamic balance gait. Am Surg 25:847, 1959
3. Tesio L, Civaschi P, Tessari L: Motion of the center of gravity of the body in clinical evaluation of gait. Am J Phys Med 64(2):57, 1985
4. d'Aubigne RM, Postel M: Functional results of hip arthroplasty with acrylic prosthesis. J Bone Joint Surg 36A:451, 1954
5. Larson CB: Rating scale for hip disabilities. Clin Orthop 31:85, 1963
6. Harris WH: Traumatic arthritis of the hip after dislocation and acetabular fractures: Treatment by mold arthroplasty. J Bone Joint Surg 51A:737, 1969
7. Vatopoulos PK, Diacomopoulos GJ, Demiris ChS, et al: Girdlestone's operation: A follow-up study. Acta Orthop Scand 47:324, 1976
8. Johnston RC, Larson CB: Results of treatment of hip disorders with cup arthroplasty. J Bone Joint Surg 51A:1461, 1969
9. Johnston RC: Clinical follow-up of total hip replacement. Clin Orthop 95:118, 1973
10. Goldie IF, Raner C: Total hip replacement with a trunnion bearing prosthesis: Biomechanical principles and preliminary clinical results. Acta Orthop Scand 50:205, 1979
11. Neumann DA, Cook TM: Effect of load and carrying position on the electromyographic activity of the gluteus medius muscle during walking. Phys Ther 65:305, 1985
12. Baldurson H: Hip replacement with the McKee-Farrar prosthesis in rheumatoid arthritis. Acta Orthop Scand 51:639, 1980
13. Niemann KMW, Mankin HJ: Fractures about the hip in an institutionalized patient population. J Bone Joint Surg 50A:1327, 1968
14. Boardman KP, Bocco F, Charnley J: An evaluation of a method of trochanteric fixation using three wires in the Charnley low friction arthroplasty. Clin Orthop 132:31, 1978

15. Brindley HH: Central dislocation arthroplasty of the hip: A follow-up study. J Bone Joint Surg 53A:1426, 1971

16. Hansen LB, Kromann B, Baekgaaard N: Uncemented two-component femoral prosthesis for the hip joint: A 50-month follow-up study. Clin Orthop 208:182, 1986

17. Stauffer RN, Smidt GL, Wadsworth JB: Clinical and biomechanical analysis of gait following Charnley total hip replacement. Clin Orthop 99:70, 1974

18. Carlsson AS: 351 total hip replacements according to Charnley: A review of complications and function. Acta Orthop Scand 52:339, 1981

19. Head WC, Paradies LH: Ipsilateral hip and knee replacements as a single surgical procedure. J Bone Joint Surg 59A:352, 1977

20. Cappozzo A: Compressive loads in the lumbar vertebral column during normal level walking. J Orthop Res 1:292, 1984

21. Gore DR, Murray MP, Gardner GM, Sepic SB: Hip function after total vs. surface replacement. Acta Orthop Scand 56:386, 1985

22. Iida H, Yamamuro T: Kinetic analysis of the center of gravity of the human body in normal and pathological gaits. J Biomech 20:987, 1987

23. Murray MP: Studies of the functional performance of patients before and after total joint replacement. Research news. Int J Rehabil Res 2:543, 1979

24. Olsson E: Gait analysis in hip and knee surgery. Department of Orthopaedic Surgery Head: Professor Ian Goldie, MD, and Physical Medicine and Rehabilitation head: Jan Ekholm, MD. Stockholm, Kongl Carolinska Medico Chirurgiska Institutet, 1986

25. Smidt GL: Hip motion and related factors in walking. Phys Ther 51:9, 1971

26. Smidt GL, Wadsworth JB: Floor reaction forces during gait: Comparison of patients with hip disease and normal subjects. Phys Ther 53:1056, 1973

27. Wadsworth JB, Smidt GL, Johnston RC: Gait characteristics of subjects with hip disease. Phys Ther 52:829, 1972

28. Arborelius MM, Carlsson AS, Nilsson BE: Oxygen intake and walking speed before and after total hip replacement. Clin Orthop 121:113, 1976

29. Jacobs NA, Skorecki J: Analysis of the vertical component of force in normal and pathological gait. J Biomech 5:11, 1972

30. Hardy AE, White P, Williams J: The treatment of femoral fractures by cast-brace and early walking: A review of seventy-nine patients. J Bone Joint Surg 61B:151, 1979

31. Murray MP, Gore DR, Brewer BF, et al: A comparison of the functional performance of patients with Charnley and Miller total hip replacements: A two-year follow-up of eight-nine cases. Acta Orthop Scand 50:563, 1979

32. Murray MP, Gore DR, Clarkson BH: Walking patterns of patients with unilateral hip pain due to osteo-arthritis and avascular necrosis. J Bone Joint Surg 53A:259, 1971

33. Marshall RN, Meyers DB, Palmer DB: Disturbance of gait due to rheumatoid disease. J Rheumatol 7:617, 1980

34. Yamamoto S, Suto Y, Kawamura H, Hashizume T, Kakurai S: Quantitative gait evaluation of hip diseases using principal component analysis. J Biomech 16:717, 1983

35. Smidt GL, Arora JS, Johnston RC: Accelerographic analysis of several types of walking. Am J Phys Med 50:285, 1971

36. Huskisson EC: Measurement of pain. Lancet 1:1127, 1974

37. Hauge MF: The gait with an ankylosed hip. Acta Orthop Scand 36:348, 1965

38. Callaghan JJ, Brand RA, Pedersen DR: Hip arthrodesis: A long-term follow-up. J Bone Joint Surg 67A:1328, 1985

39. Perrin T, Dorr LD, Perry J, et al: Functional evaluation of total hip arthroplasty with five- to ten-year follow-up evaluation. Clin Orthop 195:252, 1985
40. Carlsson AS, Josefsson G, Lindberg L: Function of fifty-seven septic, revised and healed total hip arthroplasties. Acta Orthop Scand 51:937, 1980
41. Gore DR, Murray MP, Gardner GM, Mollinger LA: Comparison of function two years after revision of failed total hip arthroplasty and primary hip arthroplasty. Clin Orthop 208:168, 1986
42. Visuri T, Honkanen R: The influence of total hip replacement on selected activities of daily living and on the use of domestic aid. Scand J Rehabil Med 10:221, 1978
43. Steven MM, Capell HA, Sturrock RD, MacGregor J: The physiological cost of gait (PCG): A new technique for evaluating nonsteroidal anti-inflammatory drugs in rheumatoid arthritis. Br J Rheumatol 22:141, 1983
44. Burton DS, Imrie SH: Total hip arthroplasty and postoperative rehabilitation. Phys Ther 53:132, 1973
45. Godges JJ, MacRae H, Longdon C, et al: The effects of two stretching procedures on hip range of motion and gait economy. J Orthop Sports Phys Ther 10(9):350, 1989
46. Spiegel JS, Paulus HE, Ward NB, et al: What are we measuring? An examination of walk time and grip strength. J Rheumatology 14(1):80–86, 1987
47. McBeath AA, Bahrke MS, Balke B: Walking efficiency before and after total hip replacement as determined by oxygen consumption. J Bone Joint Surg 62A:807, 1980
48. Waugh W, Tew M, Johnson F: Methods of evaluating the result of operations for chronic arthritis of the knee. J R Soc Med 74:343, 1981
49. Wilson FC: Total replacement of the knee in rheumatoid arthritis: Part II of a prospective study. Clin Orthop 94:58, 1973
50. Laskin RS: Total knee replacement. Orthop Clin North Am 10:223, 1979
51. Kolstad K, Wigren A, Oberg K: Gait analysis with an angle diagram technique. Application in healthy persons and in studies of Marmor knee arthroplasties. Acta Orthop 53:733, 1982
52. Skinner HB, Barrack RL, Cook SD, Haddad RJ: Joint position sense in total knee arthroplasty. J Orthop Res 1:276, 1984
53. Andersson GBJ, Andriacchi TP, Galante JO: Correlations between changes in gait and in clinical status after knee arthroplasty. Acta Orthop Scand 52:569, 1981
54. Schank JA, Herdman SJ, Bloyer RG: Physical therapy in the multidisciplinary assessment and management of osteoarthritis. Clin Ther 9:14, 1986
55. Gore DR, Murray MP, Sepic SB, Gardner GM: Correlations between objective measures of function and a clinical knee rating scale following total knee replacement. Orthopedics 9:1363, 1986
56. Collopy MC, Murray MP, Gardner GM, et al: Kinesiologic measurements of functional performance before and after geometric total knee replacement: One-year follow-up of twenty cases. Clin Orthop 126:196, 1977
57. Minns RJ, Day JB, Hardinge K: Kinesiologic and biomechanical assessment of the Charnley "load angle inlay" knee prosthesis. Eng Med 11:25, 1982
58. Kettelkamp DB, Leaverton PE, Misol S: Gait characteristics of the rheumatoid knee. Arch Surg 104:30, 1972
59. Brugioni DJ, Andriacchi TP, Rotti RA, et al: A relationship between gait, disease process, and radiographic appearance following total knee arthroplasty. p 494. In Proceedings of the Thirty-second Annual Orthopaedic Research Society, New Orleans, February 17-20, 1986
60. Johnson F, Waugh W: Evidence for compensatory gait in patients with a valgus knee deformity. Acta Orthop Belg 46:558, 1980

61. Clayton ML, Thompson R, Mack RP: Correction of alignment deformities during total knee arthroplasties: Staged soft-tissue releases. Clin Orthop 202:117, 1986
62. Gyory AN, Chao EYS, Stauffer RN: Functional evaluation of normal and pathologic knees during gait. Arch Phys Med Rehabil 57:571, 1976
63. Olsson E, Barck A: Correlations between clinical examinations and quantitative gait analysis in patients operated upon with the Gunston-Hult knee prosthesis. Scand J Rehabil Med 18:101, 1986
64. Andriacchi TP, Ogle JA, Galante JO: Walking speed as a basis for normal and abnormal gait measurements. J Biomech 10:261, 1977
65. Andriacchi TP, Galante JO, Fermier RW: The influence of total knee-replacement design on walking and stair-climbing. J Bone Joint Surg 64A:1328, 1982
66. Chao EY, Laughman RK, Stauffer RN: Biomechanical gait evaluation of pre- and postoperative total knee replacement patients. Arch Orthop Traum Surg 97:309, 1980
67. Murray MP, Gore DR, Sepic SB, Mollinger LA: Antalgic maneuvers during walking in men with unilateral knee disability. Clin Orthop 199:192, 1985
68. Seedholm BB, Dowson D, Wright V: Sear of solid phase formed high density polyethylene in relation to the life of artificial hips and knees. Wear 24:35, 1973
69. Wallbridge N, Dowson D: The walking activity of patients with artificial hip joints. Eng Med 11:95, 1982
70. Laughman RK, Stauffer RN, Ilstrup DM, Chao EYS: Functional evaluation of total knee replacement. J Orthop Res 2:307, 1984
71. Rittman N, Kettelkamp DB, Pryor P, et al: Analysis of patterns of knee motion walking for four types of total knee implants. Clin Orthop 155:111, 1981
72. Zetterlund AE, Serfass RC, Hunter RE: The effect of wearing the complete Lenox Hill derotation brace on energy expenditure during horizontal treadmill running at 161 meters per minute. Am J Sports Med 14:73, 1986
73. Weinstein JN, Andriacchi TP, Galante J: Factors influencing walking and stairclimbing following unicompartmental knee arthroplasty. J Arthroplasty 1:109, 1986
74. Smidt GL, Deusinger RH, Arora J, Albright JP: An automated accelerometry system for gait analysis. J Biomech 10:367, 1977
75. Murray MP, Gore DR, Laney WH, et al: Kinesiologic measurements of functional performance before and after double compartment Marmor knee arthroplasty. Clin Orthop 173:191, 1983
76. Brinkman JR, Perry J: Rate and range of knee motion during ambulation in healthy and arthritic subjects. Phys Ther 65:1055, 1985
77. Jakubowski S, Dubinska A: The treatment of flexion contracture of the knee joint with posterior capsulotomy in rheumatoic arthritis patients. Acta Orthop Scand 45:235, 1974
78. Simon SR, Trieshmann HW, Burdett RG, et al: Quantitative gait analysis after total knee arthroplasty for monarticular degenerative arthritis. J Bone Joint Surg 65A:605, 1983
79. Berman AT, Zarro VJ, Bosacco SJ, Israelite C: Quantitative gait analysis after unilateral or bilateral total knee replacement. J Bone Joint Surg 69A:1340, 1987
80. Landon GC, Richtsmeier K: Restoring function to the hip and knee. Geriatrics 36:125, 1981
81. Heywood AWB, Learmonth ID: Total replacement of the rheumatoid knee: A review of currently available prostheses and a follow-up of 50 operations. South Afr Med J 57:272, 1980
82. Frymoyer JW, Hoaglund FT: The role of arthrodesis in reconstruction of the knee. Clin Orthop 101:82, 1974

83. Tylkowski C, Miller G, Springfield D, et al: Gait patterns and energy expenditure of patients after resection arthrodesis of the knee. p. 310. In Proceedings of the Thirty-second Annual Orthopaedic Research Society, New Orleans, February 17-20, 1986

84. Prodromos CC, Andriacchi TP, Galante JO: A relationship between gait and clinical changes following high tibial osteotomy. J Bone Joint Surg 67A:1188, 1985

85. Corrigan B, Kannangra S: Rheumatic disease: Exercise or immobilization? Aust Fam Physician 7:1007, 1978

86. Barraclough D, Alderman WW, Popert AJ: Rehabilitation of non-walkers in rheumatoid arthritis. Rheumatol Rehabil 15:287, 1976

87. Sasaki T, Yasuda K: Clinical evaluation of the treatment of osteoarthritic knees using a newly designed wedged insole. Clin Orthop 221:181, 1987

88. Ekblom B, Lovgren O, Alderin M, et al: Effect of short-term physical training on patients with rheumatoid arthritis. I. Scand J Rheumatol 4:80, 1975

89. Moll JMH, Chesterman PJ, Meanock RI, Andrews FM: Walldius arthroplasty of the knee: Follow-up study of 51 operations. Ann Rheum Dis 32:397, 1973

90. Fouston J: Editorial: The analysis and description of human gait. Clin Biomech 2:117, 1987

91. Boobbyer GN: The long-term results of ankle arthrodesis. Acta Orthop Scand 52:107, 1981

92. Lindholm RV, Puranen J, Kinnunen P: The Moore vitallium femoral-head prosthesis in fractures of the femoral neck. Acta Orthop Scand 47:70, 1976

93. Buck P, Morrey BF, Chao EYS: The optimum position of arthrodesis of the ankle: A gait study of the knee and ankle. J Bone Joint Surg 69A:1052, 1987

94. Fjermeros H, Hagen R: Post-traumatic arthrosis in the ankle and foot treated with arthrodesis. Acta Chir Scand 133:527, 1967

95. Mazur JM, Schwartz E, Simon SR: Ankle Arthrodesis. J Bone Joint Surg 61A:964, 1979

96. Demottaz JD, Mazur JM, Thomas WH, et al: Clinical study of total ankle replacement with gait analysis: A preliminary report. J Bone Joint Surg 61A:976, 1979

97. Locke M, Perry J, Campbell J, Thomas L: Ankle and subtalar motion during gait in arthritic patients. Phys Ther 64:504, 1984

98. Scranton PE, Pedegana LR, Whitesel JP: Gait analysis: Alterations in support phase forces using supportive devices. Am J Sports Med 10:6, 1982

99. Mann RA; Biomechanical approach to the treatment of foot problems. Foot Ankle 2:205, 1982

100. Boissonnault W, Donatelli R: The influence of hallux extension on the foot during ambulation. J Orthop Sports Phys Ther 5:240, 1984

101. Clinical Orthopedics and Related Research, No. 70. JB Lippincott, Philadelphia, May-June, 1970

102. Clinical Orthopedics and Related Research, No. 142. JB Lippincott, Philadelphia, July-August, 1979

103. Clinical Orthopedics and Related Research, No. 177. JB Lippincott, Philadelphia, July-August, 1983

104. Clinical Orthopedics and Related Research, No. 181. JB Lippincott, Philadelphia, December, 1983

105. Claeys R: The analysis of ground reaction forces in pathological gait secondary to disorders of the foot. Int Orthop 7:113, 1983

106. Simkin A: The dynamic vertical force distribution during level walking under normal and rheumatic feet. Rheumatol Rehabil 20:88, 1981

107. Minns RJ, Braxford AD: Pressure under the forefoot in rheumatoid arthritis: A comparison of static and dynamic methods of assessment. Clin Orthop 187:235, 1984

108. Sharma M, Dhanendran M, Hutton WC, Corbett M: Changes in load bearing in the rheumatoid foot. Ann Rheum Dis 38:549, 1979

109. Cavanagh PR, Rodgers MM: The arch index: A useful measure from footprints. J Biomech 20:547, 1987

110. Stewart SF: Human gait and the human foot: An ethnological study of flatfoot. Part I. Clin Orthop 70:111, 1970

111. Stewart SF: Human gait and the human foot: An ethnological study of flatfoot. Part II. Clin Orthop 70:124, 1970

112. Katoh Y, Chao EYS, Morrey BF, Laughman RK: Objective technique for evaluating painful heel syndrome and its treatment. Foot Ankle 3:227, 1983

113. Barrett JP: Plantar pressure measurements: Rational shoe-wear in patients with rheumatoid arthritis. JAMA 235:1138, 1976

114. Dimonte P, Light H: Pathomechanics, gait deviations, and treatment of the rheumatoid foot. Phys Ther 62:1148, 1982

115. Ramig D, Shadle J, Watkins A, et al: The foot and sports medicine—Biomechanical foot faults as related to chondromalacia patellae. J Orthop Sports Phys Ther 2:48, 1980

116. Light LH, McLellan GE, Klenerman L: Skeletal transients on heel strike in normal walking with different footwear. J Biomech 13:477, 1980

117. Merkel KD, Katoh Y, Johnson EW, Chao EYS: Mitchell osteotomy for hallux valgus: Long term follow-up and gait analysis. Foot Ankle 3:189, 1983

118. Bohler L: The Treatment of Fractures. Grune & Stratton, Orlando, FL, 1956

119. Galasko CSB: Principles of Fracture Management. Churchill Livingstone, Edinburgh, 1984

120. Bassett CAL: The development and application of pulsed electromagnetic fields (PEMFs) for ununited fractures and arthrodeses. Orthop Clin North Am 15:61, 1984

121. Semba RT, Yasukawa K, Gustilo RB: Critical analysis of results of 53 Malgaigne fractures of the pelvis. J Trauma 23:535, 1983

122. Barnes B: Ambulation outcomes after hip fracture. Phys Ther 64:317, 1984

123. Hielema FJ: Epidemiology of hip fracture: A review with implications for the physical therapist. Phys Ther 59:1291, 1979

124. Imms FJ, MacDonald IC: Abnormalities of the gait occurring during recovery from fractures of the lower limb and their improvement during rehabilitation. Scand J Rehabil Med 10:193, 1978

125. Ceder L, Ekelund L, Inerot S, et al: Rehabilitation after hip fracture in the elderly. Acta Orthop Scand 50:681, 1979

126. Connolly JF, King P: Closed reduction and early cast-brace ambulation in the treatment of femoral fractures. J Bone Joint Surg 55A:1559, 1973

127. Connolly JF, Dehne E, LaFollette B: Closed reduction and early cast-brace ambulation in the treatment of femoral fractures. II. Results in one hundred and forty-three fractures. J Bone Joint Surg 55A:1581, 1973

128. Moll JH: The cast-brace walking treatment of open and closed femoral fractures. South Med J 66:345, 1973

129. Sarmiento A: Functional bracing of tibial and femoral shaft fractures. Clin Orthop 82:2, 1972

130. Farrell J: Nursing care of the patient in a cast brace. Nurs Clin North Am 11:717, 1976

131. Drennan DB, Locher FG, Maylahn DJ: Fractures of the tibial plateau: Treatment by closed reduction and spica cast. J Bone Joint Surg 61A:989, 1979

132. Dehne E: Ambulatory treatment of the fractured tibia. Clin Orthop 105:192, 1974

133. Brown PW: The early weight-bearing treatment of tibial shaft fractures. Clin Orthop 105:167, 1974

134. Nesbakken A, Alho A, Bjersand AJ, Jensen DK: Open tibial fractures treated with Hoffmann external fixation. Arch Orthop Trauma Surg 107:248, 1988

135. Brown PW, Urban JG: Early weight-bearing treatment of open fractures of the tibia. J Bone Joint Surg 51A:59, 1969

136. Pettine KA, Morrey BF: Osteochondral fractures of the talus: A long-term follow-up. J Bone Joint Surg 69B:89, 1987

137. Rowley DI, Norris SH, Duckworth T: A prospective trial comparing operative and manipulative treatment of ankle fractures. J Bone Joint Surg 68B:610, 1986

138. Durie ND, Shearman L: Clinical note: A simplified limb load monitor. Physiother Can 31:28, 1979

139. Carey PB, Wolf SL, Binder-Macleod SA, Bain R: Assessing the reliability of measurements from the Krusen limb load monitor to analyze temporal and loading characteristics of normal gait. Phys Ther 64:199, 1984

140. Wolf SL, Binder-Macleod SA: Use of the Krusen limb load monitor to quantify temporal and loading measurements of gait. Phys Ther 62:976, 1982

141. Beck JL, Day RW: Overuse injuries. Clin Sports Med 4:553, 1985

142. Bernau A: Long-term results following Lambrinudi arthrodesis. J Bone Joint Surg 59A:473, 1977

143. Shiavi R, Limbird T, Frazer M, et al: Helical motion analysis of the knee. II. Kinematics of uninjured and injured knees during walking and pivoting. J Biomech 20:653, 1987

144. Limbird TJ, Shiavi R, Frazer M, Borra H: EMG profiles of knee joint musculature during walking: Changes induced by anterior cruciate ligament deficiency. J Orthop Res 6:630, 1988

145. Perry J, Fox JM, Boitano MA, Skinner SR, et al: Functional evauation of the pes anserinus transfer by electromyography and gait analysis. J Bone Joint Surg 62A:973, 1980

146. Markolf KL, Bargar WL, Shoemaker SC, Amstutz HC: The role of joint load in knee stability. J Bone Joint Surg 63A:570, 1981

147. Carlsoo S, Nordstrand A: The coordination of the knee-muscles in some voluntary movements and in the gait in cases with and without knee joint injuries. Acta Chir Scand 134:423, 1968

148. Czerniecki JM, Lippert F, Olerud JE: A biomechanical evaluation of tibiofemoral rotation in anterior cruciate deficient knees during walking and running. J Orthop Sports Phys Ther 16:327, 1988

149. Dillon PZ, Updyke WF, Allen WC: Gait analysis with reference to chondromalacia patellae. J Orthop Sports Phys Ther 5:127, 1983

150. Walker HL, Schreck RC: Relationship of hyperextended gait pattern to chondro-malacia patellae. Phys Ther 55:259, 1975

151. Schult D, Adrian M, Pidco E: Effect of heel lifts on ground reaction force patterns in subjects with structural leg-length descrepancies. Phys Ther 69:663, 1989

152. Shellock FG, Mink JH, Deutsch A, Fox JM: Kinematic magnetic resonance imaging for evaluation of patellar tracking. Physician Sports Med 17:99, 1989

153. DeLacerda FG: A study of anatomical factors involved in shinsplints. J Orthop Sports Phys Ther 2:55, 1980
154. DeLacerda FG: The relationship of foot pronation, foot position, and electromyography of the anterior tibialis muscle in three subjects with different histories of shinsplints. J Orthop Sports Phys Ther 2:60, 1980
155. Lowdon A, Bader DL, Mowat AG: The effect of heel pads on the treatment of Achilles tendinitis: A double blind trial. Am J Sports Med 12:431, 1984
156. Gillies H, Chalmers J: The management of fresh ruptures of the tendo achillis. J Bone Joint Surg 52A:337, 1970
157. Benum P, Berg V, Fretheim: The strain on sutured Achilles tendons in walking cast: An EMG analysis. Eurg Surg Res 16(suppl 2):14, 1984
158. Glick JM, Gordon RB, Nishimoto D: The prevention and treatment of ankle injuries. Am J Sports Med 4:136, 1976
159. Rarick L, Bigley G, Kart R, Kart M: The measureable support of ankle joint by conventional methods of taping. J Bone Joint Surg 44A:1183, 1962
160. Laughman RK, Carr TA, Chao EY, Youdas JW: Three-dimensional kinetmatics of the taped ankle before and after exercise. Am J Sports Med 8:425, 1980
161. Carmines DV, Nunley JA, McElhaney JH: Effects of ankle taping on the motion and loading pattern of the foot for walking subjects. J Orthop Res 6:223, 1988
162. Stover CN, DeBald M: Guide to lateral ankle sprain management. Orthop Nursing 5(3):34, 1986
163. Duncan CE: A gait training suggestion for lengthening gastro-soleus muscles: Suggestion from the field. Phys Ther 69:773, 1989
164. Thomas LK, Hislop HJ, Waters RL: Physiological work performance in chronic low back disability. Phys Ther 60:407, 1980
165. Khodadadeh S, Eisenstein S, Summers B, Patrick J: Gait asymmetry in patients with chronic low back pain. Neuro Orthopedics 6:24, 1988
166. Voloshin A, Wosk J: An in vivo study of low back pain and shock absorption in the human locomotor system. J Biomech 15:21, 1982
167. Voloshin A, Wosk J: Influence of artificial shock absorbers on human gait. Clin Orthop 160:52, 1981
168. Wosk J, Voloshin AS: Low back pain: Conservative treatment with artificial shock absorbers. Arch Phys Med Rehabil 66:145, 1985
169. Keefe FJ, Hill RW: An objective approach to quantifying pain behavior and gait patterns in low back pain patients. Pain 21:153, 1985
170. Wells JA, Zipp JF, Schuette PT, McEleney J: Musculoskeletal disorders among letter carriers: A comparison of weight carrying, walking & sedentary occupations. J Occup Med 25:814, 1983
171. Thorstensson A, Carlson H, Zomlefer MR, Nilsson J: Lumbar back muscle activity in relation to trunk movements during locomotion in man. Acta Physiol Scand 116:13, 1982
172. Barash HL, Galante JO, Lambert CN, Ray RD: Spondylolisthesis and tight hamstrings. J Bone Joint Surg 52A:1319, 1970
173. Hasday CA, Passoff TL, Perry J: Gait abnormalities arising from Iatrogenic loss of lumbar fractures. Spine 8:501, 1983
174. Matsunaga T, Nakata T, Wong AC: Objective analysis of walking in a patient with ankylosing spondylitis and bilateral hip and knee fusion: A case report. Scand J Rehabil Med 18:23, 1986
175. Nicholas DD, Kratzer JH, Ofosu-Amaah S, Belcher DW: Is poliomyelitis a serious problem in developing countries? The Danfa experience. Br Med J 1:1009, 1977

176. Perry J, Barnes G, Gronley JK: The postpolio syndrome: An overuse phenomenon. Clin Orthop 233:145, 1988
177. Molbech S: Energy cost in level walking in subjects with an abnormal gait. In Evang K, Anderson KL (eds.): Physical Activity in Health and Disease. Williams & Wilkins, Baltimore, 1966
178. National Institutes of Health, Concensus Conference. Osteoporosis. JAMA 252:799, 1984
179. Hansson T, Roos B: The influence of age, height, and weight on the bone mineral content of lumbar vertebrae. Spine 5:545, 1980
180. Parfitt AM: Bone remodelling and bone loss: Understanding pathophysiology of osteoporosis. Clin Obstet Gynecol 30:789, 1987
181. Dawson-Hughes B, Li XF: Preventing osteoporosis. Evidence for diet and exercise. Geriatrics 42:76, 1987
182. Lindquiste, Bengtsson T, Hansson T, et al: Changes in bone mineral content of the axial skeleton in relation to aging and the menopause. Scand J Clin Lab Invest 43:333, 1983
183. Silverberg SJ, Lindsay R: Postmenopausal osteoporosis. Med Clin North Am 71:41, 1987
184. Lindsay R: Prevention of postmenopausal osteoporosis. Gynecol Clin North Am 14:63, 1987
185. Munnings F: Exercise and estrogen in women's health: Getting a clearer picture. Physician Sports Med 16:152, 1988
186. Notelovitz M: The role of the gynecologist in osteoporosis prevention: A clinical approach. Clin Obstet Gynecol 30:871, 1987
187. Raisz LG: Preventing osteoporosis by estrogen replacement. J Musculoskel Med 2:25, 1985
188. Dalsky GP, et al: The effect of endurance exercise training on lumbar bone mass in postmenopausal women. Med Sci Sports Ex 18(suppl):96, 1986 (abst)
189. Rundgren A, et al: Effects of a training program for elderly people on bone mineral content of the heel bone. Arch Gerontol Geriat 3:243, 1984
190. Mazur JM, Schwartz E, Simon SR: Ankle arthrodesis: Long-term follow-up with gait analysis. J Bone Joint Surg 61A:964, 1979
191. Katoh Y, Chao EYS, Laughman RK, et al: Biomechanical analysis of foot function during gait and clinical applications. Clin Orthop 177:23, 1983
192. Perry J: Contractures: A historical perspective. Clin Orthop 219:8, 1987

11 | Adult Hemiplegic Gait

Carol A. Giuliani

Normal locomotion is characterized by a smooth forward progression of the center of gravity and by well-coordinated limb movement. By contrast, the gait pattern of many hemiplegic subjects is characterized by slow, laborious, uncoordinated limb movement. A lack of selective joint control during attempted voluntary movement is usually described in terms of stereotypic movement synergies.[1] Well-controlled intralimb and interlimb coordination normally observed during locomotion is often replaced by mass limb movement patterns and by altered phasing between limbs.[1] Although the gait pattern of persons with hemiplegia is variable among subjects, clinicians frequently use the term *hemiplegic gait* to describe a characteristic pattern of body posture and limb movement observable during locomotion. Caution is urged when using these terms to describe movement because patients frequently do not fit the general characterization, and the underlying problems are often ignored in the clinical assessment.

Perry[2] hypothesized that the abnormality observed in hemiplegic gait was because of poor single-limb balance as well as difficulty controlling forward progression. She observed that subjects lacked (1) adequate shock absorption at heel strike, (2) control of momentum during stance, (3) the ability to generate force for pushoff to maintain forward propulsion, and (4) quick adequate excursion of the paretic limb during swing. Recent studies support Perry's early observations and provide some insight into the mechanisms responsible for producing gait abnormalities. This chapter presents relative kinematic, kinetic, and electromyographic (EMG) information reported on gait patterns in subjects with hemiplegia.

SPATIOTEMPORAL COMPONENTS OF GAIT

Each person has a characteristic gait. Even though spatiotemporal parameters are variable among normal subjects, these differences are small compared with differences within and among hemiplegic subjects.[3-6] Many of the differences reported in hemiplegic subjects may be because of the variability of diagnoses, amount of functional recovery, individual movement compensation acquired, and the research method used.[4,7]

One of the most consistent differences reported between normal and hemiplegic subjects is walking velocity. Subjects with hemiplegia have significantly slower walking speed, stride length, and cycle duration than normal subjects.[3,8-10] The range of average walking speed reported for hemiplegic subjects is 0.2 to 0.7 m/s compared with 1 to 1.2 m/s for normal subjects.[3,9-12] A study of 23 hemiplegic subjects reported an average strude length of 0.6 ± 0.25 m and a cycle duration of 2.3 ± 0.8 seconds.[10] These limitations in stride length and walking speed may be associated with advancing the paretic limb efficiently in swing and in shifting weight to the paretic limb in stance.[9,13]

Difficulty maintaining single-limb balance, shifting weight support between limbs, and spatiotemporal asymmetries are reported frequently by clinicians treating patients with hemiplegia. Several researchers reported an abnormal swing/stance ratio in hemiplegic subjects. Typically the stance phase was shortened and the swing phase was lengthened in the paretic limb compared with the swing and stance duration in the limb of normal subjects.[3,10,11,14,15] To compensate for these changes in the swing/stance ratio, the uninvolved limb of the hemiplegic subjects had an increased stance and decreased swing phase. Consistent with these interlimb adjustments, periods of double-limb support were longer in hemiplegic than in normal subjects.[6,9,10,14] Asymmetric steps are also characteristic of hemiplegic gait, with the paretic limb having a shorter stance time and step length than that of the uninvolved limb. Several investigators reported that the degree of asymmetry was inversely related to the degree of motor recovery[8-10] and positively related to walking speed.[6,7,10]

Many studies on hemiplegic gait are descriptive and use few subjects with differing diagnoses. Few comprehensive studies examine the temporal distance characteristics of hemiplegic gait with a homogeneous diagnostic group. Clearly, the spatiotemporal variables are the most reliable and easily measured components of gait.[3,16-18] Identifying the parameters of gait that are problematic in a hemiplegic subject will improve the ability to develop a treatment plan directed at correcting those specific parameters.[17] Documenting the changes in these variables would be useful for measuring client progress and for guiding treatment programs.

KINEMATICS

There is considerable variability in the joint kinematic patterns of hemiplegic subjects.[3-5,8,13,15,19] In contrast to the large between-subject variability, each subject appears to have a characteristic kinematic pattern clearly recognizable over steps.The variability of the joint patterns within hemiplegic subjects, however, is greater than within normal subjects.[3-6]

The kinematic pattern of the paretic limb during gait has been described as one of hip flexion, knee extension, ankle plantar flexion, and lower limb circumduction during swing; hip flexion, limited knee flexion, and ankle plantar flexion during loading; knee hyperextension during midstance; and lack of roll-off at toe-off.[2] These are common gait patterns in hemiplegia; however, subjects exhibit a wide variety of patterns, each caused by a different initial problem or compensating movement. Each patient must be examined and his or her own unique kinematic pattern identified and documented. Understanding an individual gait pattern is much more useful than having expectations of movement patterns related to diagnosis.

Limited hip, knee, and ankle range of motion resulting in a stiff-legged gait is reported frequently as characteristics of limb movement in hemiplegic gait. The limited ankle dorsiflexion observed in many patients is of particular concern and it along with limited knee flexion in swing contributes to the apparent increased length and the resulting circumduction to advance the swinging limb.[2,8] Normal patterns of ankle flexion and extension were absent in hemiplegic subjects during walking, and initial contact with the ground frequently occurred with a foot-flat or forefoot strike, rather than a normal heel-strike pattern.[3,4] Many subjects displayed knee extension in early stance instead of an energy-absorbing phase of knee flexion.[4,8,13] Ankle dorsiflexion was reduced during loading, and the rapid plantar flexion normally seen during pushoff was reduced or absent. Several investigators reported that hip flexion and extension patterns lacked the smooth trajectory and excursion commonly observed in normal subjects.[3,13,19] A lack of hip extension during terminal stance may result in a shorter stride length and decreased gait velocity reported in hemiplegic subjects.

Frequently the swing phase was initiated by flexion of the entire limb rather than by smooth sequential movements of the thigh, shank, and ankle segments.[8,13] The knee and ankle extended simultaneously and abruptly in late swing, rather than the normal knee extension with ankle dorsiflexion pattern used in preparation for heelstrike. Murray et al.[20] reported a reduced amplitude of limb movement for normal subjects during swing that was more evident at faster walking speeds.[20]

Consistent in the literature reviewed, the greatest loss of motor control of the hemiparetic limb occurs at phase transitions, that is, phases in the gait at which movement reversal is required, such as loading, foot off, and midswing. These observation may be explained by the difficulty experienced by hemiplegic subjects in performing rapid reciprocal limb movements.[21,22] Considering the functional importance of producing rapid movements, few studies investigate the effects of speed on movement patterns in subjects with hemiplegia. The effects of speed are reviewed later in this chapter. Results from the studies that were reported suggest that the demand for increased movement speed exaggerates motor dysfunction and provides a excellent method for clinical assessment and for identifying motor control deficits.

Most gait studies describe the range of angular displacement at each joint throughout the gait cycle or at critical points during the cycle. To characterize hemiplegic gait fully, we also need information about angular velocity and acceleration at each joint and about how these variables are coordinated among joints in both the paretic and nonparetic limb. Phase-plane analyses of limb kinematics, such as angle-angle or angle-velocity diagrams, would provide valuable information about the quality and coordination of limb movement in gait.[23] Generally, we display limb kinematics with each joint plotted in a time series as shown in Figure 11-1A,C. For comparison, the same values for ankle and knee displacement are plotted against each other in Figure 11-1B,D. Recently, phase-plane analyses have been used to describe abnormal walking patterns of intralimb movement of people with movement dysfunction[24,25] and of limb-pedaling patterns for hemiplegic subjects.[26] Although at first glance these plots may appear to be difficult to interpret and to quantify, they provide an excellent source for the qualitative analysis of dynamic limb control.[25]

Most frequently gait analysis is limited to studying limb movement. Movements of the trunk and pelvic girdle during locomotion also play an important role in smoothing the path of the center of gravity and minimizing energy expenditure.[27,28] Clinicians report that stroke patients frequently exhibit excessive downward rotation of the pelvis in the frontal plane during stance. This excessive pelvic movement is often attributed to gluteus medius weakness of the affected side and is associated with difficulty initiating and completing the swing phase of gait.[18] Hirschberg and Nathanson[29] reported that the timing of the gluteus medius muscle of the nonparetic side resembled that of the paretic limb; however, the average peak amplitude of gluteus medius EMG of the paretic limb was sometimes greater or less than the average peak amplitude in normal subjects.[29] Similar to the findings of Hirschberg and Nathanson, Hu[30] reported that for hemiparetic subjects with lateral pelvic drop (Trendelenburg sign), the gluteus medius onset latency was not different between sides, but the gluteus medius burst duration of the paretic side was shorter than that of the contralateral side. In addition, these subjects had an asymmetric gait characterized by a longer cycle time of paretic limb than of the contralateral limb that was attributed to a prolonged swing phase of paretic limb. It is possible that the prolonged burst duration of the gluteus medius was related to the prolonged swing duration of the contralateral limb.

KINETICS OF HEMIPLEGIC GAIT

Analysis of joint moment[5,8] and ground reaction force curves[7,31] for both limbs in hemiplegic subjects differed significantly in magnitude and shape from those of normal subjects. Boccardi et al.[5] reported from a sample of two hemiplegic subjects that these subjects had decreased joint moments at the hip, knee, and ankle and an increased number of oscillations observed in the shape of the moment curve. These deficits indicate an impaired ability to generate and grade the forces that control limb movement. In another study, Wortis et al.[31] reported

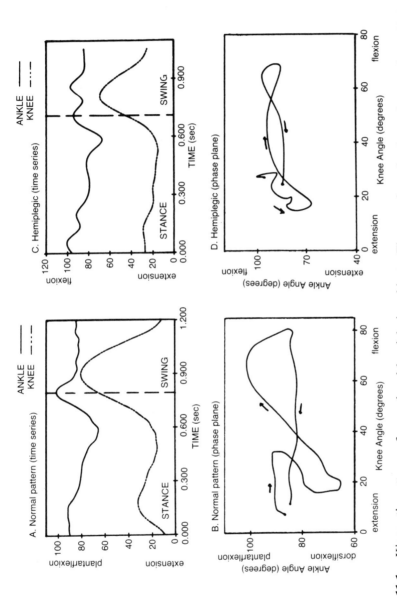

Fig. 11-1. Kinematic patterns of normal and hemiplegic subjects. These angle-angle phase plane analyses (**B & D**) provide useful information about coordination between joints that are difficult to appreciate in a time plot (**A & C**). Smooth ankle and knee flexion and extension patterns for a normal subject are shown in time plot (**A**) and in phase plane (**B**). A hemiplegic subject with abnormal ankle control and loss of knee flexion during loading (**C & D**). The smooth coordination of knee and ankle following foot contact in **D** is lacking, and increased ankle dorsiflexion with knee flexion is limited; as the knee direction changes from flexion to extension in swing, the ankle plantar flexes rather than dorsiflexes, compared with the normal pattern shown in **B**.

that hemiplegic subjects had a positive knee moment throughout stance and were missing the negative knee moment associated with a normal loading response. Consistent with the difficulty controlling forces during weight support are the reports of abnormal ground reaction force curves. Carlsöö et al.[7] suggested that hemiplegic subjects have a larger vertical component of the ground reaction force at foot strike than do normal subjects and lack the peak vertical force associated with push-off[7] (Fig. 11-2). Even though the general shape of the force curve was consistent for each subject, there was significant variability in the horizontal and vertical force components across steps.[7,31] These abnormalities in the ground reaction forces and joint moments are consistent with the kinematic deficits at foot strike, loading, and push-off. It appears that subjects with hemiplegia have difficulty controlling force parameters, especially during weight acceptance, and in transferring weight to the contralateral limb.

Producing well-coordinated movement requires the interaction of mechanical and neuromuscular systems. Patients with hemiparesis have difficulty producing and controlling muscles forces necessary for performing accurate limb movement and regulating movement speed. These deficits may be related to changes in biomechanical and neuromuscular factors that have been reported in patients with hemiparesis. Alterations in viscoelastic properties of muscles and tendons may increase muscle stiffness and passive restraint to movement.[32,33] Stiffness may also be a factor that inhibits speed of movement.[34] Muscle shortening may occur from immobilization due to spasticity or joint positioning. Animal studies have shown that muscles immobilized in a shortened position lose sarcomeres and are hypoextensible, whereas muscles that are immobilized in a lengthened position add sarcomeres and are hyperextensible.[35] These mechanical changes may affect movement patterns. Mechanisms of neural control depend on the properties of the musculoskeletal apparatus. To appreciate the

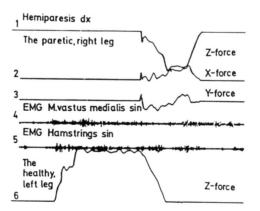

Fig. 11-2.   Ground reaction forces and EMG of both limbs in a hemiparetic subject. This patient showed a lack of initial force after footstrike and a rounded irregular peak form commonly seen in the hemiparetic limb. (From Carlsöö et al.,[7] with permission.)

effects of small mechanical changes on movement patterns, consider the effect of increasing the limb length of your arm or leg. Place a lift on one shoe or splint one finger at the interphalangeal joint and observe the effects on the accuracy of your movements. How often do you stumble or poke your finger in your eye? How long does it take you to adjust? Even though you are aware of the apparent changes made to the alter the segment length, a period of training is necessary to adjust movement patterns appropriately.

Neuromuscular changes reported in patients with hemiparesis may help clinicians understand the difficulties in motor control, as well as design appropriate treatment programs. Several researchers have reported that the muscles of hemiparetic limbs have muscle fiber atrophy predominantly of the type II or fast muscle fibers[36-38] and a hypertrophy of type I or slow fibers.[39,40] In addition to altered motor unit morphology, abnormal firing patterns were reported in subjects with hemiplegia.[41,42] Atrophy of fast fibers and a decreased rate of firing was associated with reduced force production.[41] Mechanical changes, reduced firing rates, and poor regulation of motor unit activity may help explain the difficulty in force and speed production observed in hemiparetic subjects.

MUSCLE PATTERNS

Several investigators have reported abnormalities in muscle activation during hemiplegic gait.[4,7,13,14,27,29] The most striking characteristic of muscle activity in hemiplegic subjects is the variability of muscle patterns. Although each subject has a characteristic muscle pattern, the differences among subjects are significant. An example of the variability among subjects is illustrated in Figure 11-3. Muscle patterns of the tibialis anterior (TA) and medial gastrocnemius (MG) during walking at self-selected speeds were different for each of these three subjects with hemiplegia (Fig. 11-3A–C). Although patterns varied among subjects, within-subject patterns were characteristic. As is true of the variability in kinematic and kinetic patterns, the difference may be accounted for by differences in the diagnosis, stage of recovery, and the compensatory pattern used by each subject. The amount of muscle activity (integrated EMG or root mean square value) in each muscle appears to be quite variable over trials[13,14] with the paretic limb exhibiting a lower EMG amplitude than the nonparetic limb. Although comparing the level of muscle activity across muscle and among subjects is fraught with problems, no matter what method of comparison was used, the findings are consistent that subjects with hemiplegia produce lower amplitude EMG.[13,14,31] Temporal patterns of muscle activation for hemiplegic subjects also may differ from normal subjects; however, these patterns are characteristic for each subject and consistent over trials.[13,14]

Although there are differences among subjects, some general characteristics that are consistently reported are (1) less muscle activity in the paretic limb, (2) prolonged muscle burst duration, (3) tonic rather than phasic activity at gait transitions, and (4) periods of peak muscle activity that do not coincide with

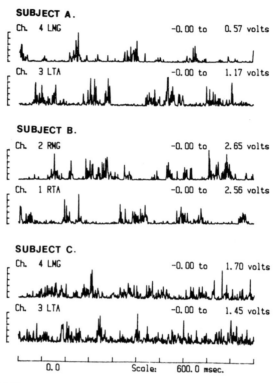

Fig. 11-3. Variability of the EMG pattern among hemiparetic subjects during walking. Subject A shows a fairly normal reciprocal pattern of flexion and extension of the TA and MG. Subject B appears to have an irregular MG pattern and greater periods of contraction between the antagonists. Subject C shows tonic activity in both muscles, with some suggestion of an underlying phasic pattern. TA, tibialis anterior; MG, medial gastrocnemius.

requirements for a normal gait pattern.[7,13,14,29,31] For example, Peat et al.[14] reported that activation of the tibialis anterior was lacking at toe-off and heel strike and that gastrocnemius activity did not peak at push-off as expected.

Knutsson and Richards[13] examined the EMG patterns in 23 hemiplegic subjects who had a stroke and three who had multiple sclerosis or brain tumor. These authors reported that an individual subject usually demonstrated one of three characteristic EMG patterns. The first pattern was characterized by premature activation of the triceps surae during early stance that was seen in 9 of the 26 subjects; the second pattern was characterized by low levels of muscle activity with a normal temporal pattern shown by seven subjects; and the third pattern, seen in four subjects, was characterized by coactivation of several muscle groups during the gait cycle. Knutsson and Richards[13] concluded that each hemiplegic subject has a unique motor control problem during locomotion reflected in the EMG pattern.[13]

SPEED-RELATED CHANGES ON GAIT PARAMETERS

As normal people increase walking speed, their cycle duration, single-limb support, and double-limb support decrease while stride length and cadence increase, and spatiotemporal symmetry between limbs is unchanged.[16,20,26,29,43,44] The peak knee-flexion moment is strongly related to walking speed, whereas angular knee displacement is fairly constant across walking speeds.[29,43] Knee flexion in the sagittal plane increases greatly, however, with running speed.[29,43] The literature on running was not included in this review because the emphasis of this publication, as well as the major clinical concerns for clients with hemiplegia, are to evaluate and improve walking.

For normal subjects, muscle patterns of the limbs remain relative constant over walking speed, with the exception of the rectus femoris. As walking speed increases, the rectus femoris peak activity shifts from knee flexion during loading to the initiation of hip flexion after midstance.[43,45] Overall, the magnitude of the EMG signal increases with increased walking speed.[43,45]

Most relevant to the study of hemiplegic locomotion is that the variability of the EMG increases at very slow walking speeds.[46] These results are important when comparing hemiplegic with normal gait. The effects of velocity on both kinematic and EMG patterns must not be overlooked. Very little research has been reported on the speed-related changes in hemiplegic gait. A study performed by Harro and Giuliani[47] that identified speed-related changes in hemiplegic gait indicated that overall hemiplegic subjects not only walk slower at a self-selected walking speed (range 0.198 to 1.096 m/sec), but they are unable to increase walking speed (range 0.305 to 1.625 m/sec) as much as normals. The mean fast walking speed for hemiplegics was slower than the mean speed for free walking in normal subjects. Patterns of joint movement and limb asymmetries, however, were found to be invariant across walking speed as was reported for normal subjects.[47]

Hemiplegic subjects were also found to have smaller amplitudes and velocities of joint movement.[7,14,47] Several investigators attribute the small step lengths and joint amplitude to a limited ability to produce selective joint movement[1,2,47] and poor balance.[2] This selectivity problem is evident when patients attempt simultaneous hip flexion with knee extension at terminal swing. Walking velocity for normal subjects is strongly correlated with stance but not with swing time, whereas walking velocity for hemiplegic subjects correlated with both stance and swing time of the hemiplegic limb. The inability of hemiplegic subjects to move their hemiplegic limb quickly through the swing phase may be an important factor that limits walking velocity. This difficulty with the duration of swing phase may be of particular interest to therapists. Much emphasis in the treatment of hemiplegic gait is placed on increasing weight-shifting ability; however, it may be equally important to improve initiation and completion of the swing phase of gait.

Subjects in Harro's study were independent ambulators who had variable levels of recovery and were tested at least 1 year following a cerebrovascular accident (CVA).[47] Walking speed was related to recovery, and positive correlations were found between the score of the motor portion of the Fugl-Meyer Motor Assessment Scale and walking velocity.[47] Subjects with poor lower limb recovery (Fugl-Meyer scores <90 percent typically had difficulty increasing walking speed compared with subjects who had good recovery (Fugl-Meyer scores ≥ 90 percent).

Brunnstrom[1] suggested that gait abnormalities resulted from the slowness of the movement itself in addition to the inability to control selected movements. This concept predicts that if hemiplegic subjects walk faster their gait should improve, and if normal subjects walk slowly they should have increased abnormalities. It is possible that normal subjects walking at the same velocity as hemiplegics would have similar gait abnormalities. Kinematic studies by Borkowski et al.[48] and by Lehmann et al.[8] addressed this question. Both groups reported increased variability of both spatiotemporal characteristics and limb movement at slow walking speeds. Some abnormalities of gait could be explained by speed alone, whereas others could not.[8,48] Lehmann et al.[8] examined the gait of subjects with hemiplegia secondary to stroke and the gait of normals matched for gender, age, height, and weight. Hemiplegic subjects walked at a self-selected speed only, and normal subjects walked at a self-selected speed and at the same speed as their matched hemiplegic subjects. Abnormalities in step length, stance, swing, and double-support duration were attributed to speed alone. Gait asymmetries that included a short step length, a prolonged stance and shortened swing duration of the unaffected limb, and a shortened stance duration of the affected limb were unique to hemiplegic gait and could be explained by speed alone.

IMPROVING GAIT IN SUBJECTS WITH HEMIPLEGIA

We know very little about changes in motor control during the recovery process following stroke. Examination of longitudinal changes in kinematic and EMG parameters of locomotion will increase our understanding of the recovery processes. Most studies to date are descriptive and lack control groups. Spontaneous changes in recovery must be identified for the therapist to identify the effects of therapeutic exercise for changing gait characteristics in patients with motor dysfunction.

Many treatments are prescribed for improving hemiplegic gait, such as proprioceptive neuromuscular facilitation, neurodevelopmental treatment, functional electrical simtulation, and, more recently, isokinetic exercises.

Few studies support the efficacy of these treatments. Efficacy research is difficult to control, yet is essential for therapists to prescribe exercise efficiently. It would be helpful for therapists to know what motor control characteristics of a subject's gait are affected, which gait characteristics are amenable to change, which are not, and which exercise may produce the desired change.[49]

Functional electric stimulation was reported to improve walking velocity, stride length, and stride time; however, Bogataj et al.[50] did not account for the effects of recovery and of practicing walking alone without such stimulation. A recent study by Winstein et al.[51] examined the effects of short-leg casting on gait characteristics, using both a casted and noncasted control group. After a 3-week period, the casted group showed significantly increased gait velocity and single-limb stance; however, foot-floor contact patterns did not change in either group. Other studies suggest that concepts of task specificity are related to the effects of exercise designed to improve hemiplegic gait. In examining the effects of resisted pelvic exercise on hemiplegic gait, for example, Trueblood et al.[52] reported that, immediately after a 15-minute exercise period, gait improved; however, measurements taken at 30 minutes after the excercise period were not significantly different from pretest results. Considerable differences were noted in individual responses to the exercise. Before we can conclude that these exercises have no effect, a longer exercise period is warranted. It may be that the pelvic exercise is not task specific enough to carry over to gait, or it is possible that more practice with the exercise is needed to observe permanent changes. Many assumptions are made about the benefits of exercises that therapists use to improve gait without benefit of the evidence to support these claims.

As an example, a commonly held belief by physical therapists is that training hemiplegic patients to shift weight in a standing position will improve their weight-shifting ability during gait. Winstein et al.[53] examined the effects of two types of standing balance training and physical therapy on hemiplegic gait. Subjects who received a program of augmented feedback for balance training had significantly better static standing symmetry than that of subjects who did not receive augmented feedback. Both groups of subjects showed improved walking velocity, cadence, stride length, and cycle time; however, asymmetric spatiotemporal patterns persisted in both groups.[53] It was concluded that improved standing balance symmetry does not necessarily lead to a concomitant reduction in asymmetries of hemiplegic gait associated with difficulty in weight shifting.

Giuliani et al.[54] examined the effects of bicycle exercise in improving gait parameters. Bicycling is a dynamic exercise; its patterns are similar to those in walking in that they require reciprocal flexion and extension movements of the hip, knee, and ankle, and alternating muscle activation of antagonists. Muscle patterns of hemiplegic subjects were more consistent with fewer periods of co-contraction during bicycle pedaling than during walking.[55] Gait characteristics of a control group and of an exercise group of hemiplegic subjects were tested before and after a 2- to 3-month home exercise program on a stationary bicycle.[54] Long-term effects of changes in muscle patterns during walking were not as dramatic as the changes between pedaling and walking. There were significant exercise effects for improved walking velocity, cycle period, and stride length. Changes in EMG patterns were not as clear and appeared to be related to patient compliance and to those muscles used in the pedaling task.[54] As similar as these behaviors may appear, the concepts of task and exercise specificity cannot be overlooked when designing treatment programs. More clinical research is needed to understand the effects of task specificity and practice for improving the characteristics of hemiplegic gait.

SUMMARY

Gait problems in patients with hemiparesis are complex and include both biomechanical and neurologic factors that may affect the ability to grade muscle force and control movement speed to produce the smooth coordinated trunk and limb movement required for efficient locomotion. Research designed to identify motor control variables of gait dysfunction and to test the efficacy of treatment to improve gait is complicated by the variability among subjects with respect to diagnosis, area of lesion, etiology of the dysfunction, functional ability, and time of recovery. Although some general characteristics of hemiparetic gait have been identified, individual differences are great, emphasizing the need for individual assessment to identify problems and design exercise programs to address those problems.

REFERENCES

1. Brunnstrom S: Recording gait patterns of adult hemiplegic patients. J Am Phys Ther Assoc 44:11, 1964
2. Perry J: The mechanics of walking in hemiplegia. Clin Orthop 63:23, 1969
3. Murray MP: Gait as a total pattern of movement. Am J Phys Med 46:290, 1967
4. Richards C, Knutsson E: Evaluation of abnormal gait patterns by intermittent-light photography and EMG. Scand J Rehabil Med 3(suppl):61, 1974
5. Boccardi S, Frigo C, Tesio L, et al: A biomechanical study of locomotion by hemiplegic patients. p 461. In Morecki LA, Fidelus K, et al (eds): Biomechanics. Vol. VII-A. University Park Press, Baltimore, 1981
6. Dewar ME, Judge G: Temporal asymmetry as a gait quality indicator. Med Biol Eng Comput 18:689, 1980
7. Carlsöö S, Dahllöf A, Holm J: Kinetic analysis of gait in patients with hemiparesis and in patients with intermittent claudication. Scand J Rehabil Med 6:166, 1974
8. Lehmann JF, Condon SM, Price R, et al: Gait abnormalities in hemiplegia: Their correction by ankle-foot orthoses. Arch Phys Med Rehabil 68:763, 1987
9. Wall JC, Ashburn A: Assessment of gait disability in hemiplegics. Scand J Rehabil Med 11:95, 1979
10. Brandstater ME, Bruin H, Gowland C, et al: Hemiplegic gait: Analysis of temporal variables. Arch Phys Med Rehabil 64:585, 1983
11. Knutsson E: Gait control in hemiparesis. Scand J Rehabil Med 13:101, 1981
12. Cocoran PJ, Jebsen RH, Brengelmann GL, et al: Effects of plastic and metal leg braces on speed and energy cost of hemiparetic ambulation. Arch Phys Med Rehabil 51:69, 1970
13. Knutsson E, Richards C: Different types of distributed motor control in gait of hemiplegic patients. Brain 102:403, 1979
14. Peat M, Dubo HIC, Winter DA, et al: Electromyographic analysis of gait: Hemiplegic locomotion. Arch Phys Med Rehabil 57:421, 1976
15. Mizrahi J, Susak Z, Heller L, et al: Variation of time-distance parameters of the stride as related to clinical gait improvement in hemiplegics. Scand J Rehabil Med 14:133, 1982
16. Murray MP, Mollinger LA, Gardner GM, et al: Kinematic and EMG patterns during slow, free, and fast walking. J Orthop Res 2:272, 1984

17. Andriacchi TP, Orgle JA, Galante JO: Walking speed as a basis for normal and abnormal gait measurements. J Biomech 10:26, 1977
18. Perry J, Giovan P, Harris L, et al: The determinants of muscle action in the hemiparetic lower extremity. Clin Orthop 131:71, 1978
19. Dimitrijevic MR, Fanganel J, Sherwood AM, et al: Activation of paralyzed leg flexors and extensors during gait in patients after stroke. Scand J Rehabil Med 13:109, 1981
20. Murray MP, Kory RC, Clarkson BH, et al: Comparison of free and fast speed walking patterns in normal men. Am J Phys Med 45:8, 1966
21. Knutsson E, Martenson A: Dynamic motor capacity in spactic paresis and its relation to prime mover dysfunction, spastic reflexes, and antagonist co-activation. Scand J Rehabil Med 12:93, 1980
22. Sahrmann SA, Norton BJ: The relationship of voluntary movement to spasticity in the upper motor neuron syndrome. Ann Neurol 2:460, 1977
23. Hershler C, Milner M: Angle-angle diagrams in the assessment of locomotion. Am J Phys Med 59:109, 1980
24. DeBruin H, Russell DJ, Latter JE, et al: Angle-angle diagrams in monitoring and quantification of gait patterns for children with cerebral palsy. Am J Phys Med 61:176, 1982
25. Winstein CJ, Garfinkle A: Qualitative dynamics of disordered human locomotiom: A preliminary investigation. J Motor Behav 21(4):373, 1989
26. Rosecrance JC: Lower extremity kinematics of stroke patients during bicycle pedalling. Phys Ther 67:769, 1987
27. Perry J: Kinesiology of lower extremity bracing. Clin Orthop 102:18, 1974
28. Inman VT, Ralston HJ, Todd F: Human Walking. Williams & Wilkins, Baltimore, 1981
29. Hirschberg CG, Nathanson M: Electromyographic recording of muscular activity in normal and spastic gaits. Arch Phys Med Rehabil 33:217, 1952
30. Hu MS: Pelvic drop in hemiplegic locomotion: A kinematic and EMG study. Master's thesis, University of North Carolina, Chapel Hill, 1988
31. Wortis SB, Marks M, Hirschberg GG, et al: Gait analysis in hemiplegia. Trans Am Neurol Assoc 76:181, 1951
32. Dietz V, Quintern J, Berger W: Electrophysiological studies of gait in spasticity and rigidity: Evidence that altered mechanical properties of muscle contribute to hypertonia. Brain 104:431, 1981
33. Knutsson E: Restraint of spastic muscle in different types of movement. p. 123. In Feldman RG, Young RR, Koella WP (eds): Spasticity: Disordered Motor Control. Yearbook Medical Publishers, Chicago, 1980
34. Tang A, Rymer WZ: Abnormal force EMG relations in paretic limbs of hemiparetic human subjects J Neurol Neurosurg Psychiatry 44:690, 1981
35. Spector SA, Simard CP, Fournier M: Architectural alterations of rat hind-limb skeletal muscles immobilized at different lengths. Exp Neurol 76:94, 1982
36. Scelsi R, Lotta G, Lommi G: Hemiplegic atrophy: Morphological findings in the anterior tibial muscle of patients with cerebral vascular accident. Acta Neuropathol (Berl) 62:324, 1984
37. Slager UT, Hsu JD, Jordan C: Histochemical and morphometric changes in muscles of stroke patients. Clin Orthop 199:159, 1985
38. Edström L: Selective changes in the sizes of red and white muscle fibers in upper motor neuron lesions and parkinsonism. J Neurol Sci 11:537, 1970
39. McComas AJ, Sica REP, Upton ARM, et al: Function changes in motoneurons of hemiparetic patients. J Neurol Neurosurg Psychiatry 36:183,

40. Chokroverty S, Reyers MG, Rubino FA, et al: Hemiplegic amyotrophy. Arch Neurol 33:104, 1976
41. Rosenfalack A, Andreassen S: Impaired regulation of force and firing pattern of single motor units in patients with spasticity. J Neurol Neurosurg Psychiatry 43:907, 1980
42. Petajan JH: Motor unit control in movement disorders. Adv Neurol 39:897, 1983
43. Kirtley C, Whittle MW, Jefferson RJ: Influence of walking speed on gait parameters. J Biomed Eng 7:282, 1985
44. Nilsson J, Thorstensson A, Halbertsma J: Changes in leg movements and muscle activity with speed of locomotion and mode of progression in humans. Acta Physiol Scand 123:457, 1985
45. Yang JF, Winter DA: Surface EMG profiles during different walking cadences in humans. EEG Clin Neurophysiol 60:485, 1985
46. Shiavi R, Bugle HJ, Limbird T: Electromyographic gait assessment: Part 2. Preliminary assessment of hemiparetic synergy patterns. J Rehabil Res Dev 24:24, 1987
47. Harro CC, Giuliani CA; Kinematic and EMG analysis of hemiplegic gait patterns during free and fast walking speeds. Neurol Rep 11(3):57, 1987
48. Borkowski RG, Craik RL, Freedman WF: An Analysis of slow walking in man. Soc Neurosci Abs. 11:705, 1985
49. Winter DA: Concerning the scientific basis for the diagnosis of pathological gait and for rehabilitation protocols. Physiother Can 17:245, 1985
50. Bogataj U, Gros N, Malezic M, et al: Restoring of gait during two to three weeks of therapy with multichannel electrical stimulation. Phys Ther 69:319, 1989
51. Winstein CJ: Short leg casts: An adjunct to gait training. Master's thesis, University of Southern California, 1984
52. Trueblood PR, Walker JM, Perry J, et al: Pelvic exercise and gait in hemiplegia. Phys Ther 69:19, 1989
53. Winstein CJ, Gardner ER, Mc Neal DR, et al: Balance training in hemiparetics. Arch Phys Med Rehabil 70:755, 1989
54. Giuliani CA, Harro CC, Rosecrance JC: The effects of bicycle pedalling on the temporal-distance and EMG characteristics of walking in hemiplegic subjects. Phys Ther 69:367, 1989
55. Giuliani CA, Harro CC, Rosecrance JC; A comparison of muscle activity during walking and pedalling in subjects with hemiplegia. Neurol Rep 12(19):81, 1988

12 | Cardiopulmonary Abnormalities

Claire Peel

Abnormalities of the cardiovascular and pulmonary systems primarily affect speed and endurance of walking, rather than gait patterns. Disorders involving the lungs, heart, or peripheral blood vessels often limit oxygen delivery to skeletal muscles that are active during walking. Without adequate oxygen, the proportion of energy generated by anaerobic metabolism increases, producing fatigue and dyspnea. Inadequate blood flow to the heart or lower extremities may also produce pain. Because of these symptoms, patients typically limit the amount of walking; the resultant physical deconditioning contributes to the patient's disability.

Walking is an important functional activity, allowing persons to move from place to place, to conduct daily activities. Cardiopulmonary abnormalities may not interfere with walking slowly on level surfaces but may interfere with activities involving higher levels of energy expenditure. Such activities include walking uphill, walking fast, or carrying loads while walking. In evaluating walking performance in persons who may have cardiopulmonary limitations, observational gait analysis is usually not helpful. Appropriate evaluation methods include measuring physiologic responses and noting signs and symptoms of cardiopulmonary limitations. Knowledge of the specific pathology and the extent of involvement is necessary to establish realistic treatment goals. Treatment programs designed to increase the efficiency of walking or to increase cardiopulmonary fitness usually result in functional improvements.

The objectives of this chapter are to discuss the following topics: (1) the role of the cardiopulmonary system in walking, (2) common disorders of the pulmonary and cardiovascular systems that affect walking performance, (3) methods to evaluate cardiopulmonary-associated gait disorders, and (4) treatment

267

strategies to improve functional walking in persons with cardiopulmonary disorders.

ROLE OF THE CARDIOPULMONARY SYSTEM
IN WALKING

Oxygen consumption, or energy expenditure, increases with walking (see Ch. 4). Oxygen consumption ($\dot{V}O_2$) is the product of cardiac output, and the difference between arterial and venous oxygen content (a-VO_2diff) (Fig. 12-1). Cardiac output can be thought of as the oxygen-delivery component, and a-VO_2diff as the oxygen-extraction component. The heart, lungs, and peripheral vessels function together to ensure adequate oxygen delivery. During activity, ventilation increases, thereby increasing the amount of oxygen per time that moves into pulmonary capillaries. The rate and force of cardiac contractions increase, increasing the amount of oxygen-rich blood delivered to the peripheral tissues. The cardiac output is shunted to active organ systems by neurally regulated alterations in resistance of peripheral blood vessels. Oxygen is then available for use by the peripheral tissues to generate energy.

In healthy adults of varied ages, walking at free or self-selected speeds is primarily an aerobic activity, which averages 30 to 50 percent of maximal oxygen consumption ($\dot{V}O_2$max).[1] The aerobic nature of free-paced walking is confirmed by respiratory exchange ratio values of less than 0.85.[2] Since oxygen delivery to tissues is adequate to meet oxygen requirements, persons are in a physiologic steady state and can continue walking for extended periods. If oxygen delivery is not adequate because of cardiopulmonary limitations, aerobic energy generation is supplemented with anaerobic metabolism to permit persons to continue walking at the same speed and intensity. The increased use of anaerobic metabolism increases blood lactate levels, leading to acidosis. Consequences include increased ventilation and subjective feelings of dyspnea and fatigue. Because of these symptoms, persons either discontinue walking activities or decrease the speed of walking to be able to walk distances required to perform functional activities.

For persons with cardiopulmonary disorders, the energy requirements of the heart during various walking activities need to be considered. Myocardial oxygen consumption ($m\dot{V}O_2$) can be estimated using the product of heart rate and systolic blood pressure.[3] For many activities, including cycling and running, $m\dot{V}O_2$ increases in a manner similar to total body $\dot{V}O_2$. For other activities, such as isometric exercise, or dynamic strengthening exercise, there is a disproportionate increase in $m\dot{V}O_2$ relative to the total body $\dot{V}O_2$. If walking is combined with isometric muscle activity, the increase in $m\dot{V}O_2$ may be considerably greater than the increase in $\dot{V}O_2$. This situation occurs when patients hold tightly on the handles of assistive devices or when they carry heavy loads during walking.

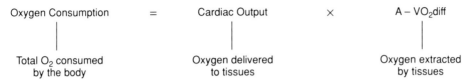

Fig. 12-1. Determinants of oxygen consumption ($\dot{V}O_2$).

ABNORMALITIES OF THE PULMONARY SYSTEM

The primary function of the pulmonary system is gas exchange between atmospheric air and circulating blood. Air moves in and out of the lungs by the process of ventilation. Minute ventilation, the total volume of air exhaled per minute, is the product of breathing rate and tidal volume. In the terminal part of the airways, or alveoli, air comes into close contact with blood flowing through the pulmonary capillaries, and diffusion of oxygen and carbon dioxide occurs. The distributions of airflow and blood flow within the lungs are not uniform, with relatively higher ventilation and blood flow in dependent lung areas. Automatic breathing is controlled by neurons located in the medulla and pons, which receive input from visceral and somatic receptors and influence respiratory muscle activity. Breathing can also be controlled voluntarily by neurons in the cerebral cortex, limbic system, and hypothalamus.[4] During activities, ventilation increases, thereby increasing the rate of airflow into and out of the lungs, as well as the amount of oxygen available for diffusion. Problems occur when there is limited ability to increase ventilation, an increased resistance to airflow, a diffusion impairment or an imbalance between the distribution of capillary blood flow and that of ventilation (Table 12-1).

Abnormalities that impair the ability to increase ventilation include respiratory muscle dysfunction and chest wall deformities. Respiratory muscle weakness or paralysis occurs in persons with cervical and thoracic spinal cord

Table 12-1. Pulmonary Abnormalities That Affect Walking Performance

Problem	Associated Conditions	Clinical Signs
Inability to increase ventilation	Respiratory muscle weakness or paralysis Chest wall deformities	Increased use of accessory breathing muscles Decreased lung volumes
Airway obstruction	Chronic bronchitis Emphysema Asthma	Decreased flow rates Increased residual volume
Diffusion impairment	Pulmonary fibrosis	Decreased PaO_2 Decreased $PaCO_2$ Shallow, rapid breathing pattern
Ventilation/ perfusion inequality	Pulmonary emboli Large airway obstruction Obstructive lung disease	Increased A-aO_2diff

injuries, muscle disease, and diseases affecting the nerve supply to the respiratory muscles. Total lung capacity, vital capacity, and inspiratory capacity are decreased in persons with these disorders. With chest wall abnormalities (including scoliosis and kyphosis), there is decreased mobility in the costovertebral joints and chest wall structures. Parts of the lung may be compressed by bony structures. These persons have difficulty taking in air because of the stiffness of the chest wall and because the alignment of respiratory muscles may be altered by the deformity. These abnormalities are examples of restrictive lung diseases, defined as conditions in which the expansion of the lungs is limited. Lung expansion also is limited in the presence of intrapulmonary structures, such as tumors or abscesses.

Another condition that results in impaired pulmonary function is obstructive lung disease, which involves an increase in resistance to airflow. Airway resistance may be increased because of excessive secretions, edema, or smooth muscle hypertrophy, which occur in bronchitis and asthma. Resistance is increased in emphysema because the radial traction supporting the small airways is lost. In obstructive lung disease, flow rates are decreased and residual volume is increased.

The extremely thin alveolar membranes and the large surface area of the lungs allow oxygen and carbon dioxide to move easily in and out of the circulating blood. Diffusion is impaired in situations in which the interstitium of the alveolar walls thicken, as in diffuse interstitial pulmonary fibrosis. The diffusion rate in decreased, and the period of contact between blood and air may not be long enough for adequate air exchange. Signs and symptoms may not be present at rest but become evident with activity.

Pulmonary abnormalities may produce changes in the regional distribution of ventilation or blood flow, or both, producing an imbalance between ventilation and profusion. Examples of extreme cases of ventilation/perfusion ($\dot{V}/\dot{Q}$) imbalance are pulmonary emboli and complete airway obstruction. A large embolus in the pulmonary circulation blocks blood flow to the lungs, allowing ventilation to occur without perfusion. Complete airway obstruction blocks airflow, permitting perfusion without ventilation. In many pulmonary diseases, including chronic bronchitis and emphysema, small areas of the lung are poorly ventilated or perfused, producing varied degrees of $\dot{V}/\dot{Q}$ inequality. The severity of inequality can be evaluated by the difference between the partial pressure of oxygen in the alveoli and the partial pressure of oxygen in arterial blood (A-aO$_2$diff).

Alterations in lung function may produce changes in the musculoskeletal system. In persons with obstructive lung disease, there is an increase in the anteroposterior diameter relative to the lateral diameter of the chest. The term *barrel chest* is used to describe thoraces of this shape.[5] Digital clubbing is seen in persons with cystic fibrosis, pulmonary fibrosis, and lung abscesses. The normal angle between the nail and the finger is lost, and the fingertips become wide and round, with a shiny appearance. Persons with pulmonary disease often assume a posture with a slightly forward head and trunk, and with the distal parts of the upper extremities stabilized. This posture facilitates breathing by means of the cervical and upper-extremity muscles.[6] The gait pattern of persons with pulmonary disease may include a forward head and trunk.

In persons with obstructive lung disease, changes in respiratory muscle function occur. Because of the increased residual volume, there is a change in the resting position of the diaphragm. At pre-inspiration, the diaphragm assumes a lower position than normal, decreasing the excursion of the muscle from pre-inspiration to end-inspiration. In both restrictive and obstructive lung diseases, the costovertebral joints often become less mobile, thereby increasing the muscle forces required for chest expansion.

Clinicians can identify persons with pulmonary abnormalities by collecting information from the medical record, listening to patient symptoms, observing the patient, and performing evaluations of chest mobility and breath sounds. Important information from the medical record includes pulmonary function testing results and arterial blood gas (ABG) values. Pulmonary function tests provide information on lung volumes and flow rates that aid in the distinction between restrictive and obstructive lung disease. Persons with restrictive disease have low lung volume, with normal flow rate, whereas persons with obstructive disease have increased residual volume and decreased flow rate.[7] An increase in $PaCO_2$ indicates that alveolar ventilation is impaired, whereas a decrease in PaO_2 indicates that oxygenation is below normal.[6]

Persons with pulmonary dysfunction typically report difficulty breathing at rest or with fairly low-level activities. These patients are usually of normal or below normal body weight and may or may not report coughing. During observation, cyanosis is often noted, which is most apparent around the lips or nail beds. Evaluation of chset mobility may indicate decreased motion from maximal expiration to maximal inspiration. Abnormal breath sounds may also be found, indicating areas of increased secretions, atelactasis, or consolidation of lung tissue.

ABNORMALITIES OF THE CARDIOVASCULAR SYSTEM

The heart and vascular system serve peripheral tissues by delivering oxygen and removing carbon dioxide and waste products. With each contraction, the left ventricle generates pressure to move oxygenated blood into the arterial system. Varied resistance at the arteriolar level allows blood to be directed to areas of the body that are metabolically active. During walking, cardiac output increases to deliver additional oxygen to active muscles. Vasodilation occurs in vessels supplying active skeletal muscles, whereas vasoconstriction occurs in less active areas. Cardiac abnormalities that interfere with walking include pathologic conditions that prevent an increase in cardiac output, and conditions that produce chest pain (Table 12-2). Peripheral vascular abnormalities that interfere with walking include atherosclerosis of peripheral vessels and abnormalities of the autonomic nervous system.

Table 12-2. Cardiovascular Abnormalities That Affect Walking Performance

Problem	Associated Conditions	Clinical Signs
Inadequate cardiac output to support activity	Myocardial infarction Cardiomyopathy Congenital heart defects Valve abnormalities Arrhythmias	Blunted or decreased SBP with activity Syncope Skin color changes
Angina	Coronary artery atherosclerosis	Facial expression indicative of pain
Lower-extremity pain with walking	Atherosclerosis of peripheral vessels	Skin changes in lower extremities
ANS dysfunction	Nervous system trauma or disease	Blunted or decreased SBP with activity Syncope Skin color changes

ANS, automatic nervous system; SBP, systolic blood pressure.

Many cardiac diseases affect the heart's ability to increase output in response to physical stress. In cases of large areas of infarction, heart muscle is replaced by fibrotic tissue, limiting the contractile ability of the heart. Cardiomyopathy, which may occur with noncardiac diseases, infections, or drug therapy, leads to a decrease in the strength of cardiac muscle. Abnormal direction of blood flow through the heart occurs with many congenital heart defects and with abnormalities of cardiac valves. With cardiac arrhythmias that produce premature beats, output may be decreased because of inadequate time for ventricular filling. A consequence of these conditions is inadequate oxygen delivery. Functional limitations vary and are related to the severity of the disease.

Signs of inadequate cardiac output include a blunted or decreasing blood pressure response during activity, changes in skin color, and incoordination. Persons may complain of dizziness, lightheadedness, and difficulty performing activities. Medical information that assists in identifying the specific problem and the extent to injury includes reports of coronary artery angiography, ventricular function, and electrocardiography (ECG). The location and extent of coronary artery occlusions and abnormal ventricular wall motion are detected by angiography. The ejection fraction, or the volume of blood ejected from the left ventricle with each contraction, may also be measured during angiography. The location and type of abnormal electrical activity are found in ECG reports.

Walking performance is limited in some persons by angina or chest pain. Angina that occurs with activity, or *exertional angina,* is thought to result from an imbalance between the oxygen requirements of the heart and the oxygen delivered to the heart. The amount of oxygen delivered to the heart may be limited because of atherosclerosis of the coronary arteries, a condition that increases the resistance to flow and limits the ability of vessels to vasodilate. Patients typically report a squeezing or pressure sensation in the chest that is fairly reproducible when a specific activity level is reached. The pain usually disappears when the activity is discontinued and when medications are taken.

Because patients with angina tend to avoid activity, a functional consequence is physical deconditioning.

Atherosclerosis in the peripheral vessels may limit blood flow to the active skeletal muscles during activities such as walking. Similar to coronary artery atherosclerosis, the resistance to flow is increased, and the capacity of the vasculature to vasodilate is limited. Typically, patients complain of leg pain after walking short distances, which is relieved by stopping the activity. Because of the discomfort, persons tend to spend less time walking and become deconditioned.

Autonomic nervous system dysfunction may result from nervous system trauma or diseases affecting the hypothalamus, spinal cord, or peripheral nerves. One consequence is an inability to distribute blood appropriately in response to stress. If vasoconstriction in inactive areas is impaired, blood supply may not be sufficient to meet the oxygen needs of active muscle. Blood accumulation, or *pooling,* may occur in dependent areas of the body, resulting in decreased venous return and cardiac output. Persons often complain of dizziness and lightheadedness, may suffer episodes of syncope, and report a decrease in activity tolerance.

FUNCTIONAL CONSEQUENCES OF CARDIOPULMONARY ABNORMALITIES

In general, the cardiopulmonary disorders that have been described affect the delivery of oxygen to working muscles during moderate to high intensity activities. Because of the relationship between $\dot{V}O_2$ and cardiac output, maximal oxygen consumption measurements are lower than normal. Impairment in $\dot{V}O_2$-max does not directly result in functional limitations because most daily activities do not involve high-intensity work levels. An important indirect consequence is that low-and moderate-level activities are performed at a higher percentage of $\dot{V}O_2$max. Because physiologic responses and subjective feelings correlate highly with percent $\dot{V}O_2$max, or relative exercise intensity, submaximal activities produce relatively high physical and psychological stresses.[8,9]

Another consequence of a low $\dot{V}O_2$max is excessive use of anaerobic metabolism for energy production at relatively low workloads. In sedentary persons, the lactate and ventilatory thresholds, which indicate an increase in anaerobic energy generation, occur at approximately 50 to 60 percent of $\dot{V}O_2$max.[10] In persons with low levels of $\dot{V}O_2$max, the workload corresponding to 50 to 60 percent of $\dot{V}O_2$max is relatively low and may occur during normal walking. Activities that involve a significant anaerobic component cannot be performed for extended periods, because the increase in blood lactate rapidly leads to fatigue.[9]

A consequence of many pulmonary disorders is an increase in the energy required for breathing. In persons with normal pulmonary function, the energy required for breathing at rest is less than 5 percent of that the total body $\dot{V}O_2$.[11] During high-level activities, the proportion increases to 20 to 30 percent.[11] In persons with lung disease that involves either airway obstruction or chest wall stiffness, or both, the forces needed to inflate the lungs are higher than normal. Consequently, breathing at rest may consume up to 25 percent of the total body $\dot{V}O_2$ and, during activities, the proportion of $\dot{V}O_2$ to support ventilation increases significantly.[12] Using a large proportion of oxygen for breathing limits the oxygen available for active skeletal muscles and other organ systems.

Limitations in the oxygen available for skeletal muscle function result in decreased walking velocity and endurance. Persons tend to walk slowly to minimize the oxygen requirement, preventing excessive anaerobic metabolism, fatigue, and pain. The duration that a person can walk at normal or fast speeds is limited. The higher energy requirements associated with walking at fast speeds may approach maximal levels and result in excessive cardiovascular and metabolic stress.

The efficiency of walking may be decreased in persons with postural adaptations related to pulmonary dysfunction. Limited trunk rotation and arm swing impair the normal energy transfer that occurs during the gait cycle.[13] With a posture involving excessive hip and trunk flexion, maintaining the upright position may require additional energy. Many persons with pulmonary disease rely on assessory breathing muscles during walking, which also increases oxygen requirements. Walking efficiency may be decreased in persons who do not have the expected activity-related increase in cardiac output. These persons are often fearful of dizziness and fainting and ambulate with short step lengths, staying near large items for support.

PHYSICAL THERAPY MANAGEMENT

The evaluation and treatment of persons with cardiopulmonary-related gait abnormalities differ from that of the typical person with musculoskeletal or neuromuscular dysfunction. Rather than concentrating on observational gait analysis, the focus of the evaluation is on physiologic responses and on signs and symptoms both during and after walking. Knowledge of the specific pathology is important to identify realistic treatment goals. Treatment programs are typically long term in nature and may include life-style changes.

EVALUATION

During the physical therapy evaluation, objective information can be collected on selected physiologic and subjective responses to walking and on walking velocity and endurance. Heart rate (HR), blood presure (BP), and respiratory rate (RR) changes occurring with free-paced walking should be documented initially to ensure appropriate responses. A patient must walk for 2 to 3 minutes to elicit steady-state responses. When walking at a comfortable speed, HR, systolic blood pressure (SBP), and RR should increase slightly, with minimal or no change in diastolic blood pressure (DBP). An excessive increase in HR or a decrease in SBP would be considered inappropriate responses.

Table 12-3. Grading Scale for Chest Pain

Grade	Degree of Pain	Definition
1	Light	Discomfort that is established, but barely perceptible (some patients speak of grade 1 or 2 discomfort as that premonitory sensation that precedes grade 1 level)
2	Light-moderate	Discomfort from which an individual can be distracted by a noncataclysmic event (it can be pain, but usually is not)
3	Moderate-severe	Discomfort or pain that prevents distraction by a pretty woman, handsome man, television show, or other consuming interest (only a tornado, earthquake, or explosion can distract an individual from grade 3 discomfort or pain)
4	Severe	The most excruciating pain experienced or imaginable

(From Pollock et al.,[14] with permission.)

Patients can estimate their subjective feelings using rating scales for angina, dyspnea, or perceived exertion (Tables 12-3 to 12-5). These scales have standardized instructions and can be used to compare a patient's responses under different conditions and over time.[14-16] Patients should be observed for changes in skin color and for signs of unsteadiness. In addition, patients should be questioned for symptoms of dizziness or lightheadedness.

If available, additional measurements that assist in identifying abnormalities include oxygen saturation, ECG, and blood lactate. Oxygen saturation can be measured noninvasively using ear lobe oximeters. This measurement is important for persons with pulmonary dysfunction because chronic oxygen desaturation can lead to right-sided heart failure.[17] Electrical activity of the heart can be recorded during activities, using radiotelemetry systems. This information is important when evaluating persons with cardiac problems because arrhythmias often occur with activity, but not at rest. Blood lactate levels can be determined fairly easily, by performing a finger stick and collecting blood in a capillary tube. Elevations in blood lactate above baseline or resting values suggest increased use of anaerobic metabolism. The associated activity level

Table 12-4. Grading Scale for Severity of Dyspnea

Class	Definition
I	Dyspnea only on severe exertion
II	Can keep pace with person of same age and body build on the level without breathlessness, but not on hills or stairs
III	Can walk a mile at own pace without dyspnea, but cannot keep up with a normal person
IV	Dyspnea present after walking about 100 yards on the level, or upon climbing one flight of stairs
V	Dyspnea present on slight exertion, such as dressing, talking, at rest

(From the Committee on Rating of Mental and Physical Impairment,[15] with permission.)

Table 12-5. Ratings of Perceived
Exertion Scale

Rating	Description
6	
7	Very, very light
8	
9	Very light
10	
11	Fairly light
12	
13	Somewhat hard
14	
15	Hard
16	
17	Very hard
18	
19	Very, very hard
20	

(From Borg,[20] with permission.)

would not be considered a steady-state level and would result in fatigue within a short period.

The measurements described can be performed with patients walking at varied speeds and under varied conditions. By documenting HR at several velocities, the minimal walking speed necessary to elicit aerobic training adaptations can be identified. To elicit cardiovascular training adaptations, the HR response needs to be in the range of 70 to 85 percent of age-predicted maximal HR.[18] The walking speed that places the least stress on the cardiovascular system can also be identified. This speed is not necessarily the slowest walking speed but is the speed associated with the lowest HR response.

The evaluation should also include an assessment of physiologic responses as the patient is performing typical walking activities. Activities may include carrying objects, such as briefcases or golf clubs; walking uphill, upstairs, and downstairs; and in varied environmental conditions. Heart rate and BP responses during functional walking are monitored to ensure the safety of the activities and to document the cardiovascular stress associated with the activity. Often the stress of the activity can be minimized by altering the walking or carrying pattern.

ESTABLISHING REALISTIC GOALS

The most important information necessary to set realistic treatment goals is knowledge of the specific pathology. With many pulmonary diseases (e.g., chronic bronchitis and emphysema) and cardiac diseases (e.g., myocardial infarction and coronary artery atherosclerosis), the damage to the tissues is irreversible. Symptoms may be improved with medications, or the rate of progression of the disease may be slowed by life-style changes. Knowledge of the primary disease process, the severity of the disease, and associated medical problems enables the therapist to predict realistic treatment interventions that will improve the client's function.

The specific pathology and the physical therapy evaluation results are viewed together. A working hypothesis is generated, linking the pathology with the clinical signs and symptoms. At this point in the decision-making process, several options are available (Fig. 12-2). The therapist is not limited to one choice and may proceed with multiple options. The patient may need to be referred to other health professionals for evaluation and treatment. Patients with inappropriate and potentially unsafe responses to activity and patients who could benefit from drug and medical therapy need to be referred for evaluation by a physician. Some abnormalities are used as compensatory mechanisms to maximize pulmonary or cardiac function. An example is the change in posture in persons with pulmonary disease, used to maximize the use of accessory breathing muscles. Changing compensatory mechanisms may not benefit such a patient.

In general, treatment objectives are directed toward improving function. Walking performance can be improved by increasing cardiopulmonary fitness, or $\dot{V}O_2$max and by increasing the efficiency of walking. An increase in $\dot{V}O_2$max allows persons to perform most walking activities with greater ease. This goal may not be realistic in persons with severe, irreversible disease. An increase in walking efficiency allows patients to perform walking activities at a lower $\dot{V}O_2$ level and consequently with less stress.

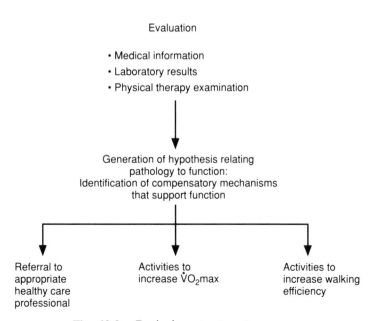

Fig. 12-2.   Designing a treatment program.

DESIGNING TREATMENT PROGRAMS

For persons who can safely perform moderate intensity aerobic exercise, improving $\dot{V}O_2$ max is often a treatment goal. Ideally, the exercise prescription is based on the results of an exercise stress test. The patient performs 30- to 40-minute sessions three to five times per week. Activities, which include walking, jogging, cycling, and swimming, involve rhythmic, continuous movements of large muscle groups. Heart rate is used as an estimate of exercise intensity. For healthy adults, HR responses averaging 70 to 85 percent of age-predicted maximal HR are necessary to improve $\dot{V}O_2$ max.[18] In persons with cardiopulmonary abnormalities, the intensity is affected by medications and by signs and symptoms. Persons taking β-adrenergic blocking agents exercise at relatively low HR levels. Persons with exercise-induced arrhythmias or angina also exercise at lower HR levels than do healthy adults. The exercise prescription should be individualized on the basis of the patient's pathology, personal interests, and activity history.

An example of the benefits of regular aerobic exercise is shown in Table 12-6. The increase in $\dot{V}O_2$ max lowers the percent $\dot{V}O_2$ max, or relative exercise intensity, for a standardized level of submaximal exercise. Before training, the relative exercise intensity for walking at 3 mph was 43 percent $\dot{V}O_2$ max; after training, the relative exercise intensity for the same work level was 38 percent $\dot{V}O_2$ max. The lower relative exercise intensity is associated with lower HR, BP, and ratings of perceived exertion. Consequently, the patient is able to handle the same workload, with less cardiovascular stress and less subjective fatigue.

Another treatment goal may be to improve walking efficiency. This goal is most appropriate for persons who do not have the capacity to exercise at sufficient intensities to improve $\dot{V}O_2$ max. An improvement in efficiency can be documented objectively by measuring $\dot{V}O_2$ before and after an intervention (Table 12-7). Methods to improve efficiency include practice and improvements in the coordination between gait and breathing patterns. Persons who perform limited walking activities often increase the efficiency of walking by beginning a regular walking program. This training adaptation has been demonstrated in studies of exercise training in persons with pulmonary disease.[19] With this population, $\dot{V}O_2$ max often does not increase in response to exercise training, but submaximal walking efficiency improves, which improves function.

Efficiency may also be improved by altering walking and breathing patterns. In some patients, the use of assistive devices or improving upright posture

Table 12-6. Changes in Ralative Exercise Intensity (percent $\overset{\circ}{V}O_2$ max) with Aerobic Exercise Training

Measurement	Pre-training	Post-training
$\dot{V}O_2$ max	28 ml/kg $\cdot$ min^{-1}	32 ml/kg $\cdot$ min^{-1}
$\dot{V}O_2$ for walking at 3 mph	12 ml/kg $\cdot$ min^{-1}	12 ml/kg $\cdot$ min^{-1}
Percent $\dot{V}O_2$ max for walking at 3 mph	43%	38%

Table 12-7. Changes in Walking Efficiency and Relative Exercise Intensity with Physical Therapy Intervention

Measurement	Pre-intervention	Post-intervention
$\dot{V}O_2$ max	23 ml/kg · min^{-1}	23 ml/kg · min^{-1}
$\dot{V}O_2$ for walking at 3 mph	15 ml/kg · min^{-1}	12 ml/kg · min^{-1}
% $\dot{V}O_2$ max for walking at 3 mph	65%	52%

may increase efficiency. Shoes with good support and shock-absorbing capabilities may also improve walking efficiency. By coordinating inspiration and expiration with stepping patterns, persons with pulmonary disease can often improve walking performance. This adaptation prevents rapid breathing patterns in which dead space ventilation is high compared with deep-breathing patterns. If equipment is not available to measure $\dot{V}O_2$ during walking, therapists can use steady-state HR responses as an indirect estimate of changes in efficiency.

SUMMARY

Abnormalities involving the heart, lungs, or peripheral blood vessels often limit the delivery of oxygen to active skeletal muscles. Walking endurance and velocity are decreased because of excessive use of anaerobic metabolism, which leads to fatigue. Cardiopulmonary abnormalities may affect walking performance in persons referred to physical therapy for problems involving the neuromuscular or musculoskeletal systems. Medical information, subjective reports, physical signs, and physiologic responses to activity are important considerations in designing appropriate treatment plans. In some cases, function can be improved by treatment programs that produce increased $\dot{V}O_2$max or increased walking efficiency.

REFERENCES

1. Waters RL, Hislop HJ, Perry J, et al: Comparative cost of walking in young and old adults. J Orthop Res 1:73, 1983
2. Waters RL, Lunsford BR, Perry J, et al: Energy-speed relationship of walking: Standard tables. J Orthop Res 6:215, 1988
3. Nelson RR, Gobel FL, Jorgensen CR, et al: Hemodynamic predictors of myocardial oxygen consumption during static and dynamic exercise. Circulation 50:1179, 1974
4. West JB: Respiratory Physiology: The Essentials. 2nd Ed. Williams & Wilkins, Baltimore, 1979
5. Lehrer S: Understanding Lung Sounds. WB Saunders, Philadelphia, 1984
6. Humberstone N: Respiratory assessment. p. 208. In Irwin S, Tecklin J (eds): Cardiopulmonary Physical Therapy. CV Mosby, St. Louis, 1985
7. West JB: Pulmonary Pathophysiology: The Essentials. 2nd Ed. Williams & Wilkins, Baltimore, 1982

8. Borg GAV: Psychophysical bases of perceived exertion. Med Sci Sports Exer 14:377, 1982

9. Astrand PO, Rodahl K: Textbook of Work Physiology. McGraw-Hill, St. Louis, 1977

10. Wasserman K, Whipp BJ, Koyal SN, et al: Anaerobic threshold and respiratory gas exchange during exercise. J Appl Physiol 35:236, 1973

11. Cherniack RM, Cerniack L, Naimark A: Respiration in Health and Disease. 2nd Ed. WB Saunders, Philadelphia, 1972

12. Levison H, Cherniack RM: Ventilatory cost of exercise in chronic obstructive pulmonary disease. J Appl Physiol 25:21, 1968

13. Inman VT, Ralston HJ, Todd F: Human Walking. Waverly Press, Baltimore, 1981

14. Pollock MJ, Wilmore JH, Fox SM: Exercise in Health and Disease: Evaluation and Prescription for Prevention and Rehabilitation. WB Saunders, Philadelphia, 1984

15. Committee on Rating of Mental and Physical Impairment: Guides to the evaluation of permanent impairment—The respiratory system. JAMA 194:919, 1965

16. Skinner JS, Hutsler R, Bergsteinova V, et al: The validity and reliability of a rating scale of perceived exertion. Med Sci Sports 5:94, 1973

17. Irwin S: Abnormal exercise physiology. p. 50. In Irwin S, Tecklin J (eds): Cardiopulmonary Physical Therapy. CV Mosby, St. Louis, 1985

18. Guidelines for Graded Exercise Testing and Exercise Prescription. American College of Sports Medicine. Lea & Febiger, Philadelphia, 1986

19. Paez PN, Phillipson EA, Masangkay M, et al: The physiologic basis of training patients with chronic airway obstruction. I. Effects of exercise training. Am Rev Respir Dis 95:944, 1967

20. Borg GAV: Perceived exertion as an indicator of somatic stress. Scand J Rehabil Med 2:92, 1970

13 | Prosthetic and Orthotic Gait

Joan E. Edelstein

Augmenting the human body with a prosthesis or orthosis markedly affects the individual's mode of travel. A prosthesis can restore bipedal gait. Similarly, an orthosis of appropriate design and construction can enable the wearer to move in a more comfortable, efficient manner than might otherwise be the case. In both instances, however, the ambulation pattern is unlikely to duplicate that of a nondisabled person. While appliances should reduce impairment to the locomotor system, rarely, if ever, do they compensate completely for the anatomic disturbance. Consequently, the task for the clinician is to recognize optimal gait with a given device, so that departures from the standard can be identified and their causes determined and, wherever possible, corrected.

PROSTHETIC GAIT PATTERNS

Walking with a prosthesis, whether partial foot, below-knee, above-knee, or hip disarticulation, requires that the wearer harmonize bodily movements with those of insensate apparatus. Clearly, the more distal the amputation, the closer the fit between prosthesis and amputation limb, the more precise the alignment, and the better the prosthetic components simulate actions of missing anatomic parts, the more natural will be the appearance of gait. Other factors contribute to locomotion as well. Physical condition is paramount. A painful amputation limb, marginal cardiopulmonary function, motion limitation because of arthritis or contracture, and central or peripheral neuropathy alter gait kinematics. Vascular disorders, such as congestive heart failure and peripheral vascular disease, restrict tissue oxygenation, reducing the walker's maximal aerobic capacity.[1] Psychological status and the adequacy of training can be inferred from the patient's ability to control the prosthesis. Wearers are apt to demonstrate different walking patterns when they are conscious of being observed in the clinic, as compared with casual gait, which typically is more relaxed when the walker does not feel on display.[2]

Of all the elements affecting locomotion, those most amenable to change relate to the device. Thus, in the description of walking patterns, emphasis is placed on prosthetic design, alignment, and fit.

Partial Foot and Syme's Amputations

Individuals with a well-healed amputation through the metatarsals or digits generally walk with minimal deviation. Unilateral amputees are likely to exhibit slight asymmetry in late stance, moving quickly from the amputated limb to spend proportionately more time on the intact one. Premature loss of the natural base of support may also hasten knee flexion in late stance, inasmuch as the floor reaction shifts behind the knee more rapidly than normal. The tendency both to abbreviate late stance and to bend the knee quickly may be reduced by a snugly fitting foot prosthesis. The socket should be attached to a firm base to substitute for the distal foot. Alternatively, the shoe itself can be stiffened by the installation of a steel plate between the inner and outer soles.

Syme's supramalleolar amputation offers the potential for quite a smooth gait, if the patient wears a well-fitting prosthesis. Without a prosthesis, walking is essentially a pivoting over the amputated limb. The short limb also causes the walker to lean laterally to the amputated side. With a prosthesis, the artificial foot enables the wearer to plantar flex in early stance to absorb shock and to achieve the stability of the foot flat phase of gait. Although the rigid keel of the solid ankle cushion heel (SACH) foot permits no dorsiflexion and the deflection plates of the Carbon Copy II or Quantum foot move very slightly into dorsiflexion, the Syme's amputee has a leg lever nearly the normal length with which to control forward movement. The final phase of stance is accomplished by passive hyperextension at the junction between the toe section and the keel or deflection plate. Optoelectronic analysis of the gait of a 5-year-old child with congenital anomaly surgically revised to the Syme level conformed to age-appropriate cadence, velocity, and gait pattern.[3]

Deviations of Syme's prosthetic gait can be caused by discomfort within the socket or by faulty foot selection or alignment. For example, if the prosthetic cushion heel is too firm, the foot will fail to absorb sufficient shock at heel contact; thus, the knee will tend to flex abnormally fast. An unduly long keel will interfere with simulated toe hyperextension in late stance. If the foot is malaligned to the prosthetic shank in excessive plantar flexion, the shank will tend to lag behind and the knee will not flex adequately. The same effect can also be caused by wearing a shoe with a heel lower than that for which the prosthetic foot was designed.

Below-Knee Amputations

Many people with below-knee amputation ambulate in a manner that defies detection of the prosthesis by the casual observer. Even some with bilateral prostheses achieve a fluent walking style. Laboratory examination of skilled walkers, however, reveals subtle departure from the nonamputee pattern. During early stance, the patient's knee bends somewhat less than normal because the prosthetic foot does not produce the controlled plantar flexion obtained naturally by eccentric contraction of the dorsiflexors. Knee flexion is also less than normal during late stance. Ordinarily, knee motion coordinates with foot motion. Unlike the anatomic foot, which plantar flexes at toe-off, the prosthetic ankle cannot move when weight has been transferred to the toe section. If the client were to allow the knee to flex to the normal extent, the torso would lower excessively, producing an inefficient, unattractive gait.[4]

Walking speed is slower,[5-8] prosthetic step length is slightly longer, and the time spent on the prosthesis is briefer than on the unimpaired limb.[9] Cadence is proportional to amputation limb length; those with shorter limbs select slower speeds.[10]

Posterior force exerted by the amputated limb is reduced substantially at heel contact, and joint moments are lower than normal. Concurrently, the sound limb generates a greater than normal dorsiflexion moment.[11] Hip extensors are more active than in the nonamputee during early and midstance; simultaneous hamstring and quadriceps activity at early stance controls knee flexion.[12,13]

The type of prosthetic foot influences knee motion and timing. As compared with the SACH component, persons wearing the single-axis foot display greater plantar flexion[14] and move more rapidly through early stance.[15] With the SACH assembly, subjects contracted hamstring and quadriceps muscles on the amputated side longer than on the intact limb.[16] Clinical observation of individuals fitted with energy-storing/energy-releasing feet, particularly the Flex-Foot and Seattle foot, manifest gait kinematics closer to that of the contralateral intact limb.[17-20] The newer feet have not overcome completely the asymmetry recorded with older components. As compared with the sound limb, the prosthetic side rises to peak load in early stance more slowly and does not achieve as high force during heel-off, but it does produce more force at toe-off.[21] Total vertical force during late stance remains less on the prosthetic side.[22]

Sagittal Plane Deviations

Gait is clinically deviant when knee flexion either is markedly limited or is excessive during stance phase.[23,24] Excessive knee flexion during early stance may be caused by any prosthetic or anatomic factor that permits the floor reaction to remain behind the knee, producing a flexion moment of force. A knee-flexion contracture exaggerates the tendency of the knee to bend. If the contracture cannot be relieved surgically or by means of active or passive exercise, the prosthetic foot should be set more anterior than customary. Anterior foot placement corresponds with posterior socket location, which, in turn, advances the floor reaction in relationship to the knee. The patient with weak quadriceps may experience knee instability or jerkiness, manifested either by excessive flexion or by conscious efforts to straighten the knee, aided by leaning forward slightly.

Prosthetically, a heel cushion or comparable element in the prosthetic foot that is too firm will fail to compress adequately, hindering plantar flexion. The knee will then be subject to the effect of the posteriorly placed floor reaction, and the foot may rotate excessively in the sagittal plane at heel contact. A shoe heel that is too high for the particular foot will also keep the floor reaction behind the knee. If the foot is aligned in dorsiflexion, the knee will be ahead of the floor reaction. Excessive flexion or anterior displacement of the socket is comparable to an uncompensated contracture. Changes in foot alignment, especially, have a profound effect on gait kinematics.[25]

The opposite deviation—insufficient knee flexion in early stance—occurs because of an anteriorly located floor reaction. Reversal of the anatomic and prosthetic causes associated with excessive flexion is the source of relative stiffness in stance. Thus, an arthritic knee or one fused in extension cannot yield at heel contact. The patient with spasticity who manifests extensor synergy will keep the knee straight in response to the distal stimulus of the floor. Rather than risking a fall, the individual with quadriceps weakness soon learns to lean forward to prevent the knee from collapsing. Anterodistal pain in the amputation limb is yet another explanation for the deviation. Because quadriceps contraction increases pressure at the "kick point," the patient avoids discomfort by extending the thigh, shortening the step, and lurching the trunk ahead. The client who is accustomed to the old-fashioned wood prosthesis, which included a thigh corset and a socket aligned vertically, may persist in the habit of walking with the knee held straight.

Among the prosthetic causes for knee flexion insufficiency are faults in suspension or in the foot. If cuff suspension is augmented by an anterior elastic fork strap, excessive strap tension will restrain knee flexion.[26] Too soft a heel cushion will hasten plantar flexion and, with it, knee extension. Heel firmness is determined by the patient's weight and vigor of walking. Both the obese person and one who strides rapidly and forcefully require a rather firm cushion. Indiscriminate switching of shoes also disturbs gait. The person who changes from a higher-heeled to a lower-heeled shoe will experience unwanted knee stability; the lower heel places the floor reaction in front of the knee. A foot aligned in plantar flexion or a socket set in inadequate flexion or placed too far posterior are other causes of insufficient knee flexion in early stance.

Knee flexion may be delayed in late stance if the floor reaction remains anterior to the joint. The patient may complain of difficulty terminating stance, likening walking to climbing up a hill. An arthrodesed or arthritic knee will not flex in late stance. Extensor synergy may persist as long as any part of the limb touches the floor. By the time of late stance, the walker has transferred weight from the heel so that the firmness of the heel cushion is no longer a consideration. Instead, the location of the distal tip of the keel, or similar component, determines the ease of knee flexion. An unduly long keel retains the floor reaction in front of the knee, hampering flexion, as will a shoe with a heel lower than that for which the prosthesis was designed. A foot set in plantar flexion or a socket lacking proper flexion impedes knee flexion in early and late stance. The older type of prosthesis obliged the wearer to keep the knee relatively extended throughout much of stance phase. At late stance, the wearer tended to lean against the leather check straps that joined the back of the thigh corset to the posterior socket brim. The contemporary patellar tendon-bearing socket does not need such straps; nevertheless, someone who has learned to rely on the straps may continue to keep the knee extended as if the straps were there.

Once again, the opposite deviation can be caused by contrary prosthetic and anatomic elements. If the floor reaction passes too far behind the knee, the walker may comment that the knee is dropping off into space. An uncompensated knee-flexion contracture may be responsible for this complaint. A prosthetic foot that is too short or one having too short a keel will also cause premature knee flexion. Children are likely to demonstrate early knee flexion; if the youngster has outgrown the original shoes and is now wearing a pair of new, longer shoes, the prosthetic foot and keel have become functionally too short. A shoe with a heel higher than appropriate for the particular prosthetic foot may be at fault. A foot aligned in dorsiflexion or a socket that is too far anterior or excessively flexed are other possibilities. All such errors reduce the distance that body weight must travel forward before losing the major base of support.

Frontal Plane Deviations

The wearer of a below-knee prosthesis may exhibit excessive frontal motion of the prosthetic brim at midstance. Movement occurs when the rigid plastic of the prosthesis pushes the yielding skin and subcutaneous tissue of the leg. Although the ideal arrangement would be to eliminate all motion, the dissimilar materials of the prosthesis-skin interface stymie this goal. Patients who wear an elastic sleeve suspension, however, experience less proximal movement because the fabric holds the prosthesis very snugly and masks any incipient motion. At midstance, all weight is loaded onto the prosthesis eccentrically. The foot must be aligned medial to the socket so that motion that does occur is least uncomfortable. Medial foot placement causes the prosthetic brim to shift laterally, gapping laterally and compressing the proximomedial tissues. These structures, composed chiefly of the flat pes anserinus tendons, tolerate pressure reasonably well. Pressure is exerted concurrently on the distolateral aspect of the amputation limb, where the severed end of the fibula may not be very tolerant of intermittent loading. Inseting the foot also minimizes the walking base, thereby reducing the tendency toward unsightly, fatiguing lateral trunk flexion.

Excessive foot inset, however, increases lateral thrust of the brim and may result in discomfort, especially at the end of the fibula. Foot outset is to be avoided because this malalignment compels the patient to walk with medial thrust of the brim. Such displacement impacts on the sensitive fibular head proximally and on the tibial end. In addition, the amputee will exhibit a wide-based gait with lateral flexion of the trunk. Table 13-1 summarizes the gait deviations observed among below-knee amputees.

Knee Disarticulations and Above-Knee Amputations

Absence of the anatomic foot and knee compromises gait considerably. Patients with disarticulation or amputation at or above the knee are apt to limp noticeably. These patients lack the skeletal, motor, and sensory functions of the distal structures and, in comparison with the below-knee amputee, must transport an artificial limb perceived as being rather heavy. Prosthetic weight, while less than the anatomic segment, is often considered a burden because the prosthesis is imperfectly united to the body and lacks normal neuromuscular control. Objective testing, however, suggests that changes in prosthetic foot

Table 13-1. Below-Knee Prosthetic Gait Analysis

Deviation	Prosthetic Causes	Anatomic Causes
Excessive knee flexion in early stance	Insufficient plantar flexion Stiff heel cushion or plantar bumper Excessive socket flexion Socket malaligned too far anteriorly Excessive posterior placement of cuff tabs	Knee flexion contracture Weak quadriceps
Insufficient knee flexion in early stance	Excessive plantar flexion Soft heel cushion or plantar bumper Insufficient socket flexion Socket malaligned too far posteriorly	Pain at anterodistal aspect of amputated limb Weak quadriceps Extensor spasticity Knee arthritis
Excessive lateral thrust	Excessive inset of foot Excessive socket adduction	
Medial thrust	Outset of foot Insufficient socket adduction	
Early knee flexion in late stance "drop off"	Insufficient plantar flexion Distal end of keel or toe break misplaced posteriorly Soft dorsiflexion stop Excessive socket flexion Socket malaligned too far anteriorly Excessive posterior placement of cuff tabs	Knee flexion contracture
Delayed knee flexion in late stance "walking uphill"	Excessive plantar flexion Distal end of keel or toe break misplaced anteriorly Stiff dorsiflexion stop Insufficient socket flexion Socket malaligned too far posteriorly	Extensor spasticity Knee arthritis

(Adapted from Edelstein,[76] with permission.)

weight do not alter stride length, knee motion, or velocity,[27] while alteration in shank weight does affect cadence; a shank with a relatively proximal center of mass is associated with a briefer prosthetic swing.[28] Socket material contributes to prosthetic weight and to gait kinematics; wearing a flexible socket was associated with less deviant gait than with the rigid one.[29]

Young adults using above-knee prostheses tend to select a comfortable walking speed that is slower than that chosen by nondisabled peers.[30-32] Elderly dysvascular amputees usually walk considerably slower than healthy age mates.[33] Juvenile subjects also choose slower speeds.[34,35] When skilled prosthesis users walk, velocity may approach that of normal subjects; however, stance phase on the prosthesis is shorter.[36]

Other gait characteristics are altered by above-knee amputation. The upper torso of the prosthesis wearer not only rotates through a greater than normal amplitude but also demonstrates asymmetric rotations. The pelvis tends to rise on the side of the swinging prosthesis, rather than lower, as seen in the nonamputee. The pelvis may contribute to prosthetic swing, compensating for lack of active push-off by the prosthesis.[37] Knee action is decidedly different. In contrast to the intact knee, which flexes in early stance to decrease upward displacement of the body's center of mass, the amputee cannot permit knee flexion, lacking the quadriceps effectiveness that would normally control flexion.[38] Distal factors are also at work. The heel cushion or similar posterior resilient portion of the prosthetic foot does not permit fine control of plantar flexion during early stance. This departure from normal gait, aggravted by deficiencies in the artificial knee, compels the sound limb to compensate for the inadequacies on the prosthetic side. Gait thus becomes quite asymmetric.[39]

The discrepancy between sound and prosthetic sides is exaggerated when the individual walks on uneven terrain, runs, climbs, jumps, and engages in other ambulatory pursuits. Nevertheless, a very few persons move so gracefully, subconsciously compensating for the inherent biomechanical deficiencies, that passersby may not be aware of the prosthesis.

Sagittal Plane Deviations

Gait abnormalities in the sagittal plane representing marked departure from optimal performance include (1) foot slap, (2) uneven heel rise, (3) terminal swing impact, and (4) uneven step length.

Foot Slap. In early stance, this gait abnormality results from faulty selection or adjustment of the prosthetic foot. With proper componentry, the client should be able to compress the posterior portion of the foot at heel contact. Compression permits the entire sole to contact the ground to stabilize the walker. The rate of compression should be similar to that of plantar flexion on the sound side. If the heel cushion is unduly soft, it yields too rapidly. If the shoe sole is leather, the foot will slap noisily onto the floor. Although foot slap does not endanger the patient, it contributes to gait asymmetry.

Uneven Heel Rise. This deviation is asymmetric shank motion at the beginning of swing phase. The heel is seen to rise too high or too low compared with action of the sound limb. Maladjustment of the knee unit is at fault. If the friction mechanism in the unit does not dampen the pendular action of the shank enough, the shank will swing higher than normal. For the patient with a sliding friction unit, even if the unit is well adjusted for the wearer's usual cadence, more rapid gait will cause high heel rise because sliding friction units do not compensate for changes in walking velocity. By contrast, a fluid-controlled mechanism, whether hydraulic (oil) or pneumatic (air), if properly regulated for the user's customary speed, will increase damping automatically when the walker increases the pace of ambulation. Hydraulic control can maintain reasonably symmetric heel rise during fast walking.[40,41]

Many knee units also have an internal or external extension aid. If the aid does not resist shank motion in early stance, the result will be high heel rise. Looseness of the friction mechanism or tightness of the extension aid will have the opposite effect, namely, low heel rise. Finally, if the patient uses excessive vigor to flex the hip on the amputated side, the initial impulse will cause the knee to flex too much and the heel to rise too high.

Terminal Swing Impact. This problem refers to the appearance, and sometimes the sound, of the shank passing through late swing too rapidly. Insufficient friction or a tight extension aid creates the deviation. The insecure patient may insist on retaining this abnormality because the tremor and noise of impact signal that the prosthetic knee is extended fully and the prosthesis is therefore safe for weightbearing.

Uneven Step Length. This gait abnormality, usually with the prosthetic limb taking the longer step, is observed during swing phase. A well-fitted and trained patient may be able to walk with steps of equal length; however, step-length discrepancy is very common and is virtually always associated with uneven timing, reflecting the dissimilar weight and control of the two limbs. Unless step lengths or timing differ markedly, no corrective action need be taken. The major prosthetic error is incorrect friction adjustment. If friction is insufficient, the patient tends to hurl the prosthesis forward a greater distance than is taken with the sound limb. Socket discomfort compels the amputee to minimize stance time on the prosthesis, exaggerating prosthetic swing time and distance. The principal anatomic cause of uneven step length and timing is a hip flexion contracture on the amputated side that interferes with forward motion of the sound limb.

Frontal Plane Deviations

Several typical aberrations occur in the frontal plane or include motion in that plane: (1) abduction, (2) lateral trunk flexion, (3) circumduction, and (4) vaulting.

Abduction. This problem occurs through the gait cycle. The walker maintains an abnormally wide base by keeping the hip on the amputated side abducted. Although the average walking base of the nonamputee is 5 cm (2 in.),[24] many who wear a knee disarticulation or above-knee prosthesis prefer to widen the base slightly. Excessive width, however, dissipates energy by compelling the patient to oscillate markedly in the frontal plane in an effort to shift the torso to the stance limb. A socket that produces discomfort in the perineum or that does not provide adequate force with its lateral wall may be at fault. For those who wear a pelvic band, the mechanical hip joint may have been bent into abduction. The knee unit may be misset in excessive valgity, thereby widening the base. A prosthesis that is too long obliges the wearer to abduct it. Length may be the result of too much material in the thigh or shank sections or may be caused by a socket that is so snug that the patient cannot lodge the amputation limb properly. In the absence of prosthetic causes for abduction, the client's insecurity while walking may be the explanation. Intuitively, one broadens the base when confronting uncertain circumstances. A hip abduction contracture also places the limb too far laterally.

Lateral Trunk Flexion. During early stance, lateral trunk flexion may be seen as the subject transfers weight onto the prosthesis. The same socket, pelvic joint, knee unit, and anatomic problems contributing to abduction also produce lateral flexion. Limited cinematic evidence suggests that the ischial containment socket design reduces, but does not eliminate, lateral flexion.[42] Prosthesis length has different consequences, however. While an unduly long prosthesis compels the wearer to abduct it, a prosthesis that is too short forces the amputee to bend the trunk toward the prosthetic side. The prosthesis may have been shortened intentionally to compensate for a manually locked knee unit; during swing phase, 1-cm ($\frac{1}{2}$-in.) shortening permits the prosthesis to clear the floor. Outgrowing the prosthesis is a common phenomenon among juvenile amputees; lateral flexion indicates that the current prosthesis needs lengthening or replacement with a longer one.[43] A short prosthesis, in addition to forcing the wearer to bend the trunk laterally, also contributes to pain in the low back, hips, and knee.[44]

Circumduction. This aberration is the composite frontal and sagittal movement seen in swing phase when the walker swings the prosthesis in a semicircle. The fundamental cause of circumduction is excessive prosthetic length, because of too much material in the thigh or shank sections, socket misfit, or faulty knee motion. The knee will not swing properly if the extension aid is too taut or the knee friction is inadequate or excessive. Insufficient friction permits the shank to swing rapidly to reach extension prematurely. Excessive friction tends to maintain the knee extended. Paradoxically, with regard to the socket, if it is too snug, the prosthesis is effectively too long because the amputation limb cannot settle deeply enough; however, if the socket is too large and the suspension is poor, the prosthesis will lower during swing phase, creating transient length.

Vaulting. An alternate maneuver in swing phase is vaulting. The walker exaggerates plantar flexion of the sound limb to aid prosthetic swing. As with circumduction, vaulting is a response to excessive permanent or transient length. Transient length, in which the prosthetic knee fails to flex properly, may be produced by inadequate friction or looseness of the extension aid.[45] While the elderly client is apt to cope with a long prosthesis by circumducting, the young, agile walker will discover that vaulting readily achieves clearance. The deviation places substantial demand on the intact triceps surae, raising the entire body. The athletic client may also find that vaulting compensates for lack of toe push-off in the prosthetic foot,[46] particularly when moving rapidly.

Transverse Plane Deviations

The wearer may exhibit gait asymmetry because of (1) foot rotation on heel contact, or (2) whip.

Foot Rotation on Heel Contact. This deviation can upset the patient's balance, as the prosthetic foot fails to ease into plantar flexion at the appropriate time. The delay allows the floor reaction to remain behind the knee, exerting a flexion moment of force. Rotation is caused by a heel cushion or plantar bumper that is too firm in relationship to the force the amputee applies to the prosthesis.

Whip. This problem occurs at heel-off and immediately thereafter. The shank should move in the line of progression; however, if the socket does not fit well or the knee bolt is malrotated, the shank and foot will swing internally (medial whip) or externally (lateral whip) in late stance. An internally rotated knee bolt is associated with medial whip. Optimizing thigh axial torque should reduce whip.[47]

Table 13-2 summarizes gait deviations associated with above-knee prosthetic use.

Hip Disarticulation and Hemipelvectomy

The bulkiness of the hip disarticulation and hemipelvectomy prostheses, as well as the need to control mechanical hip, knee, and foot components with movements of the torso mitigate against normal gait kinematics. The functional sequence when walking with a hip disarticulation prosthesis differs from that employed with other prostheses. At heel contact, the wearer causes the hip to flex approximately 15° by pelvic and torso motion. The knee is extended by virtue of its stable alignment. At midstance, the knee remains fully extended. In late stance, the hip and knee flex slightly as the client tilts the pelvis to contact an elastic bumper behind the hip joint.[48] Very similar kinematics are displayed by those wearing hemipelvectomy prostheses.[49] The amputee loads the prosthesis with less force than recorded with those wearing below-knee or above-knee prostheses. Unlike the normal biphasic pattern during normal stance, the individual with hip disarticulation has a single peak of axial force later in stance.[50] Comfortable walking speed is substantially slower than that of age mates of young patients with high amputations.[51]

Under the best of circumstances, the wearer is likely to vault, exaggerating plantar flexion of the sound ankle to aid prosthetic swing-phase clearance, even though the prosthesis is intentionally shorter than the contralateral limb. Many deviations associated with above-knee prostheses, such as foot flap or rotation, uneven heel rise, terminal impact, whips, and lateral trunk flexion, are exhibited by some persons with high amputations. The basic causes are the same for both types of prosthesis, particularly poor heel cushion selection, improper knee adjustment or alignment, and shortness of the prosthesis.

Table 13-2. Above-Knee Prosthetic Gait Analysis

Deviation	Prosthetic Causes	Anatomic Causes
Lateral trunk bending	Short prosthesis Inadequate lateral wall adduction Sharp or excessively high medial wall Malalignment in abduction	Weak abductors Abduction contracture Hip pain Very short amputation limb Instability
Wide walking base (abducted gait)	Long prosthesis Excessive abduction of hip joint Inadequate lateral wall adduction Sharp or excessively high medial wall Malalignment in abduction	Abduction contracture Adductor tissue roll Instability
Circumduction	Long prosthesis Excessive stiffness of knee unit Inadequate suspension Small socket Excessive plantarflexion	Abduction contracture Poor knee control
Medial (lateral) whip	Faulty socket contour Malrotation of knee unit	
Rotation of foot on heel strike	Stiff heel cushion or plantar bumper Malrotation of foot	
Uneven heel rise	Inadequate knee friction Lax or taut extension aid	
Terminal swing impact	Insufficient knee friction Taut extension aid	Excessively forceful hip flexion
Foot slap	Soft heel cushion or plantar bumper	
Uneven step length	Faulty socket contour Inadequate knee friction Lax or taut extension aid	Weak hip musculature Hip flexion contracture Instability
Lordosis	Inadequate support from posterior brim Inadequate socket flexion	Hip flexion contracture Weak hip extensors
Vaulting	Long prosthesis Inadequate suspension Inadequate knee friction Excessive plantar flexion Small socket	Walking speed exceeding that for which friction in a sliding friction knee unit was adjusted

(Adapted from Edelstein,[76] with permission.)

ORTHOTIC GAIT PATTERNS

An orthosis imposes forces that may restrict or assist motion. As with a prosthesis, wearing an orthosis requires that the patient coordinate bodily motions with the appliance. Common to both types of device are the importance of suitable components and adequate fit; the patient's cardiopulmonary and neurologic status and psychological outlook likewise influence performance with an orthosis. Training also affects the appearance and ease of walking with the device.

Unlike a prosthesis, however, the orthosis is worn over the limb; consequently, underlying motor behavior and articular function affect gait. Another dissimilarity between appliances is that an orthosis always adds weight to the limb, in contrast to a prosthesis, which weighs less than the missing anatomic portion.

When evaluating the client's gait, one should distinguish between restrictions imposed by the orthosis that are necessary for the wearer's performance and those that diminish function and detract from appearance. Examples of the former are knee locks needed to prevent collapse or a posterior ankle stop used to gain clearance during swing phase. Features that hamper performance relate to poor fit and alignment or insufficiency of orthotic control. Deviations are the outcome of orthotic and anatomic interaction in which the orthosis either fails to compensate for physical disorder or introduces unwanted forces.

Orthotic gait deviations share many characteristics with their prosthetic counterparts. The fundamental biomechanical principles that govern prosthetic gait, particularly the relationship of the floor reaction to a given joint, also apply to ambulation with orthoses. Many of the same disorders may be observed by watching wearers of either device.[52] Observational gait analysis, a convenient technique, however, is only moderately reliable.[53] Consequently, alternate means of assessing the patient are desirable, such as measuring heart rate and walking speed under various orthotic conditions.[54]

Sagittal Plane Deviations

Abnormalities in the sagittal plane include (1) inadequate dorsiflexion control, (2) knee instability, (3) knee hyperextension, and (4) trunk flexion.

Inadequate Dorsiflexion Control. This abnormality encompasses both toe drag during swing phase and foot slap early in stance, deviations that occur together. The swing-phase deviation may cause the patient to stumble. The orthosis fails to compensate for dorsiflexor weakness or extensor spasticity, although it is unlikely that an orthosis can replace the effect of paralyzed anterior muscles completely.[55] When a plastic orthosis, such as the posterior leaf spring ankle-foot orthosis, fails to support the weight of the wearer's foot, the patient is likely to drag the toes during swing phase and slap the foot at early stance.[56] An inadequate metal spring in a dorsiflexion spring assist or a posterior ankle stop that does not limit motion to the neutral position has the same effects.[57] Ordinarily, the spring assist is associated with more dorsiflexion in swing phase than is the rigid stop.[58] A unilateral orthosis that simulates dorsiflexor activity causes compensatory alteration in performance of the unbraced limb.[59]

Knee Instability. This deviation during stance phase can be very serious, for if the knee collapses suddenly, the patient may fall. The knee-ankle-foot orthosis should counteract quadriceps weakness with a knee lock or a knee joint offset, so that its axis is appreciably posterior to the floor reaction at heel contact. Optimal knee stabilizing force is achieved by a lock complemented by anterior bands immediately above and below the knee[60] or by a single broad anterior tibial band.[61] Orthotic restriction of the knees decreases shank motion but does not affect trunk and thigh orientation during crutch walking.[62] If the patient has a knee-flexion contracture, an adjustable knee lock must be selected so that the orthosis can be aligned to conform to the angle of contracture.[52]

Some people can manage to control knee instability with an ankle-foot orthosis having an anterior tibial band and an anterior dorsiflexion stop at the ankle. The dorsiflexion stop, whether metal or the trimline of a plastic solid ankle-foot orthosis, creates an extension moment at the knee, particularly when the ankle is stopped in slight plantar flexion.[63] An anterior ankle stop controls knee instability by causing the floor reaction to move forward.[64]

Rather than stabilizing the paralyzed knee, an ankle-foot orthosis can induce buckling. A rigid posterior ankle stop tends to destabilize the knee during early stance. In order to avoid collapse, the patient is apt to take shorter steps.[65] Aligning the uprights in dorsiflexion exaggerates the knee destabilizing effect.[66] Knee instability may also be caused an ankle-foot orthosis with an insert, if the insert is placed in a shoe having a heel higher than that for which the orthosis was designed.[67] Instability of the knee is thus the result of incorrect orthotic prescription, construction, or use.

Knee Hyperextension. This aberration during early and midstance may result as the paralyzed or deranged knee sinks backward. The maneuver may be intentional, to avert buckling. By leaning forward and perhaps pressing on the thigh, the orthosis wearer ensures that the knee will not bend even though the floor reaction is posterior. Hyperextension is sometimes observed in those who have pes equinus who attempt to place the entire sole on the floor. Restraint or compensation of the ankle deformity is indicated to prevent the gait deviation. The patient with central neuropathy who manifests extensor synergy will also tend to extend the entire limb upon contact with the floor. Repetition of this deviant pattern may eventuate in painful strain of knee ligaments.

A knee-ankle-foot orthosis should have the hyperextension stop of the knee joint set at neutral position. A lock may also be needed. A calf band and distal thigh band shaped rather shallowly provide anteriorly directed force to oppose the tendency of the knee to move posteriorly. Broad plastic bands in plastic/metal orthoses, however, do not offer more effective control of hyperextension than do the narrower bands in a leather/metal brace.[68]

Just as some deficiencies of ankle-foot orthoses can cause knee instability, other orthotic problems may fail to control genu recurvatum. If the floor reaction remains in front of the knee, as is often the case in patients having cerebral palsy or cerebrovascular accident, the knee will hyperextend.[69] The hinged ankle-foot orthosis, which permits ankle dorsiflexion, is more effective in restraining knee hyperextension than the plastic solid ankle orthosis,[70] which, in turn, is better than a rigid metal ankle-foot orthosis.[71]

Trunk Flexion. This deviation during early stance may complement knee hyperextension as a means of coping with quadriceps weakness. Forward lean places the weight line in front of the knee, preventing the joint from bending. The deviation may point to the need for a knee-ankle-foot orthosis with a knee lock. The posterior ankle stop and the knee stop should both limit knee motion to the neutral position.

Frontal Plane Deviations

Gait disturbances that occur solely or principally in the frontal plane include (1) abduction, (2) lateral trunk flexion, (3) circumduction, (4) hip hiking, and (5) vaulting.

Abduction. This gait disturbance of the hip produces a wide base during swing and stance phases. The medial upright of a knee-ankle-foot orthosis may be too high, impinging into the perineum. A unilateral orthosis equipped with a knee lock requires a 1-cm ($\frac{1}{2}$-in.) lift on the contralateral shoe; otherwise, the patient will keep the braced limb abducted because that side is functionally longer. The client fitted with bilateral orthoses having knee locks will also abduct when performing the two-point or four-point gait pattern because the locks prevent knee flexion during swing phase. The pelvic joint of a hip-knee-ankle-foot orthosis may have been abducted; this orientation is sometimes intentional to avoid contact between the medial uprights in a pair of orthoses. The client's confidence in orthotic stability may be bolstered by the use of sturdier materials in the orthoses or by the addition of crutches or other walking aids.

Lateral Trunk Flexion. This deviation during early stance is a means of maintaining the torso over the supporting limb in the absence of hip abductor muscle contraction or in the presence of hip abduction contracture or hip dislocation. The deviation may be produced by excessive height of the medial upright of the knee-ankle-foot orthosis or by abduction of the hip joint of a hip-knee-ankle-foot orthosis. The patient with a short leg who lacks an appropriate shoe lift will lean toward the short side. In the absence of correctable orthotic deficiencies, the gait deviation can be eliminated by the use of a cane in the contralateral hand.[72]

Circumduction. This swing-phase aberration is comparable in appearance and in pathomechanics to the prosthetic namesake. It is a means of advancing the limb while avoiding hip flexion. The unilateral hip-knee-ankle-foot orthosis having a hip lock or the single knee-ankle-foot orthosis with a knee lock should be compensated by a lift on the opposite shoe, so that the wearer can swing the braced limb forward. Similarly, a patient with fixed pes equinus needs a lift on the other shoe. Another cause of excessive limb length in swing phase is a dorsiflexion spring assist or plantar stop that does not control the ankle as intended.

Hip Hiking. This gait abnormality refers to elevation of the pelvis during swing phase. It is a somewhat vigorous alternative to circumduction used when the limb is functionally too long because of engagement of a hip or knee lock or malfunctioning plantar stop or dorsiflexion spring assist. Hiking may also be employed by the person with equinus deformity with or without extensor synergy.

Vaulting. Another option during swing phase is vaulting. To clear the braced limb, the patient exaggerates plantar flexion on the contralateral side. Once again, the orthotic side is functionally longer, and correction of orthotic faults or a lift on the opposite shoe is indicated.

Transverse Plane Deviations

The orthosis wearer may exhibit abnormal rotations, including (1) internal or external hip rotation, or (2) excessive medial or lateral foot contact.

Both deviations can occur at any time during the gait cycle and, in the absence of muscle imbalance or joint deformity, indicate malalignment of the orthosis. Whether plastic/metal or leather/metal, the orthosis should be congruent with the client's degree of tibial torsion and subtalar alignment. Otherwise, the limb will be forced into malrotation within the orthosis. Malrotation of the foot and ankle may suggest the need for a medial longitudinal arch support or heel cup,[73] a foot orthosis extending just behind the metatarsal heads and having medial and lateral walls,[74] or medial and lateral uprights.[75] Table 13-3 summarizes common deviations associated with gait patterns of individuals wearing orthoses.

Table 13-3. Orthotic Gait Analysis

Deviation	Orthotic Causes	Anatomic Causes
Lateral trunk bending	Excessive height of medial upright of KAFO Excessive abduction of hip joint Insufficient shoe lift to compensate for leg shortening	Weak abductors Abduction contracture Dislocated hip Hip pain Instability
Hip hiking	Hip or knee lock uncompensated by contralateral shoe lift Pes equinus uncompensated by contralateral shoe lift Inadequate plantar flexion stop or dorsiflexion spring	Weak hip flexors Hip extensor spasticity
Internal (external) hip rotation	Transverse plane malalignment	Weak lateral (medial) hip musculature
Circumduction	Hip or knee lock uncompensated by contralateral shoe lift Pes equinus uncompensated by contralateral shoe lift Inadequate plantar flexion stop or dorsiflexion spring	Weak hip flexors Abduction contracture

(continued)

Table 13-3. (*continued*)

Deviation	Orthotic Causes	Anatomic Causes
Wide walking base	Excessive height of medial upright of KAFO Excessive abduction of hip joint Knee lock uncompensated by contralateral shoe lift	Weak abductors Abduction contracture Instability Genu valgum
Excessive medial (lateral) foot contact	Transverse plane malalignment	Weak invertors (evertors) Pes valgus (varus) Genu valgum (varum)
Anterior trunk bending	Inadequate knee lock	Weak quadriceps
Posterior bending		Weak hip extensors
Lordosis	Inadequate support from the brim of a weight-relieving KAFO	Hip flexion contracture Weak hip extensors
Hyperextended knee	Genu recurvatum inadequately controlled by plantar stop and excessively concave calf band Pes equinus uncompensated by contralateral shoe lift	Weak quadriceps Lax knee ligaments Extensor spasticity
Knee instability	Inadequate knee lock Inadequate dorsiflexion stop	Knee flexion contracture Weak quadriceps
Inadequate dorsiflexion control	Inadequate plantar flexion stop or dorsiflexion spring	Weak dorsiflexors Extensor spasticity
Vaulting	Hip or knee lock uncompensated by contralateral shoe lift Pes equinus uncompensated by contralateral shoe lift Inadequate plantar flexion stop or dorsiflexion spring	Weak hip flexors Abduction contracture

(Adapted from Edelstein,[77] with permission.)
KAFO, knee-ankle-foot orthosis

SUMMARY

An orthosis or prosthesis can contribute substantially to the wearer's ability to walk comfortably, efficiently, and attractively. While it is unrealistic to expect an appliance to eliminate underlying physical disorders, one can expect that the wearer will walk at least as well as other persons with the same diagnosis.

Prosthetic gait patterns depend on the level of amputation and on the person's physical and psychological condition. The adequacy of the prosthesis, in terms of design, fit, and alignment, influences walking and is most amenable to change. Rather than comparing the amputee's gait to that of a nondisabled person, analysis should focus on marked departures from the pattern displayed by a skilled wearer. Partial foot and Syme's amputees with proper prostheses walk very well. Those with more proximal amputation share common ambulatory features, such as slower pace, longer prosthetic step, and briefer time on the prosthesis. The insensate artificial foot, regardless of design, does not produce neurologically controlled plantar flexion in early stance and cannot plantar flex in late stance. The below-knee amputee may exhibit deviations in the sagittal and frontal planes relating to faulty knee control. Wearers of knee disarticulation and above-knee prostheses, lacking normal quadriceps action, are obliged to keep the prosthetic knee extended throughout early and midstance. Sagittal deviations pertain to foot and knee action. Frontal abnormalities reflect abnormal hip motion or maneuvers to obtain clearance during swing phase. Analysis of transverse plane kinematics may reveal gait asymmetry because of poor foot adjustment or failure of the prosthesis to swing in the line of progression. Walking with a hip disarticulation or hemipelvectomy prosthesis differs appreciably from the normal pattern. Many gait deviations noted for above-knee amputees are also seen with those having higher levels of amputation.

An orthosis may impose gait deviation in order to ensure the client's stability, as in the case of a knee lock. A poorly designed or fitted device causes additional abnormalities in the walking pattern. Many of the sagittal and frontal plane deviations observed with amputees are repeated by orthosis wearers, for the same fundamental biomechanical reasons.

Gait analysis of patients wearing prostheses and orthoses is a valuable clinical procedure. The goal is not normal walking, but rather optimal performance within the wearer's anatomic limitations.

REFERENCES

1. Bowker JH, Kazim M: Biomechanics of ambulation. p. 272. In Moore WS, Malone JM (eds): Lower Extremity Amputation. WB Saunders, Philadelphia, 1989
2. Mensch G, Ellis PM: Physical Therapy Management of Lower Extremity Amputations. Aspen, Rockville, MD, 1986
3. Sutherland DH: Gait Disorders in Childhood and Adolescence. Williams & Wilkins, Baltimore, 1984
4. Breakey J: Gait of unilateral below-knee emputees. Orthot Prosthet 30:17, 1976
5. Ganguli S, Bose KS, Datta SR: Optimal speed of walking in the BK amputee-PTB prosthesis system. Med Life Sci Eng 1:1, 1975
6. Ganguli S, Mukherjee P, Chakrabarty S: Preliminary observations on normal and rehabilitee cadence. Biomed Eng 9:149, 1974
7. Nielsen DH, Shurr DG, Golden JC, et al: Comparison of energy cost and gait efficiency during ambulation in below-knee amputees using different prosthetic feet: A preliminary report. J Prosthet Orthot 1:24, 1988

8. Skinner HB, Effeny DJ: Gait analysis in amputees. Am J Phys Med 64:82, 1985
9. Robinson JL, Smidt GL, Arora JS: Accelographic, temporal, and distance gait factors in below-knee amputes. Phys Ther 57:898, 1977
10. Gonzalez EG, Corcoran PH, Reyes RL: Energy expenditure in below-knee amputes: Correlation with stump length. Arch Phys Med Rehabil 55:111, 1974
11. Lewallen R, Quanbury AO, Ross K, et al: A biomechanical study of normal and amputee gait. p. 587. In Winter D, Norman R, Wells R, et al (eds): Biomechanics. Vol. IX-A. Human Kinetics, Champaign, IL, 1985
12. Inman VT, Ralston HJ, Todd F: Human Walking. Williams & Wilkins, Baltimore, 1981
13. Winter DS, Sienko SE: Biomechanics of below-knee amputee gait. J Biomech 21:361, 1988
14. Doane NE, Holt LE: A comparison of the SACH and single axis foot in the gait of unilateral below-knee amputes. Prosthet Orthot Int 7:33, 1983
15. Goh JCH, Solomonidis SE, Spence WD, et al: Biomechanical evaluation of SACH and uniaxial feet. Prosthet Orthot Int 8:147, 1984
16. Culham EG, Peat M, Newell E: Below-knee amputation: A comparison of the effect of the SACH and single-axis foot on electromyographic patterns during locomotion. Prosthet Orthot Int 10:15, 1986
17. Edelstein JE: Prosthetic feet: State of the art. Phys Ther 68:1874, 1988
18. Michael J: Energy storing feet: A clinical comparison. Clin Prosthet Orthot 11:154, 1987
19. Murray DD, Hartvikson WJ, Anton H, et al: With a spring in one's step. Clin Orthot Prosthet 12:128, 1988
20. Wing DC, Hittenberger DA: Energy-storing prosthetic feet. Arch Phys Med Rehabil 70:330, 1989
21. Menard MR, Murray DD: Subjective and objective analysis of an energy-storing prosthetic foot. J Prosthet Orthot 1:220, 1988
22. Wagner J, Sienko S, Supan T, et al: Motion analysis of SACH vs. Flex-Foot in moderately active below-knee amputes. Clin Prosthet Orthot 11:55, 1987
23. Engstrom B, Van de Ven C: Physiotherapy for Amputees: The Roehampton Approach. Churchill Livingstone, New York, 1985
24. Staff, Prosthetics and Orthotics. Lower-Limb Prosthetics. New York University Post-Graduate Medical School, New York, 1990
25. Hannah RE, Morrison JB: Prostheses alignment: Effect on gait of persons with below-knee amputations. Arch Phys Med Rehabil 65:159, 1984
26. Sanders GT: Lower Limb Amputations: A Guide to Rehabilitation. FA Davis, Philadelphia, 1986
27. Godfrey, CH, Bret R, Jousse AT: Foot mass effect on gait in the prosthetic limb. Arch Phys Med Rehabil 58:268, 1977
28. Tashman S, Hicks R, Jendrzejczyk DJ: Evaluation of a prosthetic shank with variable inertial properties. Clin Prosthet Orthot 9:23, 1985
29. Krebs DE, Tashman S: Kinematic and kinetic comparison of the conventional and ISNY above-knee socket. Clin Prosthet Orthot 9:28, 1985
30. James U, Oberg K: Prosthetic gait pattern in unilateral above-knee amputes. Scand J Rehabil Med 5:35, 1973
31. Murray MP, Sepic SB, Gardner GM, et al: Gait patterns of above-knee amputes using constant-friction knee components. Bull Prosthet Res 17:35, 1980
32. Otis JC, Lane JM, Kroll MA: Energy cost during gait in osteosarcoma patients after resection and knee replacement and after above-the-knee amputation. J Bone Joint Surg 67A:606, 1985

33. Beekman CE, Axtell LA: Prosthetic use in elderly patients with dysvascular above-knee and through-knee amputations. Phys Ther 67:1510, 1987
34. Gage JR, Hicks R: Gait analysis in prosthetics. Clin Prosthet Orthot 9:17, 1985
35. Hoy MG, Whiting WC, Zernicke RF: Stride kinematics and knee joint kinetics of child amputee gait. Arch Phys Med Rehabil 63:74, 1982
36. Zuniga EN, Leavitt LA, Calvert JC, et al: Gait patterns in above-knee amputees. Arch Phys Med Rehabil 53:373, 1972
37. Capozzo A, Figura F, Gazzani F, et al: Angular displacements in the upper body of AK amputees during level walking. Prosthet Orthot Int 6:131, 1982
38. Oberg KET, Kamwendo K: Knee components for the above-knee amputation. p. 152. In Murdoch G, Donovan RG (eds): Amputation Surgery and Lower Limb Prosthetics. Blackwell, London, 1988
39. Eberhart HD, Elftman H, Inman VT: The locomotor mechanism of the amputee. p. 472. In Klopsteg PE, Wilson PD (eds): Human Limbs and Their Substitutes. McGraw-Hill, New York, 1954
40. Godfrey CM, Jousse AT, Brett R, et al: A comparison of some gait characteristics with six knee joints. Orthot Prosthet 29:33, 1975
41. Murray MP, Mollinger LA, Sepic SB et al: Gait patterns in above-knee amputee patients: Hydraulic swing control vs constant-friction knee components. Arch Phys Med Rehabil 64:339, 1983
42. Flandry F, Beskin J, Chambers RB, et al: The effect of the CAT-CAM above-knee prosthesis on functional rehabilitation. Clin Orthop 239:246, 1989
43. Friberg O: Biomechanical significance of the correct length of lower limb prostheses: A clinical and radiological study. Prosthet Orthot Int 8:124, 1984
44. Ogg HL: Gait analysis for lower-extremity child amputees. J Am Phys Ther Assoc 45:940, 1965
45. Murphy EF: The swing phase of walking with above-knee prostheses. Bull Prosthet Res 10(1):5, 1964
46. Seligman A: Causes and corrections of deviations in gait by the above-knee amputee. Phys Ther Rev 32:126, 1952
47. Ishai G, Bar A, Susak Z: Effects of alignment variables on thigh axial torque during swing phase in AK amputee gait. Prosthet Orthot Int 7:41, 1983
48. Radcliffe CW: The biomechanics of the Canadian-type hip-disarticulation prosthesis. Artif Limbs 4:29, 1957
49. Iwakura H, Abe M, Fujinaga H, et al: Locomotion of the hemipelvectomy amputee. Prosthet Orthot Int 3:111, 1979
50. Solomonidis SE, Laughran AJ, Taylor J, et al: Biomechanics of the hip disarticulation prosthesis. Prosthet Orthot Int 1:13, 1977
51. Nowroozi F, Salvanelli ML, Gerber LH: Energy expenditure in hip disarticulation and hemipelvectomy amputees. Arch Phys Med Rehabil 64:300, 1983
52. Staff, Prosthetics and Orthotics. Lower-Limb Orthotics. New York University Post-Graduate Medical School, New York, 1986
53. Krebs DE, Edelstein JE, Fishman S: Reliability of kinematic gait analysis. Phys Ther 65:1027, 1985
54. Stallard J, Rose GK, Tait JH, et al: Assessment of orthoses by means of speed and heart rate. J Med Eng Technol 2:22, 1978
55. Lehmann JF, Ko MJ, deLateur BJ: Double-stopped ankle-foot orthosis in flaccid peroneal and tibial paralysis: Evaluation of function. Arch Phys Med Rehabil 61:536, 1980
56. Lehmann JF, Esselman PC, Ko MJ, et al: Plastic ankle-foot orthoses: Evaluation of function. Arch Phys Med Rehabil 64:402, 1983

57. Hale S, Wall JC: The effects of different ankle-foot orthoses on the kinematics of hemiplegic gait. Orthot Prosthet 41:40, 1987

58. Lee K, Johnston R: Biomechanical comparison of 90-degree plantar-flexion stop and dorsiflexion-assist ankle braces. Arch Phys Med Rehabil 54:302, 1973

59. Opara C, Levangie P, Nelson D: Effects of selected assistive devices on normal distance gait characteristics. Phys Ther 65:1188, 1985

60. Lehmann JF, Warren CG: Restraining forces in various designs of knee ankle orthoses: Their placement and effect on the anatomical knee joint. Arch Phys Med Rehabil 57:430, 1976

61. Lehmann JF, Warren CG, Hertling D, et al: Craig-Scott orthosis: A biomechanical and functional evaluation. Arch Phys Med Rehabil 57:438, 1976

62. Wells RP: The kinematics and energy variations of swing-through crutch gait. J Biomech 12:579, 1979

63. Lehmann JF: Biomechanics of ankle-foot orthoses: Prescription and design. Arch Phys Med Rehabil 60:200, 1979

64. Lehmann JF, Condon SM, deLateur BJ: Ankle-foot orthoses: Effect on gait abnormalities in tibial nerve paralysis. Arch Phys Med Rehabil 66:212, 1985

65. Lee K, Johnston R: Effect of below-knee bracing on knee movement: Biomechanical analysis. Arch Phys Med Rehabil 55:179, 1974

66. Lehmann JF, Ko MJ, deLateur BJ: Knee moments: Origin in normal ambulation and their modification by double-stopped ankle-foot orthoses. Arch Phys Med Rehabil 63:345, 1982

67. Cook TM, Cozzens B: The effects of heel height and ankle-foot-orthosis configuration on weight line location: A demonstration of principles. Orthot Prosthet 30:43, 1976

68. Krebs DE, Edelstein JE, Fishman S: Comparison of plastic/metal and leather/metal knee-ankle-foot orthoses. Am J Phys Med Rehabil 67:175, 1988

69. Stallard J: Assessment of the mechanical function of orthoses by force vector visualisation. Physiotherapy 73:398, 1987

70. Middleton EA, Hurley GRB, McIlwain JS: The role of rigid and hinged polypropylene ankle-foot-orthoses in the management of cerebral palsy: A case study. Prosthet Orthot Int 12:129, 1988

71. Smith AE, Quigley M, Waters R: Kinematic comparison of the BiCAAL orthosis and the rigid polypropylene orthosis in stroke patients. Orthot Prosthet 36:49, 1982

72. Blount WP: Don't throw away the cane. J Bone Joint Surg 38A:695, 1956

73. Scranton P, Pedegana L, Whitesel J: Gait analysis: Alterations in support phase forces using supportive devices. Am J Sports Med 10:6, 1982

74. Burkett L, Kohrt W, Buchbinder R: Effects of shoes and foot orthotics on VO_2 and selected frontal plane knee kinematics. Med Sci Sports Exerc 17:158, 1985

75. Burdett RG, Borello-France D, Blatchly C, et al: Gait comparison of subjects with hemiplegia walking unbraced, with ankle-foot orthosis, and with Air-Stirrup brace. Phys Ther 68:1197, 1988

76. Edelstein JE: Prosthetic assessment and management. Chapter 20. In O'Sullivan SB, Schmitz TJ (eds.): Physical Rehabilitation: Assessment and Treatment Procedures. 2nd Ed. FA Davis, Philadelphia, 1988

77. Edelstein JE: Orthotic assessment and management. Chapter 27. In O'Sullivan SB, Schmitz TJ (eds.): Physical Rehabilitation: Assessment and Treatment Procedures. 2nd Ed. FA Davis, Philadelphia, 1988

14 | Gait Assessment and Training in Clinical Practice

Gary L. Smidt

PERSPECTIVE ON GAIT TRAINING

I define ideal gait as walking (1) in a smooth, rhythmic, and symmetric manner; (2) while using minimal physiologic energy; (3) without experiencing symptoms; and (4) without the aid of assistive devices. Ideal gait may be a realistic ultimate goal for some patients and not for others. The severity and nature of the musculoskeletal abnormality, among many factors, influence the prognostic outlook for gait. To this end, what part should training the patient in walking play, if at all?

In the case of postoperative care for lower-extremity and trunk problems, gait training is typically provided while patients are in the hospital but, following discharge, patients are often left to themselves for making progress in walking. The tacit assumption of this self-restoration approach is that gait will instinctively improve in concert with decrease in symptoms, decrease in pathology, and improvement in physiologic function. Reciprocally, another dogmatic view is that walking alone improves isolated function, such as muscle strength and joint motion.

A progression of gait training toward normal has been suggested.[1] Another has recommended tape on the floor in large gridlike fashion to help train the patient to walk with a narrower base and more equal step lengths.[2] The use of quotas in gait training, similar in concept to muscle strength training, has been effectively used.[3] Chapter 4 on energy costs and Chapter 12 on cardiopulmonary abnormalities present gait-training considerations within a physiologic context and, in so doing, have demonstrated that patients can improve their cardiovascular efficiency by walking. In the case of musculoskeletal and neuromuscular abnormalities, the effects and benefits of gait training have not been demonstrated convincingly.

It may very well be that patients instinctively alter their gait either toward or away from the ideal, depending on personal preference. Rose[4] pointed out that, in one study,[5] some patients with above-knee prostheses walked with a limp. When the knee mechanism was adjusted in an attempt to eliminate the limp, the knee mechanism became damaged, and patients returned to a limping gait. The reversion to the limp was thought to indicate that the overriding instinctively preferred option was to walk with low energy consumption. Therefore, "force feeding" the gait of patients toward an ideal gait may not be the best approach for some musculoskeletal abnormalities. James and Brubaker[6] provided another example. On examination, a patient was found to have moderate bilateral tibial torsion and to walk with her toes outward. She was instructed to run with her toes straight ahead. As a consequence, she developed knee pain, symptoms believed to be caused by excessive strain on the capsular structures of the knees. The pain disappeared when the patient ran in her natural out-toed gait. However, a controversy does exist because some investigators indicate that, left to themselves, patients may not select the best gait for themselves; in fact, the self-preferred gait may be detrimental, adversely affecting the body structures.

In an experimental study of arthritic patients, feedback for step lengths during walking was used to alter foot placement symmetry in a positive way.[7] The highest pitched tones were associated with the longest step lengths. The mean pretraining step length difference was 9.4 percent. Following one 20-minute training session consisting of audiofeedback (instantaneous feedback of results) during walking and description of results for one sequence of walking (delayed knowledge of results), patients were able to walk with improved step length and step time symmetry. This study simply indicates that patients can be trained to walk in a symmetric manner. It could be that gait training for patients needs to progress through stages from development of a "perceptual trace" or designed movement pattern, and then repeatedly practice until the movement becomes a "memory trace." Finally, as knowledge of results and preplanning diminish, the response becomes "learned."[8]

It appears reasonable to assume that, in the main, patients with musculoskeletal abnormalities must instinctively adapt a gait according to a rank-order hierarchy of personal preference: (1) alleviate or reduce pain, (2) minimize energy cost, (3) use no assistive device, and (4) achieve symmetric and smooth body movement. Since personal preferences vary, the rank-order priorities may selectively vary among patients. Patients with neuromuscular abnormalities may function with a different set of priorities. Furthermore, it seems reasonable that the top gait training goals would be to walk without pain and assistive devices. Once these goals are accomplished and some residual internal body malfunction precludes attainment of an ideal gait pattern, it may be necessary to choose between relative minimal energy expenditure and esthetics (e.g., symmetry and smoothness of movement). I believe that the added external forces and timing requirements imposed by walking aids necessitate independent gait-training considerations for each of the many types of assisted gait. This section provides a framework for understanding gait training; it is intended to prompt clinical investigation and reports to help clarify the effects of various gait-training methods for various types of patients and conditions.

PERSPECTIVE ON GAIT ASSESSMENT

Impairment (impaired function) and disability (impaired ability to perform job related functions) in the broad context encompass three areas: physical, mental, and social.[9] Walking is largely a physical function. However, this physical function can logically be affected by physical, mental, and social factors. Within the context of impairment, does gait assessment have diagnostic value? Some say no,[10] while Winter[11,12] has strongly promulgated the diagnostic value of gait assessment, particularly kinetics. Rose[4] is less enthusiastic about the clinical value of kinetics.

It appears implausible to identify a disease entity from an assessment of gait. The most sophisticated gait-analysis system involving three-dimensional kinematic analyses coupled with force-plate data can provide calculated resultant joint forces and moments. However, even with a three-dimensional mathematical analysis (e.g., inverse dynamics approach), there are far more unknowns than equations, so the joint forces and moments provide a less than comprehensive "real-life" representation. Electromyography (EMG) can help estimate which muscles are contributing to the joint moment. However, apart from invasive measures that are clearly unacceptable in clinical practice, kinetic analyses provide no information concerning the status of biologic elements or pathology—the cornerstone of medical diagnosis. Still, it should be acknowledged that medical diagnoses such a osteoarthritis, cerebral hemorrhage, or fracture do not in themselves reflect the functional capacity or ability of the patient. Meaningful information concerning the patient's functional capacity, including gait, is a matter separate from the medical diagnosis but one that is nonetheless of utmost clinical importance. It is critical to bear in mind that gait assessment can provide information concerning such things as hypo- and hyper-joint mobility, forces, muscle activity, energy expenditure, and asymmetry. However, we must constantly bear in mind that gait assessment provides information for a limited single, albeit common, highly relevant, and complex, motor function.

Since gait assessment is important yet limited in scope, it stands to reason that assessment should be combined and related with results from other clinical tests and the clinical examination. For example, a patient who walks with decreased knee extension (an effect) at early stance phase may be influenced by many of factors. These factors must be identified from the clinical examination or other clinical tests. Some potential causes might be a hamstring contracture, weak quadriceps, effusion, bone malformation, or flexor spasticity, to name a few. Also, the information gathered from the gait assessment and other tests must be interpreted in view of the clinical problem identified. If, for example, the primary problem identified in the clinical examination is a flexion contracture and the plan of action calls for some form of hamstring elongation procedure (e.g., exercise or surgical), the gait abnormality (decreased knee extension during early stance) must be re-evaluated in gait assessment to determine whether improvement in isolated knee extension motion is transferred to the global function of walking. In this simple example, kinetics (moment of force or strength) is often less important than kinematics (acquisition of joint motion) because a person can walk normally with considerably less than normal strength[13] (e.g., quadriceps) but cannot walk normally without complete knee extension motion. Step time and step length asymmetries will likely reflect this abnormality as well.

From this simple example, we can see that gait assessment was useful in several distinctive ways. First, an indication of physical impairment was provided by the recognition that deficient knee extension during early stance was a deviation from normal. Second, the recognition or measurement of the knee extension deficit during gait in conjunction with the information garnered from the clinical examination combined to permit identification of the clinical dysfunction problem. Recognition of the hypomobility during the gait assessment could also cue or direct the clinician toward the knee joint for the clinical examination. In many cases, the information gained from the gait assessment might also be combined usefully with results from pathology laboratories, radiography, magnetic resonance imaging (MRI), and other medical tests to aid in the cause of movement dysfunction. Third, the determination of whether a patient's walking ability has improved, remained status quo, or diminished is worthwhile clinically, irrespective of the medical diagnosis. Changes in walking ability, whether from carefully controlled treatment intervention or from mysterious unknown causes (physical, mental, or social), should be considered for clinical relevancy.

In closing this section, I remind the reader that gait assessment is a useful tool in many ways conceptually analogous to the Minnesota Multiphasic Personality Inventory (MMPI) in the psychological domain: "MMPI's publishers say the test shouldn't be used alone to diagnose psychological problems . . . ; it should be given in conjunction with other tests."[11,13] So it should be with gait assessment in the diagnostic process. The data provided by gait assessment have not been shown to be pathognomonic. Some of the earlier mentioned medical and physical therapy tests, including passive and active joint motion, muscle strength, pain, spasm, tenderness, and motor and sensory function, are but a few that might be considered judiciously. The purpose and value of clinical gait assessment are outlined in Table 14-1.

Table 14-1. Clinical Gait Assessment

Purpose	Value
Aid in physical dysfunction problem solving	Combine and associate data with other tests
Aid in confirming medical diagnosis	Help clarify therapeutic efficacy and clinical disease course
Help determine physical impairment deviation from normal	

CLINICAL GAIT ASSESSMENT ESSENTIALS

There is a need for increased clarity and standardization in reporting a patient's walking performance. This section is intended to aid in satisfying this need, so that a clinician's written reports in the clinical record and the investigators results can be easily understood. A clear understanding is essential to represent the patient's ability accurately at assessment, for making comparisons with other patients, and most importantly to be able to follow up gait assessments to replicate the method and make justifiable statements about the patient's change in walking ability.

The following elements are relevant to the entire spectrum of gait-assessment situations ranging from the time-constrained clinical environment to the high-technology laboratory. Some basic elements are absolutely critical for inclusion:

1. Age, height, weight, sex
Comment: Age is measured in years, height in centimeters (cm), and weight in kilograms (kg).
2. Medical diagnosis
3. Footware
Comment: The type of shoe and composition of the soles and heels should be presented. Ideally, the same footware should be worn in follow-up clinical gait assessments. The confounding influences of various types of footware the patient can be avoided by having the patient walk unshod (barefoot).
4. Orthosis or prosthesis
Comment: The type of device should be identified. Also indicate on which lower extremity or both it (they) is (are) worn. Refer to Chapter 13 (Prosthetic and Orthotic Gait) for details.
5. Standing posture
Comment: In neuromuscular and musculoskeletal abnormalities, the abnormal gait pattern is sometimes an extension of what is observed in standing posture. For example, the patient may stand with the trunk and head leaning to the left, with the left hip and knee flexed. The description of the gait assessment may reflect this postural abnormality.
6. Type of assisted gait and walking aid used
Comment: The type of walking aid used (e.g., Lofstrand crutch, conventional cane) should be identified. Often in the literature and in clinical notes,

a patient is described as walking with one cane, with two crutches, and so forth—nonspecific information that does not permit accurate conceptualization and subsequent replication of the assisted gait used by the patient. The patient could have the cane in either hand, also several timing and location combinations are possible for the cane and foot placement during the assisted cane gait. The *A system* for various assisted gait is described in Chapter 7. A more complete and accurate description follows: using conventional wooden crutches, the patient walked with a delayed three-point gait, right foot (i.e., the right foot was the lead foot). This brief description permits a precise, ready conceptualization of the assisted gait. The classification system for types of assisted gait can also be viewed as a progression from most to least external assistance used. The progression of assisted gaits is outlined below:

    A. Four-point crutch gait
    B. Delayed five-point gait with walker
    C. Delayed three-point gait with two crutches
    D. Three-point gait with walker
    E. Three-point gait with two crutches
    F. Delayed three-point gait with two canes
    G. Three-point gait with two canes
    H. Delayed two-point gait with crutch
    I. Delayed two-point gait with cane
    J. Two-point gait with crutch
    K. Two-point gait with cane
    L. Walk with assistive device
   7. Walking velocity

   Comment: In Chapter 1 and elsewhere in this volume, the point has repeatedly been made that most gait parameters are influenced by walking velocity. The clinician can develop observational skills in reporting the forward velocity, such as slow and fast (see Ch. 1) or with a stopwatch and designated walking distance, the walking velocity can be objectively reported in centimeters per second (cm/s). From the literature, it is apparent that two walking velocities should be obtained: (a) the patient's preferred, self-selected velocity, and (b) the fastest rate at which the patient can walk safely and comfortably. Cadence can be reported on an optional basis but should never be reported instead of walking velocity. An extreme negative example supports this admonition: a person could use a cadence of two steps per second while walking in one spot (walking in place).

OBSERVATIONAL ANALYSIS

   Because the clinical questions being posed are incredibly diverse, it seems most fruitful to present some key suggestions in reporting information obtained from an observational analysis of gait. The start of this section is directed toward the clinician, whose time is limited, and for whom the resources at hand are a stopwatch, a measured walking distance, floor markings, and visual transducers (the eyes). Several gait profiles and observational analysis approaches have been reported.[12,15-19] Two significant problems exist with these approaches. First, they tend to be complex and time-consuming. The average clinician cannot justify spending large blocks of time performing an observational gait analysis. Second, some approaches[16,18] include kinetic factors. The problem here is that forces cannot be seen. Therefore, observational analyses should include only temporal and distance factors, orientation of body segments, and movement of body segments. Forces and moments of force and cardiovascular factors cannot be measured with the eye.

TEMPORAL AND DISTANCE FACTORS

Step times and lengths are the factors of choice. For clinical purposes, it is impractical to consider all the available factors. Step times and lengths should be individually assessed, with the examiner viewing the walking patient from the side. Obviously, the focus should be on the feet. The step is best designated by the lead foot. For example, a left step is in reality a step bounded by the trailing right foot and the lead left foot. The step length and time from foot-floor contact on one side to foot-floor contact on the other side. In this way, asymmetries can be reported as follows: left step length is greater than the right, and right step time is faster than the left. Simple methods using floor markings, grid pattern,[20] and foot switches[21] will permit acquisition of objective data.

Kinematics

Data are available in the literature that provide patterns and magnitudes of body movement during normal gait. Some are linear-type movements, such as the vertical path of the head during gait, while others are angular movement pathways, such as sagittal plane knee motion during the cycle. With knowledge of the magnitude and pattern of these movements, deviations from normal can be identified by observational analysis. As a general rule, linear and angular movements in the sagittal plane can best be viewed from the side and frontal plane movement from the front or back. Transverse movements are best viewed from the top but, for practical purposes, a side, front, or back view can be used effectively. Again, the eye can best see movement in terms of displacement as opposed to velocity and acceleration. Linear displacement or tracking one body reference through the cycle is easier than tracking angular displacement, which requires tracking two body segments and conceptualizing an intervening angle.

Normal movement patterns for some key regions of the body are illustrated in Figure 14-1 and 14-2. The stance and swing phases are each divided into three equal segments. To facilitate recording while performing an observational analysis, a notation scheme is provided (Fig. 14-3 and 14-4). (The scheme can be applied to additional movement patterns identified by the clinician that are not included in Figs. 14-1 and 14-2.) The decision to be made by the clinician is

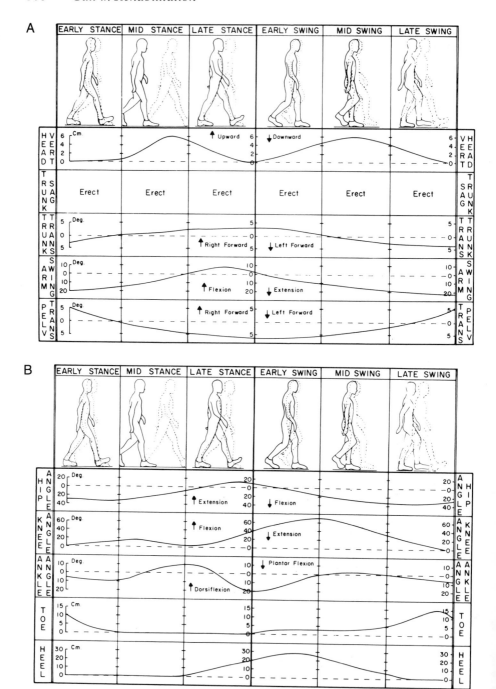

Fig. 14-1. Normal gait profile: sagittal view. **(A)** head to pelvis. **(B)** Hip to foot. (Figs. 14-1 through 14-4 by Gary Smidt, courtesy of the University of Iowa Physical Therapy Program.)

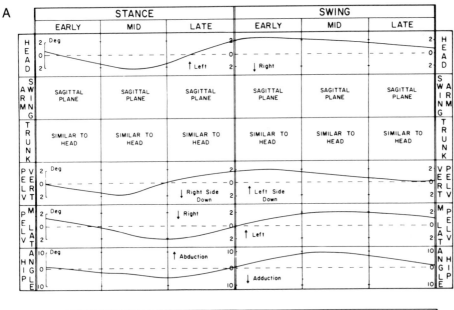

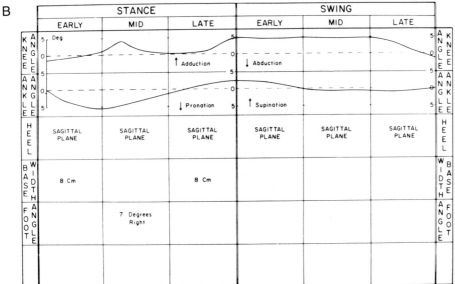

Fig. 14-2. Normal gait profile: coronal view. **(A)** Head to hip. **(B)** Knee to foot. (Courtesy of the University of Iowa Physical Therapy Program.).

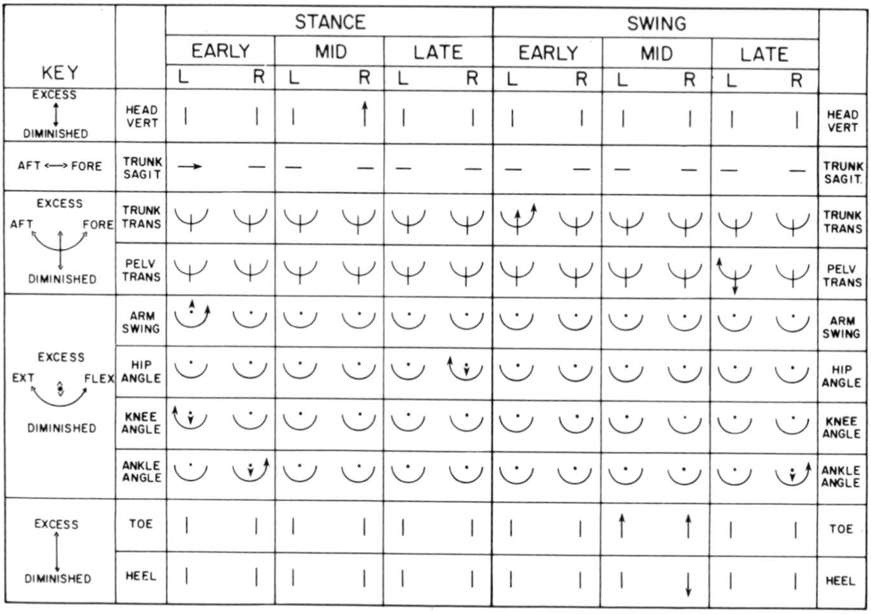

Fig. 14-3. Observational analysis scheme for gait: sagittal view. Illustrative definitions for notations shown, starting at the top and progressing downward:

Head Vert: Excessive head elevation during midstance on the right foot.

Trunk Sagit: Excessive forward movement of trunk during early stance on the left foot.

Trunk Trans: Excessive forward trunk axial rotation during early swing of the left foot.

Pelv Trans: Decreased posterior pelvic axial rotation during late swing of the left foot.

Arm Swing: Excessive upper-extremity flexion during early stance on the left foot.

Hip Angle: Decreased hip extension during late stance on the right foot.

Knee Angle: Decreased knee extension during early stance on the left foot.

Ankle Angle: Decreased dorsiflexion of ankle during late swing and early stance on the right foot.

Toe: Excessive toe elevation during midswing bilaterally.

Heel: Diminished heel elevation during midswing on right.

(Courtesy of the University of Iowa Physical Therapy Program.)

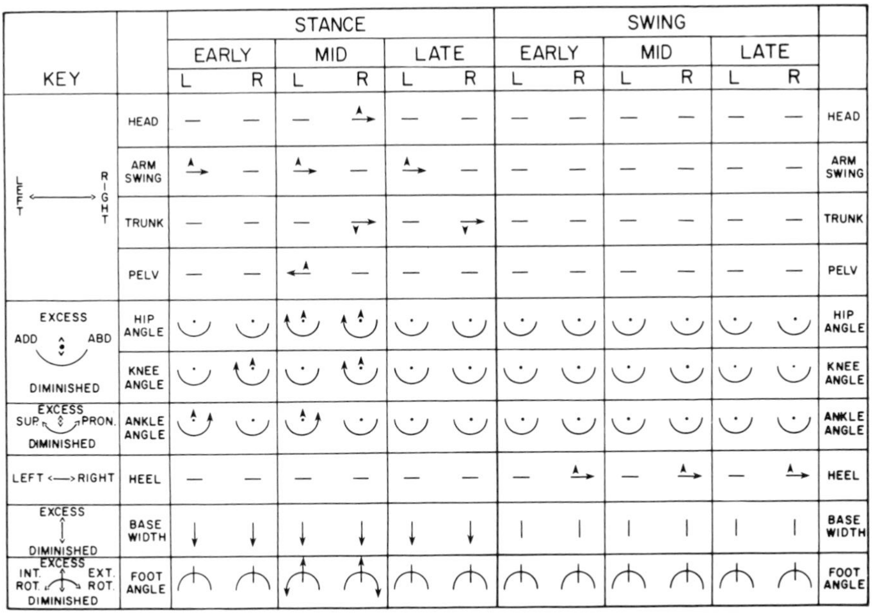

KEY		STANCE						SWING						
		EARLY		MID		LATE		EARLY		MID		LATE		
		L	R	L	R	L	R	L	R	L	R	L	R	
	HEAD	—	—	—	▲→	—	—	—	—	—	—	—	—	HEAD
LEFT ←→ RIGHT	ARM SWING	▲→	—	▲→	—	▲→	—	—	—	—	—	—	—	ARM SWING
	TRUNK	—	—	—	→▼	—	→▼	—	—	—	—	—	—	TRUNK
	PELV	—	—	←▲	—	—	—	—	—	—	—	—	—	PELV
EXCESS ADD ▲ ABD / DIMINISHED	HIP ANGLE	⌣	⌣	⌣	⌣	⌣	⌣	⌣	⌣	⌣	⌣	⌣	⌣	HIP ANGLE
	KNEE ANGLE	⌣	⌣	⌣	⌣	⌣	⌣	⌣	⌣	⌣	⌣	⌣	⌣	KNEE ANGLE
EXCESS SUP. ↕ PRON. DIMINISHED	ANKLE ANGLE	⌣	⌣	⌣	⌣	⌣	⌣	⌣	⌣	⌣	⌣	⌣	⌣	ANKLE ANGLE
LEFT ←→ RIGHT	HEEL	—	—	—	—	—	—	—	▲→	—	▲→	—	▲→	HEEL
EXCESS ↑ DIMINISHED	BASE WIDTH	↓	↓	↓	↓	↓	↓	|	|	|	|	|	|	BASE WIDTH
EXCESS INT. ROT. / EXT. ROT. DIMINISHED	FOOT ANGLE	⌒	⌒	⌒	⌒	⌒	⌒	⌒	⌒	⌒	⌒	⌒	⌒	FOOT ANGLE

Fig. 14-4. Observational analysis scheme for gait: coronal view. Illustrative definitions for notations shown, starting at the top and working downward:

Head: Excessive movement of head to right during midstance on the right foot.

Arm Swing: Excessive lateral arm swing to the right during entire stance phase on the left foot.

Trunk: Diminished lateral movement of the trunk to the right during mid- and late stance on the right foot.

Pelv: Excessive lateral movement of the pelvis to the left during midstance on the left foot.

Hip Angle: Excessive hip adduction during midstance bilaterally.

Knee Angle: Excessive adduction (varus) movement during early and midstance on the right foot.

Ankle Angle: Excessive ankle pronation during early and midstance on the left foot.

Heel: Excessive lateral movement (circumduction) during the entire swing phase on the right foot.

Base Width: Diminished base of gait during stance for each step (bilateral).

Foot Angle: Excessive external rotation (outward) foot placement during midstance on right foot and excessive internal rotation (inward) foot placement during midstance on the left foot.

(Courtesy of the University of Iowa Physical Therapy Program.)

whether a patient exhibits too much or too little motion during a particular phase of the gait cycle. In the crudest sense, the movement deviation from normal should be associated with either stance or swing phase on either the right or left side. Most people should be able to associate the movement abnormality with three divisions for stance phase (early, mid, or late) or swing (early, mid, or late) for a designated side (e.g., decreased knee flexion during midstance on the right). Only a few of the most obvious and most important gait deviations should be reported.

Pain

The location, nature, and intensity of the pain experienced during walking should be related to a part of the gait cycle as explained earlier (e.g., late stance, midswing).

Cardiovascular

Resting heart rate and postwalking heart rate can be used to provide an indication of the patient's response to the exercise (see Ch. 12.)

SMIDT NUMBER

The application of high technology toward the understanding of gait and attempts toward clinical relevance has paradoxically yielded one simple factor, which seems to be the most meaningful and useful indicator of walking ability. That factor is *forward walking velocity*. Self-selected walking velocity and the patient's maximum walking velocity have repeatedly been demonstrated as useful and important.

For the purpose of quantifying gait impairment and for use in future clinical studies, preferred walking velocity and maximum walking velocity have been combined in a simple equation to provide the *Smidt Number* (SN):

$$SN = MV + PV$$

where MV is maximum forward walking velocity (cm/s) and PV is the preferred or self-selected walking velocity (cm/s).
To determine MV:

The timed period is for a minimum of three strides (six steps)
The timed period begins and ends with the patient walking at a steady rate
The verbal instructions are: "Please walk forward at your fastest reasonable rate."

To determine PV:

The timed period is for a minimum of three strides (six steps)
The timed period begins and ends with the patient walking at a steady rate
The verbal instructions are: "Please walk forward at your preferred walking speed."

Rationale

Normal walking requires the ability to walk at a reasonable self-selected velocity as well as at a demonstrably maximum velocity that is considerably faster than the self-selected rate. Pathologic gait may be manifested by a decrease in either or both maximum and self-selected rates.

Classification for Reporting

For purposes of reporting, the calculated numerical value for the SN as well as proposed descriptors analogous to those used for the manual muscle test (e.g., normal, good, fair, poor, and zero) is based on data for self-selected velocity[22] and fast walking velocity.[23] The highest possible SN is 3 SD above the mean. The lowermost margin of the normal range is 1 SD below the mean, and the lowermost margin for the normal minus grade for gait is 2 SD below the mean. The balance of the numerical range is equally divided to accommodate the levels from good plus downward to poor minus and zero. The classification or rating scale appropriate for the SN is shown in Table 14-2. Therefore, in a broad sense, the SN range for normal gait is 215 and above, good 140 to 214, fair 65 to 114, and poor 1 to 64.

Table 14-2. Smidt Number Rating Scale

Grade for Gait	Range for SN
Normal	N = 285 and above
Normal minus	N⁻ = 215–284
Good plus	G⁺ = 190–214
Good	G = 165–189
Good minus	G⁻ = 140–164
Fair plus	F⁺ = 115–139
Fair	F = 90–114
Fair minus	F⁻ = 65–89
Poor plus	P⁺ = 40–64
Poor	P = 15–39
Poor minus	P⁻ = 1–14
Zero	O = 0 (unable to walk)

SAMPLE CLINICAL REPORT ON GAIT

A 68-year-old man with osteoarthritis whose height was 180 cm and weight 90 kg was evaluated. He wore leather solid shoes and was able to stand erect with a cane in his right hand. His average preferred forward velocity was slow at 50 cm/s while walking with a delay two-point assisted cane (conventional wooden) gait, right hand-left foot. His maximum walking velocity was 70 cm/s. Therefore his Smidt Number is 120 or a grade fair plus. The patient was able to walk 20 m. His left step time was considerably slower than the right. This patient demonstrated an excessively wide base; on the left side, he displayed decreased ankle dorsiflexion at early stance and excessive pelvic transverse rotation to the right during midstance. He complained of sharp pain at the left hip during midstance on the left. His cardiovascular response to walking was normal.

DEFINITION OF LIMP

In the reading done for this book, I frequently encountered the term *limp* but failed to encounter a definition in the parlance of accepted terminology used for temporal and distance factors. For universal as well as technical understanding, I propose the following definition for a limp.

Limp: While walking, the step times or step lengths or both are unequal.

SUMMARY

This chapter provides a perspective on gait assessment and training in the clinical context. An observational analysis approach and associated notation scheme for rapid clinical recording is illustrated. A sample clinical report using a proposed format is provided. Finally, an equation with rationale, instructions, and interpretation of the Smidt Number is presented for clinical use.

REFERENCES

1. Heap MF: Relearning to walk. Physiother Rev 23:208, 1943
2. Jims SC: Foot placement pattern: An aid gait training. Phys Ther 57:286, 1977
3. Doleys DM, Crocker M, Patton D: Response of patients with chronic pain to exercise quotas. Phys Ther 62:1111, 1982
4. Rose GK: Clinical gait assessment: A personal view. J Med Eng Technol 7:273, 1983
5. University of California Prosthetic Research Project. Fundamental Studies of Human Locomotion and other Information Relating to the Design of Artificial Limbs. National Research Council, Washington, DC, 1947
6. James SL, Brubaker CE: Running mechanics. JAMA 221:1014, 1972
7. McGraw ML: Development of a Measurement Tool and a Method for Gait Training

and Gait Assessment of Patients with Asymmetry of Step Lengths. Master's thesis. Physical Therapy Graduate Program, University of Iowa, 1977

8. Adams JA: A closed loop theory of motor learning. J Motor Behav 3:111, 1970
9. LeRoy RE: Assessment of disabilities. Med J Aust 1:635, 1980
10. Brand RA, Crowninshield RD: Comment on criterion for patient evaluation tools. J Biomech 16:655, 1983
11. Winter DA: The locomotion laboratory as a clinical assessment system. Med Prog Technol 4:95, 1976
12. Winter DA: Concerning the scientific basis for the diagnosis of pathological gait and for rehabilitation protocols. Physiother Can 37:245, 1985
13. Smidt GL, Arora JS, Johnston RC: Accelerographic analysis of several types of walking. Am J Phys Med 50:285, 1971
14. The Wall Street Journal, September 13, 1989, p 8
15. Brunnstrom S: Recording gait patterns of adult hemiplegic patients. Phys Ther 44:11, 1964
16. Koerner I: Observation of Huamn Gait, A Study Guide to Accompany Videocassettes. Health Sciences Audiovisual Education. University of Alberta, Edmonton, Alberta, Canada, July 1984
17. Olney SJ, Elkin ND, Lowe PJ, et al: An ambulation profile for clinical gait evaluation. Physiother Can 31:85, 1979
18. Professional Staff Association of Rancho Los Amigos Hospital Inc. Normal and Pathological Gait Syllabus. Downey, California, 1981
19. Tracy KB, Montague EC, Gabriel RP, et al: Computer-assisted diagnosis of orthopedic gait disorders. Phys Ther 59:268, 1979
20. Robinson JL, Smidt GL: Quantitative gait evaluation in the clinic. Phys Ther 61:351, 1981
21. Wall JC, Charteris J, Hoare HW: An automated on-line system for measuring the temporal patterns of foot/floor contact. J Med Eng Technol 2:187, 1978
22. Finley FR, Cody KA: Locomotor characteristics of urban pediatricians. Arch Phys Med Rehabil 51:423, 1970
23. Murray MP, Kory RC, Clarkson BH: Alking patterns in healty old men. J Gerontol 24:169, 1969

SUGGESTED READING

Smidt GL: Biomechanical analysis of knee flexion and extension. J Biomech 6: 79, 1973

Index

Page numbers followed by *f* indicate figures; these followed by *t* indicate tables.